INFLAMMATION
Fundamental Mechanisms

INFLAMMATION

Fundamental Mechanisms

Editor

Klaus Ley

La Jolla Institute for Allergy and Immunology, USA

World Scientific

NEW JERSEY • LONDON • SINGAPORE • BEIJING • SHANGHAI • HONG KONG • TAIPEI • CHENNAI • TOKYO

Published by

World Scientific Publishing Co. Pte. Ltd.

5 Toh Tuck Link, Singapore 596224

USA office: 27 Warren Street, Suite 401-402, Hackensack, NJ 07601

UK office: 57 Shelton Street, Covent Garden, London WC2H 9HE

Library of Congress Cataloging-in-Publication Data
Names: Ley, Klaus, 1957– editor.
Title: Inflammation : fundamental mechanisms / edited by Klaus Ley.
Other titles: Inflammation (Ley)
Description: New Jersey : World Scientific, 2018. | Includes bibliographical references and index.
Identifiers: LCCN 2017058719 | ISBN 9789813109438 (hardcover : alk. paper)
Subjects: | MESH: Inflammation--physiopathology
Classification: LCC RB131 | NLM QZ 150 | DDC 616/.0473--dc23
LC record available at https://lccn.loc.gov/2017058719

British Library Cataloguing-in-Publication Data
A catalogue record for this book is available from the British Library.

For any available supplementary material, please visit
http://www.worldscientific.com/worldscibooks/10.1142/10028#t=suppl

Typeset by Stallion Press
Email: enquiries@stallionpress.com

Contents

Chapter 1

TNF Superfamily in Inflammation

Marisol Veny*, Richard Virgen-Slane*
and Carl F. Ware*

1. Introduction

1.1. *Discovery of TNF and lymphotoxin*

Studies of the tumor necrosis factor superfamily (TNFSF) can be traced back to the 1800s, when it was found that acute inflammation induced by bacterial extracts could trigger necrosis of tumors. Nearly two centuries later, activated lymphocytes in culture were shown to produce a cytotoxic factor for tumor cells,[1] named Lymphotoxin (LT)[2] and macrophages secreted a cytotoxin that caused hemorrhagic necrosis of tumors, named Tumor Necrosis Factor (TNF).[1–3] Although these host-derived anti-tumor factors were greeted with great enthusiasm, knowledge of their true physiologic functions awaited advances in protein chemistry and molecular biology.

*Infectious and Inflammatory Diseases Center, Sanford Burnham Prebys Medical Discovery Institute, 10901 N. Torrey Pines Road, La Jolla, CA 92037, USA.

The cloning of the genes for LT[4–6] and TNF[7–10] revealed significant shared sequence homology.[4,11,9] Additionally, the recombinant proteins displayed similar biological activities[4,9] and bound the same two cell surface receptors, now referred to as TNFR1 and TNFR2.[12–17] Thus, LT and TNF were recognized as the founding members of a superfamily of homologous ligands, and their specific cell surface receptors forming the TNF receptor superfamily. The similarities in TNF and LT and their receptors suggested redundancy of function.[18] This outlook changed with the discovery of two important differences in the properties of TNF and LT. The first key difference, which prompted the renaming of LT (also called TNFβ) to LTα, was its interaction to form a novel ligand with lymphotoxin-β (LTβ) forming a heterotrimeric complex $LT\alpha_1\beta_2$.[1,9] Later, a receptor specific for $LT\alpha_1\beta_2$, but not TNF, was discovered and named the LTβ receptor (LTβR).[20] The second major finding was that mice deficient in either one of the genes LTα, LTβ, or LTβR fail to develop lymph nodes and other secondary lymphoid organs.[21–23]

Several more receptors (Table 1) and ligands (Table 2) were discovered as members of these superfamilies, revealing the scope of these ligand–receptors in animal physiology. Among the receptors critical for immune responses include CD27,[24] CD40,[25] CD30,[26] OX40,[27] 4-1BB,[28] and Fas.[29] Members of the TNFRSF also play important roles in the physiology of skin, bone, and nervous system, and orthologous genes were found in the genomes of large DNA viruses including poxvirus[30] and herpesviruses.

1.2 *Description of TNFSF proteins*

1.2.1. *TNFSF ligands*

With the exception of TL1A[31] and FasL,[32] the expression of TNFSF ligands is restricted to cells of the immune system, including dendritic cells (DC), activated lymphocytes, and myeloid cells. TNF-related cytokines are type II transmembrane proteins with short cytoplasmic tails (15–25 amino acids) and larger extracellular regions (~150 amino acids). They contain a signature β-sheet sandwich, known as the TNF homology domain, which facilitates

Table 1. TNFSF receptors.

TNF Receptor Superfamily			
	Chromosomal location		
Gene Name/Alias	Human	Mouse	Gene Symbol
TNFR1, p55-60	12p13.2	ch6 (60.55 cM)	TNFRSF1A
TNFR2, p75-80	1p36 3-36.2	ch4 (75.5 cM)	TNFRSF1B
LTβR	12p13	ch6 (60.4 cM)	LTβR
OX40	1p36	ch4(79.4 cM)	TNFRSF4
CD40	20q12-q13.2	ch2 (97.0 cM)	CD40
FAS, CD95	10q24.1	ch19(23.0 cM)	TNFRSF6
DcR3	20q13	unknown	TNFRSF6B
CD27	12p13	ch6 (60.35)	TNFRSF7
CD30	1p36	ch4 (75.5 cM)	TNFRSF8
4-1BB	1p36	ch4 (75.5 cM)	TNFRSF9
TRAILR-1, DR4	8p21	unknown	TNRSF10A
TRAIL-R2, DR5	8p22-p21	ch14(D1)	TNFRSF10B
TRALLR3, DcRl	8p22-p21	ch7 (69.6 cM)	TNFRSF10C
TRAILR4, DcR2	8p21	ch7 (69.6 cM)	TNFRSF10D
RANK, TRANCE-R	18q22.1	ch1	TNFRSF11A
OPG, TR1	8q24	ch15	TNFRSF11B
FN14	16p13.3	ch17	TNFRSF12A
TRAMP, DR3, LARD	1p36.3	ch4 (E1)	TNFRSF25
TACI	17p11.2	ch11	TNFRSF13B
BAFFR	22q13.1-q13.31	ch15	TNFRSF13C
HVEM, HveA, ATAR	136.3-p36.3	ch4	TNFRSF14
P75NTR, NGFR	17q12-q22	ch11 (55.6 cM)	TNFRSF16
BCMA	16pl3.1	ch16(B3)	TNFRSF17
AITR, GITR	1p36.3	ch4(E)	TNFRSF18
RELT	11q13.2	unknown	TNFRSF19L
TROY, TAJ	13q12.11-q12.3	ch14	TNFRSF19
EDAR	2q11-q13	ch10	EDAR1
EDA2R	Xq11.1	chX	EDA2R
DR6	6p12.2-21.1	ch17	TNFRSF21
IGFLR1,Tmem149	19q13.12	ch7	IGFLR1

Table 2. TNFSF ligands.

TNF Superfamily			
	Chromosomal location		
Gene Name/Alias	Human	Mouse	Gene Symbol
TNF	6p21.3	ch17 (19.06 cM)	TNFSF1A
LTα	6p21.3	ch17 (19.06 cM)	TNFSF1B
LTβ	6p21.3	ch17 (19.06 cM)	TNFSF3
OX40-L	1q25	ch1 (84.90 cM)	TNFSF4
CD40-L,CD154	Xq26	chX (18.0 cM)	TNFSF5
Fas-L	1q23	ch1 (85.0 cM)	TNFSF6
CD27-L, CD70	19p13	ch17(20.0 cM)	TNFSF7
CD30-L,CD153	9q33	ch4 (32.20 cM)	TNFSF8
4-1BB-L	19p13	ch17(20.0 cM)	TNFSF9
TRAIL	3q26	ch3	TNFSF10
RANK-L, TRANCE	13q14	ch14 (45.0 cM)	TNFSF11
TWEAK	17p13	ch11	TNFSF12
APRIL/TALL2	17p13.1	ch13	TNFSF13
BAFF, BLYS, TALL1	13q32-q34	ch8 (3 cM)	TNFSF13B
LIGHT	19p13.3	ch17(D-E1)	TNFSF14
TL1A	9q33	ch4 (31.80 cM)	TNFSF15
GITRL, AITRL	1q23	unknown	TNFSF18
EDA1	Xq12-q13.1	chX (37.0 cM)	EDA1
EDA2	Xq12-q13.1	cX(37.0 cM)	EDA2

trimer formation and receptor binding. The ligands have highly conserved tertiary structures,[33–37] despite only limited sequence homology (<35%). Linker regions between the β stands are variable and form specific contacts with the receptors. Many TNFSF ligands can form homotrimers, and some also assemble as heterotrimers; examples of the latter group are LTα with LTβ[19] and APRIL with BAFF.[38] Alternatively spliced variants of TNFSF ligands produce molecules with additional functionalities. These include the fusion of TWEAK and APRIL to form TWE-PRIL[39] and the cytosolic form of LIGHT.[40]

1.2.2. *TNF receptors superfamily*

Unlike the ligands, TNFRSF expression is not restricted to cells of the immune system. The ligand-binding extracellular region of the receptors contains a cysteine-rich domain which is typically composed of six cysteine residues forming three disulfide bonds. Most TNFRSF members are type I transmembrane glycoproteins (extracellular N-terminus) and can be further segregated into two groups based on whether the intracellular domain (i) contains a death domain (DD) or (ii) binds TRAFs directly. Several TNFRSF members (e.g., TRAILR3) are membrane anchored via a glycolipid linkage that binds ligand but does not propagate signaling, and some receptors can be proteolytically released to generate soluble forms.

1.2.3. *Ligand-receptor binding models*

While TNFSF receptor–ligand binding is in general monotypic, some members have multiple partners[41] with non-redundant cellular responses that are unique for each ligand–receptor pair. The binding affinities are in the high picomolar to low nanomolar range. TNFRSF members are activated by aggregation, which is induced physiologically by interaction with their trimeric ligands. This activating mechanism not only explains why bivalent anti-TNFR antibodies can act as receptor agonists[42] but also clarifies why overexpression of TNFR, which has a propensity to self-associate,[43] results in ligand-independent signaling.

Signaling through ligand–receptor complexes can be influenced by the physical state of the ligand, whether membrane-bound or secreted (e.g., TNF). For example, membrane FasL induces apoptosis in peripheral T cells, but this activity is blocked by the secreted protein.[44] Changes in the expression of TNFSF members in response to environmental factors can also affect signaling. This has been observed for FasL expressed on endothelial cells, which is downregulated in response to TNF during inflammation. This is particularly important in inflammation, because under normal conditions, FasL induces leukocyte apoptosis to prevent tissue infiltration.[45] Further regulation of TNFR signaling is achieved by controlling ligand availability. Thus, decoy receptors such as DCR1, DCR2, DCR3, and OPG can inhibit signaling by sequestering the ligands.[46]

The interaction between a TNFSF ligand and its cognate receptor induces one of two outcomes: the cell will either undergo apoptosis via formation of the death-inducing signaling complex (DISC) or activate transcription factors to promote survival. How this is achieved will be discussed in the signaling pathways section further below.

1.2.4. *The lymphotoxin and tumor necrosis factor network*

The complexity of interactions and outcomes of the TNFSF members is well exemplified by the network that LT and TNF form with their different receptors (Figure 1).

TNF, LTα, LTβ, and LIGHT define the immediate group of TNF-related ligands that bind four cognate cell surface receptors with distinct but shared specificities. TNF and LTα both bind two receptors, TNFR1 and TNFR2. The heterotrimeric LT$\alpha_1\beta_2$ complex binds the LTβR, which also binds LIGHT. LIGHT also engages HVEM (Herpesvirus entry mediator; TNFRSF14), which acts as a ligand for Ig superfamily members, BTLA and CD160.[47] Two distinct human herpesviruses, herpes simplex virus and cytomegalovirus (CMV), target the HVEM-BTLA pathway using different mechanisms (Fig. 1).[48,49]

This pattern of shared utilization of ligands and receptors together with bidirectional signaling defines a complex co-stimulatory and inhibitory network. HVEM forms a switch between positive cosignaling through LIGHT-HVEM interaction and inhibitory signaling through B- and T-lymphocyte attenuator (BTLA). LIGHT and LTα bind HVEM at a distinct site from BTLA and CD160, yet all four ligands can activate the HVEM-NF-κB pathway to promote cell survival and differentiation.[50] In contrast, reverse signaling by HVEM engagement of BTLA restricts T and B cell proliferation by a direct inhibitory mechanism via the ITIM module in BTLA that recruits SHP1/2 tyrosine phosphatase, limiting antigen receptor activation.[51,52] UL144 of human CMV binds BTLA, but not LIGHT

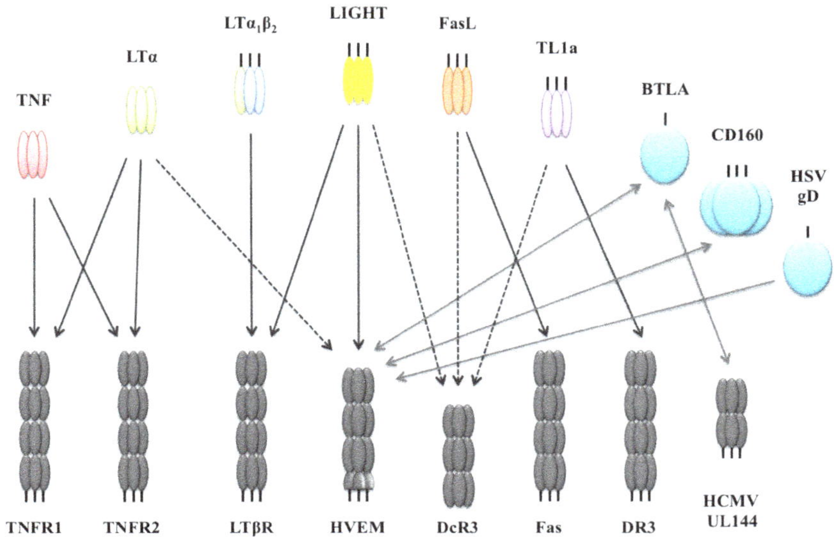

Fig. 1. The lymphotoxin and TNF network. Signaling network formed between TNF, LTα, LTβ, LIGHT, and cognate receptors. The network is characterized by the complexity of interactions due to the cross-utilization of ligands and receptors. The network increases in complexity (i) as non-TNF superfamily members (BTLA and CD160) interact with HVEM, (ii) as BTLA also interacts with the UL144 viral protein from the human cytomegalovirus (HCMV) that shares significant sequence homology with HVEM, and (iii) as another viral protein, HSV gD, is also able to bind HVEM. Fas ligand and TL1A are included in the network due to their sharing of decoy receptor-3 (DcR3). Shaded background shows ligands in the network that are not part of the TNFSF. Arrows determine direction of signal, some of them being bidirectional signaling pathways. Dashed lines represent interactions that occur in humans, but not mice.

or CD160, selectively mimicking the inhibitory pathway of HVEM-BTLA.

The broad range of immunologic processes controlled by this network is extensive, ranging from the development and homeostasis of lymphoid organs to the mobilization of innate defense systems and cosignaling activity promoting adaptive immune responses.[53–55] All these specific functions are dependent upon the integration of signals transduced following receptor activation.

1.3. Signaling pathways

1.3.1. The TNF-TNFR pathway

TNF can induce apoptosis upon ligation of TNFR1. Although TNFα also binds to TNFR2, this receptor lacks a DD and therefore cannot induce apoptosis. Upon TNFR1 activation, the intracellular DD recruits TNFR-associated death domain (TRADD) and Fas-associated death domain (FADD) proteins. In turn, FADD recruits procaspases 8 and 10 via their death effector domains (DED) to form the multi-protein complex DISC. DISC activates caspase 8, which induces apoptosis by activating the effector caspases 3, 6, and 7. FasL binding to Fas can also induce this mechanism of apoptosis (Figure 2).

Although apoptosis is the default pathway initiated by activation of TNFRSF members, cells are able to avoid death by synthesizing anti-apoptotic factors. Expression of these survival factors is mediated by the five-member NF-κB family, which comprises RelA, RelB, c-Rel, p50/NF-κB1, and p52/NF-κB2. Formation of active factors requires proteasome-dependent maturation of NF-κB1 and NF-κB2 from their respective inactive forms, p105[57] and p100.[58] In unstimulated cells, homodimers and heterodimers of NF-κB family members are sequestered in the cytosol by inhibitory proteins such as IκB (inhibitor of NF-κB). Receptor activation induces degradation of IκB and unmasking the NF-κB nuclear localization motifs that allow nuclear translocation and subsequent activation of transcription.[59]

TNFR1 ligation by TNF stimulates the canonical NF-κB pathway through activation of the IκB kinase (IKK) complex, which comprises IKKα, IKKβ, and NEMO (Figure 2). This process is initiated by TRADD, which recruits TRAF2, cIAP1/2 (via TRAF2), and receptor-interacting protein kinase 1 (RIPK1). This assembly of proteins is called signaling complex I. Lysine 63 (K63)-linked polyubiquitination of RIPK1 and TRAF2 by the E3 ligases cIAP1/2 or of TRAF2 by UeV1A and Ubc13 recruits the linear ubiquitin assembly complex (LUBAC), composed of HOIL-1, HOIP, and SHARPIN. TRAF2 and RIPK1 undergo linearly linked polyubiquitination by LUBAC, which then recruits IKK and targets NEMO for linear polyubiquitination. This allows the recruitment of IKK

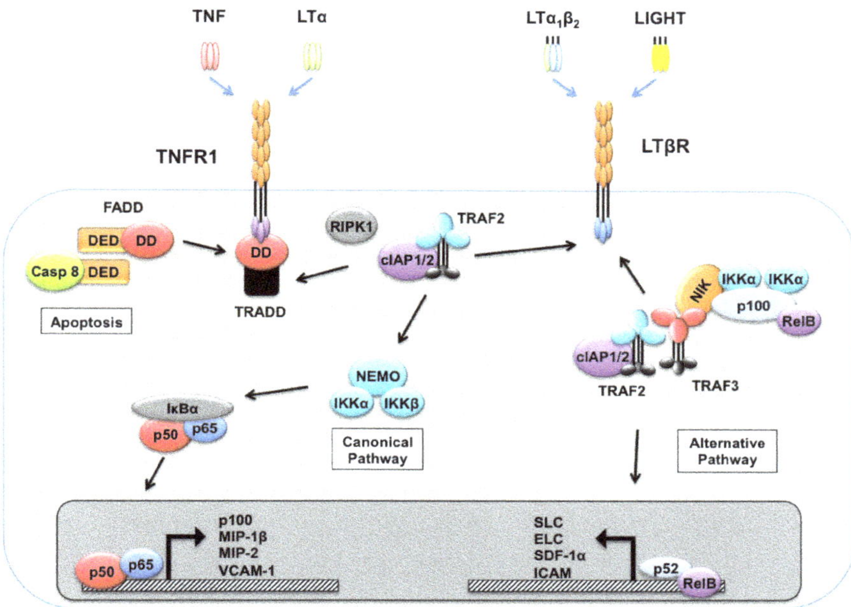

Fig. 2. TNFRSF signaling and NF-κB. TNFR1 DD recruits TRADD upon receptor activation by TNF or LTα. TRADD promotes apoptosis through formation of DISC, which is composed of FADD and caspase 8. The canonical NF-κB pathway is also activated by TRADD recruitment of RIPK1, TRAF2, and cIAP1/2. Downstream activation of the NEMO/IKKα/IKKβ complex leads to the translocation of the p50:p65 NF-κB complex to the nucleus upon the degradation of IκBα. LTβR activation by LIGHT or $LT\alpha_1\beta_2$ directly recruits the TRAF2:cIAP1/2 complex to activate the canonical NF-κB pathway. The alternative NF-κB pathway is repressed in the unstimulated cell by the TRAF2:TRAF3:cIAP1/2 complex, which targets NIK proteasome-dependent degradation. Allosteric inhibition of the TRAF2:TRAF3:cIAP1/2 complex upon LTβR activation leads to the accumulation of NIK.[56] NIK activates IKKα, which leads to proteolytic processing of p100 into p52. The translocation of the p52:RelB complex to the nucleus activates transcription. Genes activated by NF-κB include chemokines (e.g., MIP-1β, MIP-2, SLC, ELC, and SDF-1α) and adhesion molecules (e.g., VCAM-1 and ICAM).

activating kinases, transforming growth factor (TGF)-β activating kinase 1 (TAK1), TAK1-binding protein (TAB)-2 (TAB2), and TAB2. NEMO is then phosphorylated and activated by TAK1. The activated IKK complex phosphorylates IκB, resulting in its ubiquitin-dependent degradation and allowing the release and nuclear translocation of NF-κB1. Genes activated by NF-κB1 include cellular inhibitor of apoptosis (XIAP) and FLICE inhibitory protein (FLIP), which block apoptosis.

The transcription factor activating protein 1 (AP-1) is activated by TNFR1. This pathway is initiated upon activation of TAK1 by TNFR1, which stimulates MAPK kinase kinases (MAP3Ks), JNK, and p38 to phosphorylate c-Jun and ATF2. This induces formation of the c-Jun/ATF2 heterodimer, which is also known as AP-1.

The apoptosis and survival signaling pathways described here are shared by other TNFSF receptors. For example, activation of Fas by FasL also leads to FADD-mediated recruitment of TRADD and activation of NF-κB and AP-1. Additionally, TNFR2 activates NF-κB1 via a similar mechanism; however, it does so without recruiting TRADD since it is able to directly recruit TRAF2.

1.3.2. *LTβR signaling and the alternative NF-κB pathway*

LTβR signal transduction differs from TNFR1 signaling in three ways. First, LTβR does not contain the DD present in other TNFRSF members, instead it activates NF-κB1 by directly recruiting TRAF2. Second, dimerization of LTβR by $LT\alpha_1\beta_2$[60] or LIGHT[61] is necessary and sufficient for signaling. Third, LTβR can initiate an alternative NF-κB signaling pathway that leads to activation of NF-κB2 (Fig. 2). The alternative NF-κB signaling pathway is repressed in unstimulated cells via the depletion of cellular pools of the NF-κB inducer NIK by the E3 ubiquitin ligase complex, which contains TRAF2, TRAF3, and cIAP1/2. Upon LTβR activation, the E3 ligase complex is recruited to and sequestered by the receptor. This allows NIK to accumulate and subsequently phosphorylate and activate IKKα. IKKα then phosphorylates and targets p100 for proteasomal processing into p52. Interestingly, TNFR2, but not TNFR1, can activate NF-κB2 via this alternative pathway. Other TNFSF receptors that can activate the alternative NF-κB signaling pathway include CD40,[62] BAFF-R,[63] RANK,[64] TWEAK,[65] and CD27.[66]

Signaling pathways activated by TNFSF ligand–receptor interactions contribute to many critical cellular processes such as activation, growth, survival, and apoptosis. It is therefore not surprising that the TNFSF members play a prominent role in the cascade of events activated in response to an inflammatory insult.

2. TNFSF and inflammation

2.1. *Acute inflammation*

Some of the earliest events in the acute inflammatory response are changes in endothelial activation, vascular permeability, cell adhesion, cell recruitment, and neutrophil activation. Each of these events is influenced by members of the TNFSF.

Cytokines such as TNF and IL-1β were among the first factors shown to influence activation of endothelial cells (ECs) and recruitment of leukocytes to sites of inflammation.[67,68] The cytokines affect both cell types, resulting in a dramatic increase in the adhesion of leukocytes to the endothelium. Although slightly less effective than TNF, LT released by the injured tissue acts similarly on ECs to increase expression of cell adhesion molecules (CAM) such as ICAM-1, VCAM-1, and E-selectin and by promoting chemokine production,[69] culminating in elevated leukocyte adhesion.[70] Both TNF and LT activate NADPH oxidase and induce the production of ROS in EC and neutrophils.[69,71] Since these early studies, a growing number of TNFSF members have been shown to activate EC and thus promote leukocyte adhesion and diapedesis.

Binding of CD40L to CD40 on EC induces cell surface expression of E-selectin and ICAM-1. VCAM-1 is not induced by CD40L-mediated activation alone, but it is synergistically induced by TNF and CD40L. In this case, the contribution of CD40L could be secondary to TNF-induced activation of EC, because CD40 expression is negligible in healthy human vessels and increases under inflammatory conditions.[72,73] CD40L expressed by activated platelets markedly upregulates CAM expression and IL-8 and MCP-1 chemokine secretion by human umbilical cord endothelial cells (HUVEC).[74]

LIGHT is able to upregulate CAM, IL-8, and COX-2 expression in HUVEC through its interaction with LTβR and HVEM.[75] Similar to the findings with CD40L, expression of LIGHT by activated platelets increases their adhesion to HUVEC, and the interaction is reduced by the addition of a blocking anti-LIGHT monoclonal antibody.[76] Furthermore, both soluble and membrane LIGHT expressed by activated lymphocytes can induce expression of ICAM-1 and IL-8 by HUVEC. This is also blocked by treatment with an anti-LIGHT antibody.[77]

TRANCE (RANKL, TNFSF11) induces expression of ICAM-1 and VCAM-1 and production of ROS in EC through NF-κB activation.[78] Moreover, TRANCE induces vascular hyperpermeability, leukocyte recruitment, and angiogenesis *in vivo*. These effects are mediated by nitric oxide (NO) produced by EC eNOS.[79]

TRAIL stimulates eNOS phosphorylation in HUVEC with consequent NO production and prostanoid synthesis.[80] However, the effects of TRAIL are unusual in that it can induce HUVEC proliferation, but it cannot trigger NF-κB activation and increased expression of CAM.[81] TWEAK plays a role in EC activation by increasing expression of E-selectin and ICAM-1, thereby enhancing leukocyte adhesion.[82]

Interestingly, DcR3, a decoy receptor for TL1A, FasL, and LIGHT, has been shown to upregulate CAM expression and IL-8 production in EC, most likely through reverse signaling via an unidentified novel ligand.[83]

The activation of EC by TNF or other TNFSF members is mediated by TNFRSF signaling, NF-κB and AP-1 activation, as detailed above, and synthesis of adhesion molecules and chemokines.[71] Both canonical and alternative activation of NF-κB downstream of TNFR and LTβR have been shown to contribute to the induction of CAM and chemokines in activated EC.[84]

As might be expected from their function, increased expression of TNFSF members that contribute to EC activation usually correlates with endothelial dysfunction and an increased risk of atherosclerosis and coronary disease.[74,85–89]

Not all TNFSF members interacting with EC induce cell activation. For example, FasL:Fas interactions can induce apoptosis, as explained in the previous section. Under physiological conditions, FasL expressed by EC maintains homeostasis by inducing apoptosis of Fas^+ leukocytes adhering to the vasculature. During inflammation, however, TNF downregulates FasL expression by EC, thereby facilitating leukocyte diapedesis and recruitment into the tissue.[45] In addition, soluble FasL is a potent neutrophil chemoattractant despite being unable to activate or induce apoptosis in these cells.[90]

TNFSF members continue to influence neutrophil activation once they have migrated into the tissue. Neutrophils express a number of TNFSF receptors, including TNFR1, TNFR2, Fas, LTβR, RANK, TRAIL-R2, and TRAIL-R3.[91] As mentioned above, TNF and LT induce NADPH oxidase activation and ROS production in neutrophils.[69,71] In addition, both cytokines enhance neutrophil phagocytic ability and weakly stimulate degranulation.[92,93]

LIGHT is also able to enhance the phagocytic ability of neutrophils and monocytes. LIGHT signaling through HVEM stimulates their bactericidal activity by enhancing production of NO, ROS, and the proinflammatory cytokines IL-8 and TNF.[94]

Resolution of inflammation is tightly linked with timed neutrophil apoptosis. However, delayed neutrophil apoptosis is a common observation in non-resolving chronic inflammatory states due to the persistence of proinflammatory mediators at sites of inflammation.

TNFR1, Fas, and TRAIL-R2 are the DD-containing TNFSF receptors expressed by neutrophils. TNF plays a modest role in inducing neutrophil apoptosis, since signaling through TNFR2 and subsequent NF-κB-mediated induction of pro-survival signals overrides the pro-apoptotic signals.[95] Moreover, the role of TNF in apoptosis depends not only on the ratio of TNFR1 and TNFR2 but also on the concentration of TNF present, in that low concentrations favor neutrophil survival and high concentrations induce apoptosis.[96]

After extravasation into tissues, neutrophils downregulate TNFR1 while maintaining expression of Fas,[97] pointing to a role for Fas in induction of neutrophil apoptosis and resolution of inflammation. However, although the apoptosis rate of activated inflammatory neutrophils *in vitro* is higher than that of non-activated circulating neutrophils, membrane Fas levels are comparable and Fas sensitivity is equivalent in both populations.[98] Thus, once neutrophils have migrated into tissue they remain sensitive to Fas-induced apoptosis, and it is the combined influence of the inflammatory milieu (especially cytokines and growth factors) and availability of FasL that determines the apoptotic response. Finally, FasL is expressed by tissue-infiltrating monocytes/macrophages and is able to induce Fas-mediated apoptosis of neutrophils.[99,100]

TRAIL induces neutrophil apoptosis without activating NF-κB or inducing a chemotactic response[101] and plays an important role in the elimination of senescent neutrophils.[102] This is consistent with studies showing increased neutrophil survival and delayed inflammation resolution in TRAIL$^{-/-}$ mice.[103–105] These studies establish an important role for TRAIL in the apoptotic removal of neutrophils to ensure prompt resolution of inflammation.

In contrast, OX40L-activated signaling is anti-apoptotic and promotes the survival of neutrophils once they have migrated into tissue.[106]

LIGHT has been shown to contribute to the resolution of inflammation in several mouse models. In a wound healing model, LIGHT$^{-/-}$ mice showed delayed healing, and in some cases the wounds became chronically inflamed. It was proposed that LIGHT deficiency caused a redox imbalance that created an inflammatory environment with increased numbers of immune cells that remained at the wound site much longer than was observed in control mice.[107,108] In another wound healing study, LIGHT induced apoptosis of macrophages. Removal of macrophages once they have engulfed apoptotic neutrophils is an important step in the resolution of inflammation.[109] LIGHT:LTβR signaling also promotes healing in an asthma model. In this case, LIGHT induced expression of TGF-β and IL-13 by macrophages and eosinophils, respectively, which promoted fibrosis and airway remodeling.[110]

In a mouse experimental autoimmune encephalomyelitis (EAE) model of multiple sclerosis (MS), LIGHT levels were increased dramatically during the recovery phase of the disease. Radioresistant cells in the central nervous system were suggested to be the source.

The mechanism of action proposed for this model was that LIGHT suppressed the activity of inflammatory cells, especially macrophages/microglial cells, and thus promoted the resolution of the nervous system inflammation.[111] In an inflammatory bowel disease (IBD) model, LIGHT-deficient mice failed to recover the loss in body weight induced by administration of dextran sulfate sodium. Although the mechanism for this effect was not completely elucidated, the authors proposed a model similar to that in the wound healing and EAE models. In this case, LIGHT could affect the survival of fibroblasts responsible for the increased IL-6 levels observed in the colons of colitic LIGHT$^{-/-}$ mice.[112]

The ability of many TNFSF molecules to promote neutrophil apoptosis suggests that they might be useful therapeutic agents for the resolution of inflammation. However, a likely side effect of long-term treatment with such agents is immunosuppression. For this reason, it would be preferable to target proinflammatory mediators that prolong the lifespan of neutrophils in order to resolve the acute inflammation.

2.2. *Chronic inflammation and autoimmunity*

Failure to resolve acute inflammatory responses invariably leads to chronic, non-resolving inflammation. In previous sections, we discussed the impact of TNFSF molecules on EC and innate immune cell activation at the first stages of acute inflammation. However, the adaptive immune system plays an important role in maintaining the proinflammatory milieu. Lymphocytes express nearly all TNFSF members, and the functions of these proteins are best characterized in the context of chronic inflammation.

Activation of the adaptive immune system requires antigen presentation, which takes place predominantly in lymph nodes. Although lymph nodes are normal in TNF$^{-/-}$ mice, follicular dendritic cells, primary B cell follicles, and germinal centers do not develop properly.[113] Recent work has also highlighted the importance of TNF in the development of spleen fibroblastic reticular cells.[114] Even though TNF is not essential for lymph node development, overexpression of

TNF is able to drive maturation of lymph node stromal cells and formation of secondary lymph nodes in the absence of LTi cells. TNF overexpression re-establishes normal splenic architecture in the absence of LTβR signaling, but is unable to bypass the requirement for LTβR for secondary lymph node development.[115]

LT–LTβR signaling is required for the development of lymph nodes, as clearly demonstrated by the partial or complete lymph node deficiency in $LT\beta R^{-/-}$, $LT\alpha^{-/-}$, and $LT\beta^{-/-}$ mice.[54] LIGHT is not essential for lymph node development, although it does play a role when $LT\alpha_1\beta_2$ is absent.[116,117] LIGHT may play a role in inflammation-associated lymph node hypertrophy, however, by affecting the migration of B and T cells.[118] Indeed, LIGHT reverse signaling has previously been shown to affect T cell migration *in vitro* and *in vivo*.[119]

The RANK/RANKL axis is essential for lymph node development. Animals deficient in this axis fail to develop lymph nodes and have defects in Peyer's patches and the spleen. RANKL and LT are expressed by LTi cells, and RANKL is induced in lymphoid-tissue organizer (LTo) cells via LTβR signaling. Thus, RANKL is thought to be instrumental in the accumulation of LTi and B cells for lymph node formation.[120]

Naïve T cells migrate to lymph nodes through high endothelial venules (HEV), which are formed by specialized EC expressing a set of glycans collectively known as peripheral lymph node addressin (PNAd). PNAd facilitates the entry of naïve T cells into the lymph node by interacting with L-selectin expressed on the T cells. Maintenance of the HEV phenotype requires continuous homeostatic signaling, without which both PNAd expression and EC morphology are disrupted.[121] LT–LTβR signaling is required not only for the development of lymph nodes but also for their maintenance. Blockade of LTβR signaling reduces the cellularity of lymph nodes and prevents the development of collagen-induced arthritis. Although these effects probably resulted from several different mechanisms, expression of PNAd and MAdCAM in mucosal lymph nodes was decreased, as was the expression of sulfotransferases and fucosyltransferases required for PNAd synthesis. Signaling via

LT-LTβR, but not TNF, maintains the display of addressins and optimal functioning of HEV, and consequently supports naïve T cell migration into the lymph nodes.[122]

Another mechanism by which TNFSF members affect chronic inflammatory diseases is by promoting the formation of ectopic lymphoid structures. *De novo* formation of these tertiary lymphoid tissues is thought to occur through the same steps involved in the development of secondary lymph nodes. Thus, the adult counterpart of LTi cells or activated B, T, or DC are responsible for production of $LT\alpha_1\beta_2$[123] or LIGHT,[124] initial recruitment of cells, and organization of the lymphoid tissue. These structures resemble secondary lymph nodes, but they develop during inflammation and support antigen presentation and activation of reactive T cells. Thus, targeting of these lymphoid structures has been proposed as a therapeutic strategy for a wide spectrum of inflammatory and autoimmune disorders, including Crohn's disease, rheumatoid arthritis,[125] Sjögren's syndrome, autoimmune thyroiditis, myasthenia gravis, chronic bacterial infection, atherosclerotic plaques, chronic inflammatory liver disease, diabetes,[124] and MS.[126]

In addition to their roles in the development and homeostatic maintenance of lymphoid structures, many TNFSF receptors and ligands play important roles in controlling the activation of T, B, and antigen-presenting cells. Indeed, after the B7-CD28 superfamily, the second major group of T cell costimulatory receptors consists of several TNFSF members; 4-1BBL, OX40L, CD70, GITRL,[127] and TL1A,[128] with 4-1BBL having the most potent effects. CD30L and LIGHT are also involved in T cell proliferation and activation.[129,130]

Additionally, some TNFRSF are expressed in T regulatory (Treg) cells, playing relevant roles in their maturation and functionality. TNFR2, GITR, and OX40 are required for the development of Treg cells in the thymus.[131] In mature Treg, TNFR2 ligation induces their proliferation and enhances their suppressive ability.[132] DR3 activation induces Treg cell expansion but dampens their suppressive function exacerbating inflammation.[133,134]

DC maturation is induced by engagement of CD40L and LIGHT expressed by lymphocytes.[135,136] The subsequent upregulation of

CD86 expression and IL-12 secretion allows DC to prime T cells more efficiently.

TNFSF members play an essential role in B cell maturation and activation. BAFF and APRIL are required for B cell survival, maturation, and, together with CD40L and OX40L, class switch recombination.[137] CD40L is particularly important for the differentiation of B cells into antibody-secreting plasma cells. IL-4 and CD40L synergize to induce expression of cytidine deaminase, an enzyme necessary for class switch recombination.[138] CD40L synergizes with another cytokine, IL-21, to upregulate expression of the transcription factor Blimp-1, a master regulator of mature B cell differentiation into plasma cells.[139] The survival factors BAFF and APRIL are required for the long-term maintenance of plasma cell populations. LIGHT can also act as a costimulatory molecule for CD40L-induced human B cell proliferation.[140] Interestingly, mice with T cell-specific overexpression of LIGHT have an enlarged IgA^+ cell population in the intestinal lamina propria as well as increased serum IgA levels.[141]

$LT\alpha_3$ and $LT\alpha_1\beta_2$ signaling through LTβR play a crucial role in driving T cell-dependent and -independent IgA production. Ablation of LTα in $ROR\gamma t^+$ cells decreases IgA production in the gut and, as a consequence, induces a marked change in the gut microbiota.[142,143]

Polymorphisms in TNFSF genes have been associated with diverse human diseases.[52,144] It is not the objective of this chapter to exhaustively discuss associations between all TNFSF members and human inflammatory diseases. Instead, we focus on two prominent inflammatory disorders that have been associated with several members of the TNFSF: rheumatoid arthritis (RA) and IBD.

2.3. *TNFSF signatures in human pathologies*

2.3.1. *Rheumatoid arthritis*

Rheumatoid arthritis is a chronic inflammatory disorder of the joints, initially causing swelling and eventually leading to bone erosion and joint deformation. Early work implicated synovial macrophage-derived TNF as an effector molecule responsible for inducing the characteristic symptoms of RA. This observation led to the development of anti-TNF therapies that were first tested in clinical trials with RA patients[145] (discussed further below).

Several other members of the TNFSF have been associated with RA, and most of these are found at increased levels in the serum, circulating cells, or synovial fluid of RA patients. They include CD70, CD30L, CD40L, OX40, 4-1BBL, Fas, and BAFF. In contrast, FasL expression is extremely low in the inflamed joints, which could explain the prolonged survival of synoviocytes. However, other studies have found increased expression of soluble FasL, which, in contrast to the membrane form, has a detrimental effect on disease by inducing proliferation of synovial fibroblasts.[146]

TRAIL is also considered to have a beneficial effect on RA. The disease is exacerbated by blockade or deficiency of TRAIL but ameliorated by enforced expression in the joint. This effect is probably mediated by ligation of the death receptor DR5 and induction of apoptosis in fibroblasts-like synoviocytes.[147]

In addition to deregulated expression of TNFSF members, polymorphisms in their genes have also been linked to RA. One report implicated a polymorphic variant of TNF,[148] even though an earlier analysis had found the same association in Latin American populations but not in the global population.[149] Interestingly, a polymorphism in TNFRSF14 (HVEM) has been associated with both RA and celiac disease[150] and was found to be protective for RA.[151] In contrast, variants of TNFRSF9 (4-1BB)[152] and CD40[153] are associated with an increased risk for development of RA.

2.3.2. *Inflammatory bowel disease*

IBD is a group of chronic inflammatory disorders that can affect the entire digestive tract but are most frequently associated with the small intestine and colon. The most common forms of IBD are Crohn's disease and ulcerative colitis. Similar to its history in RA, TNF expression was detected at elevated levels in IBD patients more than 20 years ago.[154] Although not all studies have reported increased TNF expression in the involved intestinal mucosa or serum of affected patients, the efficacy of TNF-targeting agents in IBD therapy is unequivocal.[155] The pathological effects of TNF in IBD are mediated through several different mechanisms. One example is the induction of apoptosis in intestinal epithelial cells, which compromises the intestinal barrier function. The resulting breach allows lumenal microbiota to cross the barrier and promote inflammation. Notably, almost all of the immune cell types infiltrating the mucosa of IBD patients are able to produce TNF, thus exacerbating the immune response.

Other members of the TNFSF, including TL1A and FasL, are upregulated in the peripheral blood and/or inflamed intestinal lamina propria of IBD patients. TL1A synthesis is increased in lamina propria-infiltrating cells, and the number of $TL1A^+$ cells correlates with the severity of inflammation.[156] Similarly, FasL is upregulated in patients with active Crohn's disease and ulcerative colitis. Given the similar roles of FasL and TNF in promoting apoptosis, it has been proposed that FasL increases the intestinal barrier permeability by inducing epithelial cell apoptosis. However, several studies have shown that epithelial cells and lymphocytes in the inflamed intestine have enhanced resistance to Fas-mediated apoptosis. Another mechanism by which FasL could play a role in IBD is through reverse signaling. This is supported by the observation that ligation of FasL in activated lymphocytes enhances their proliferation, suggesting they could play a role in perpetuating inflammation.[155]

LIGHT is overexpressed in the inflamed intestinal mucosa and may contribute to IBD pathology by increasing T cell activation.[157,158]

Interestingly, DcR3, the soluble decoy receptor for TL1A, FasL, and LIGHT, is expressed at high levels in the inflamed mucosa and serum of Crohn's disease and ulcerative colitis patients.[159,160] Upregulation of DcR3 is considered to be a protective mechanism in IBD, similar to the upregulation of Foxp3 and other anti-inflammatory molecules.

Expression of TRAIL is differentially regulated in the mucosal cell populations of IBD patients, being downregulated in epithelial cells and upregulated in infiltrating mononuclear cells.[161] In addition, TRAIL may play a role in the fibrostenosing complications observed in Crohn's disease patients by affecting the apoptosis/proliferation balance of intestinal fibroblasts.[162]

Another TNFSF member, TWEAK, is found at elevated levels in the mucosa of ulcerative colitis and Crohn's disease patients, although the functional significance of this observation has yet to be elucidated.[163]

Finally, CD40L is overexpressed in T cells isolated from the inflamed mucosa of IBD patients. Additionally, *in vitro* activation of peripheral blood T cells from these patients upregulates cell surface expression of CD40L levels.[164]

Alleles of several TNFSF ligands and receptors have been associated with an increased risk for IBD. TNF polymorphisms have been reported as risk factors in small studies with specific populations. Although other studies have found no such correlation with the incidence of IBD, a potential association with patient response to anti-TNF therapy was detected.[165] Interestingly, broader meta-analyses of genome-wide association scans in IBD did not detect TNF as a risk locus, but did identify associations with other TNFSF ligands (FasL, GITRL, and TL1A) and receptors (HVEM, GITR, OX-40, 4-1BB, CD40, and DcR3).[166]

Although the IBD6 risk locus maps to 19p, which contains the LIGHT gene, no further association between LIGHT polymorphisms and disease have been reported. Other potential susceptibility candidates in the IBD6 locus have been identified.[167]

2.4. *Experimental models and the TNFSF as drug targets*

One of the key lines of evidence implicating TNF as a main player in inflammation came from studies showing that TNF and TNFR knockout mice display impaired inflammatory responses.[168] More importantly, results from these early studies have been substantiated by the efficacy of anti-TNF agents in the treatment of human inflammatory disorders (discussed in next section).

Other important models for the study of human inflammatory disorders include mice overexpressing TNF due to deletion of the regulatory ARE elements in TNF mRNA. These mice spontaneously develop arthritis and Crohn's-like ileitis.[169] Overexpression of LIGHT, OX40L, TL1A, and CD40L on T cells also leads to the spontaneous development of intestinal inflammation.[141,170,171] Mice with deficiencies in these TNFSF molecules are typically protected from inflammatory disease. Collectively, observations with the genetically modified mice confirm the important roles of TNFSF members in mediating inflammation *in vivo*.

Even more valuable and informative are the models in which animals with inflammatory diseases are treated with antibodies or soluble receptors targeting TNFSF members. In most cases, the treatments resulted in significant amelioration of the disease. Some of these models are summarized in Table 3, with a focus again on RA and IBD.

Given that TNFSF members play diverse roles in the immune response, it is not surprising that blocking their functions affects multiple immune mechanisms. The models summarized in Table 3 underscore some common mechanisms affected by blockade of the TNFSF member and/or improvement of the chronic inflammatory process. From the *in vivo* models, we can not determine whether these mechanisms are the cause or consequence of the attenuation of the inflammation; however, from *in vitro* data we know the role that TNFSF members play in directly driving some of the observed effects.

One effect of TNFSF blockade is a decrease in antigen-specific antibodies, especially in the RA models. This may result from interference with several disease mechanisms. For example, several TNFSF are important for the maintenance of lymph node architecture and function. Additionally, some family members are critical for B cell function, particularly their survival, maturation, and differentiation, as well as for antibody production by plasma cells. However, we should not rule out indirect effects of TNFSF blockade on T helper cells or myeloid cells involved in B cell maturation and function. Thus, blockade of some family members would affect the development of germinal centers and thus impair class switching, affinity maturation, and, ultimately, the production of pathological antibodies.

Table 3. Summary of mouse models for RA and IBD where a TNFSF member has been targeted.

TNFSF Targeting in RA and IBD mouse models				
Human disease	Mouse model	TNFSF targeting strategy	Effect	References
Arthritis	Collagen-induced arthritis	TNFR1-IgG1	Ameliorates	[172]
		TNFR2-IgG1	Ameliorates	[173]
		Anti-LTα	Ameliorates	[174]
		LTβR-Ig fusion protein	Ameliorates	[175]
		Anti-CD70	Ameliorates	[176]
		Anti-OX40L	Ameliorates	[177]
		Agonistic Anti-4-1BB	Ameliorates	[178]
		Anti-CD40L	Ameliorates	[179]
		CD40 antisense oligonucleotides	Ameliorates	[180]
		Anti-TL1A	Ameliorates	[181]
		BAFF virus	Ameliorates	[182]
		FasL virus	Ameliorates	[183]
		TRAIL virus	Ameliorates	[184]
	IL-1b-induced arthritis (rabbit)	TRAIL virus	Ameliorates	[185]
		rTRAIL	Ameliorates	[186]
	SCID-HuRAg	Anti-human Fas	Ameliorates	[187]
Inflammatory bowel disease	IL-10$^{-/-}$	Anti-TNF	Ameliorates	[188]
	Acute DSS colitis	Anti-TNF	Aggravates	[189]
	CD45RBhi transfer colitis	Anti-TNF	Prevented	[190]
		Anti-TNF and TNFR-Fc	No effect in treating	[190]

(Continued)

Table 3. (*Continued*)

TNFSF Targeting in RA and IBD mouse models

Human disease	Mouse model	TNFSF targeting strategy	Effect	References
	Chronic DSS colitis	Anti-TL1A	Ameliorates	[191]
		OX40-Ig	Ameliorates	[192]
		Anti-TNF	Ameliorates	[189]
	Th1-type TNBS colitis	LTβR-Ig fusion protein	No effect	[193]
	Th2-dominant TNBS colitis	LTβR-Ig fusion protein	Ameliorates	[193]
	CD45RBhi transfer colitis and TNBS colitis	Anti-CD70	Ameliorates	[194]
	TNBS colitis and IL-$2^{-/-}$mice	OX40-Ig	Ameliorates	[195]
	Acute and chronic DSS colitis	CD30-Ig	Ameliorates	[196]
	a-CD3 injection	CD30-Ig	Ameliorates	[197]
	TNFΔARE	Anti-TNF	Ameliorates	[198]
	CD45RBhi transfer colitis	Anti-TNF and LTβR-Ig fusion protein	Ameliorates	[199]
		Anti-OX40L	Ameliorates	[200, 201]
		Anti-CD40L	Ameliorates	[202, 203]
	TNBS colitis	Agonistic Anti-4-1BB	Ameliorates	[204]
		CD40 antisense oligonucleotides	Ameliorates	[205]

A hallmark of the resolution phase of inflammation is decreased production of cytokines. Blockade of TNFSF members reduces the levels of many proinflammatory cytokines, especially IFNγ, TNF, IL-6, IL-2, and IL-17. In some cases, increased numbers of Treg cells and levels of anti-inflammatory cytokines such as IL-10 are also observed. These profound effects are perhaps not surprising given that most TNFSF members play a role in immune cell activation and thus in the expression and secretion of cytokines. Importantly, TNFSF members are critical T cell costimulatory receptors, promoting their differentiation, proliferation, and cytokine production. Indeed, T cells are one of the main contributors of cytokine production in chronic inflammation.[206,207]

Another commonly observed feature of mouse IBD and rheumatoid arthritis models treated with TNFSF blockers is the reduced number of tissue-infiltrating T cells. One potential explanation for this effect is inhibition of EC activation and migration of immune cells into tissue, which is highly dependent on TNFSF members, as described above. In addition, blockade of TNFSF members involved in T cell proliferation and/or apoptosis could contribute to the reduced T cell numbers in these mouse models.

TNFRSF agonists have also been shown to have beneficial effects on inflammatory disease, most notably FasL and TRAIL. Agonists to these TNFRSF molecules are particularly effective in the collagen-induced arthritis model, which is characterized by a dramatic proliferation of fibroblast-like synoviocytes. Disease amelioration has been observed in animals following viral vector-induced overexpression of FasL or TRAIL, injection of recombinant FasL or TRAIL, and injection of agonist antibodies to the receptors Fas and TRAILR. Induction of Fas[183,187] and TRAILR[184–186] signaling not only induces synoviocyte apoptosis but also reduces the number of tissue-infiltrating T cells and the production of cytokines in this model.

Another interesting mechanism by which TNFRSF agonists reduce inflammation is illustrated by the effects of 4-1BB agonists in the hapten-derivatized protein with TNBS (2,4,6-trinitrobenzenesulfonic acid) model of colitis and the collagen-induced arthritis model. Here, treatment with the agonists ameliorates disease through expansion of a regulatory T cell population that counteracts CD4 T cell proliferation and production of cytokines.[178,204]

Since anti-TNF therapy has proven success in the clinic, current efforts are focused on reducing their side effects and improving efficacy. One objective is to facilitate administration of the agents, since current anti-TNF therapies must be injected intravenously or subcutaneously. To this end, orally active anti-TNF antibodies have been developed, and they have shown efficacy in two murine models of IBD.[208] Several approaches are being taken to develop IBD treatments that directly block TNF synthesis by pathogenic cells in the intestine. One method used microspheres to deliver TNF antisense oligonucleotides to colonic macrophages.[209] Another study used *Lactococcus lactis* engineered to secrete TNF-neutralizing nanobodies. This treatment was effective in two mouse models of IBD and did not interfere with immunity against *Salmonella*, suggesting that it could be a safe and effective treatment for human IBD.[210]

3. Targeting TNFSF in the clinic

3.1. *TNF inhibitors*

The first successful trial of an anti-TNF antibody (infliximab) was performed in 1994 and examined its efficacy in RA.[211] To date, five TNF inhibitors have been approved for clinical use[144] in RA, Crohn's disease, ulcerative colitis, psoriasis, juvenile idiopathic arthritis, psoriatic arthritis, and ankylosing spondylitis (Table 4).

Many cell types, both hematopoietic and nonhematopoietic, are able to produce TNF. However, lymphocytes and macrophages are likely to be the primary sources of TNF in autoimmune diseases.[212] As mentioned, TNF in its transmembrane form can be proteolytically cleaved to generate the soluble form. The presence of two forms of TNF is particularly relevant from a therapeutic viewpoint because the inhibitors can target the TNF-producing cells by binding to cell surface TNF and also act as scavengers by binding to the soluble form. Thus, TNF inhibitors act as competitive antagonists by blocking both the soluble and membrane forms of TNF from engaging their receptors.

The TNF inhibitors infliximab, adalimumab, certolizumab, golimumab, and etanercept are all structurally based on the IgG1 subclass antibody. The N-terminus of IgG1 antibodies contains an

Table 4. Clinical indications for TNF inhibitors.

TNF inhibitors in the Clinic				
Drug	Commercial name	Indications	Contraindication	No effect
Etanercept	Enbrel	RA, Ps, PsA, AS	MS	IBD, SLE, OA
Infiiximab	Remicade	RA, Ps, PsA, AS, IBD	MS	SLE, OA
Adalimumab	Humira	RA, Ps, PsA, AS, IBD	MS	SLE, OA
Golimumab	Simponi	RA, Ps, PsA, AS, IBD	MS	SLE, OA
Certolizumab	Cimzia	RA, Ps, PsA, AS,IBD	MS	SLE, OA

Note: RA, rheumatoid arthritis; Ps, psoriasis; PsA, psoriatic arthritis; AS, ankylosing spondylitis; IBD, inflammatory bowel disease including Crohn's disease and ulcerative colitis; MS, multiple sclerosis; SLE, systemic lupus erythematosus; OA, osteoarthritis.
Source: Adapted from Ref. [144].

antigen-binding variable domain and the C-terminal domain (Fc) provides the effector activity.[213] However, each of these inhibitors has different physical and functional properties, including specificity, valence, effector function, pharmacokinetics, and antigenicity. Infliximab is a humanized mouse antibody, while adalimumab and golimumab are fully human IgG1 molecules. Etanercept is a fusion protein of the TNFR2 with the Fc fragment of IgG1 and is the only TNF inhibitor that also inhibits LTα. Interestingly, and in contrast to etanercept, the fusion protein generated with TNFR1 (onercept) failed in clinical trials, although the mechanism underlying this disparity is unknown.[214]

In addition to competitive antagonism, other effector mechanisms for TNF inhibitors have been described. Cross-linking of membrane TNF is thought to induce an intracellular signaling cascade.[215] Complement-dependent cytotoxicity and antibody-dependent cell-mediated cytotoxicity are additional potential mechanisms of action of some TNF inhibitors.[216,217] IgG1 strongly activates complement through C1q binding and engages Fc receptors, enabling the elimination of TNF-expressing inflammatory cells. However, the efficacy of certolizumab, a Fab' (Fc-less) fragment PEGylated to increase its half-life, provides a strong argument that the primary mode of action of these drugs is direct antagonism.

Although TNF inhibitors are in broad use for many inflammatory disorders, their efficacy varies with the disease pathology (see Table 4). Significant heterogeneity is also observed in the response of patients with a specific condition. Moreover, there are several autoimmune and inflammatory disorders for which TNF inhibitors are ineffective, including systemic lupus erythematosus (SLE), Sjögren's syndrome, and osteoarthritis. TNF inhibitors are contraindicated in MS patients because they promote the onset of and/or exacerbate disease symptoms. Recent evidence from genome-wide analyses identified a genetic variant of TNFR1 (rs1800693) that is associated with an increased risk for MS. Carriers of this variant have higher levels of a soluble form of TNFR1 that appears to mimic the effect of TNF inhibitors in MS.[218]

Several mechanisms could explain the differing efficacies of infliximab and etanercept. Infliximab binds to the monomeric and trimeric forms of both soluble and membrane TNF. In contrast, etanercept binds only to unstable complexes with soluble TNF, which could contribute to an undesirable prolongation of the half-life of circulating TNF.[219] Furthermore, in contrast to infliximab, etanercept is unable to induce lymphocyte apoptosis.[217] Finally, etanercept also binds LTα which could be playing a protective role in IBD helping in the production of IgA.[142,143,220]

Unfortunately, TNF inhibitors have several recognized side effects, including increased risk for infections (especially reactivation of latent tuberculosis),[221,222] lymphoma, demyelinating disease,[223,224] and induction of autoantibodies or anti-drug antibodies.

Despite the proven efficacy of TNF inhibitors, more than 30% of treated RA and IBD patients show no clinical response.[225] Other patients show an initial response to therapy but become refractory to treatment or intolerant to administration over time. Anti-drug antibodies are believed to be the primary cause of the response failure. All of the TNF inhibitors (antibodies and chimeric TNF receptors) are protein-based and can evoke anti-drug immune responses, even the inhibitors of human origin. Notably, anti-drug antibodies generated by treated patients can effectively alter the clinical response by sequestering the drug and reducing its half-life.[226,227] Increasing the inhibitor dose or switching inhibitors has been reported to overcome this complication in some patients.[228] These negative aspects of the anti-TNF therapy are the main drivers for the proposal of targeting others in inflammatory diseases.

3.2. *Other TNFSF targets*

As previously described, other members of the TNFSF and TNFRSF have been broadly implicated in inflammatory disorders. We have already explained that the trimeric structure of TNFSF ligands promotes the clustering of the receptors that in turns activate the signaling pathway. Indeed, specific bivalent antibodies can also trigger TNFRSF clustering, inducing its activation in a similar manner as the native ligand. This feature of the TNFRSF poses specific antibodies as potential drugs.

Other than the anti-TNF agents, two biologics directed to TNFSF members have been approved, and 13 more are under clinical development for the treatment of inflammatory disorders (Table 5).

Denosumab, an antagonistic human anti-RANKL antibody, was approved in 2010 for the treatment of osteoporosis and is currently in phase III trials for the treatment of RA. A pilot phase I/II study will be initiated in the near future to assess the safety and efficacy of denosumab for the treatment of bone loss in children with rheumatic disorders receiving glucocorticoids.

Belimumab is an antagonistic human anti-BAFF antibody that was approved in 2011 for the treatment of a subset of patients with SLE. This antibody was first tested in RA patients and showed only a modest therapeutic effect in phase II trials, leading to its discontinuation for RA.

Table 5. Biologics targeting TNFSF in clinical trials for inflammatory disorders.

TNFSF in Clinical Trials					
TNFSF member	Biologic (trade name)	Type of agent	Activity of biologic	Indications	Stage of development
LTα	Pateclizumab	Human LTα-targeting antibody	Depleting and antagonist	RA	Phase II
TNF	TNF kinoid	Recombinant TNF carrier (self-immunization)	Antagonist	RA,Crohn's disease	Phase II
	ESBA105	Humanized scFv TNF-specific antibody	Antagonist	Uveitis	Phase II
LTβ/LIGHT	Baminercept	Human LTβR-Ig fusion protein	Antagonist	RA, Sjögren's syndrome	Phase II
	SAR252067	Human LIGHT-specific antibody	Antagonist	IBD	Phase I
OX40L	Oxelumab	Human OX40L-specific antibody	Antagonist	Asthma	Phase II
CD40L	ASKP1240/4D1	Human CD40-specific antibody	Antagonist	Transplantation/ psoriasis	Phase I/II
RANKL	Denosumab	Human RANKL-specific antibody	Antagonist	RA	Phase III
TWEAK	BIIB023	Humanized TWEAK-specific antibody	Antagonist	RA, lupus nephritis	Phase I/II
BAFF	Belimumab	Human BAFF-specific antibody	Antagonist	RA	Phase II
	Tabalumab	Human BAFF-specific antibody	Antagonist	SLE, RA, MS	Phase II/III
	Blisibimod	Human BAFF-binding peptibody Ig	Antagonist	SLE	Phase II/III
BAFF/APRIL	Ataricept	Human TACI-Ig fusion proteion	Antagonist	SLE, RA, MS	Phase II/III

Source: Adapted from Refs. [144, 229].

Although clinical trials have also been performed with targeted therapies against other TNFSF members, the trials were suspended due to severe side effects. For example, an anti-CD40L antibody was associated with thromboembolism.[230] Current efforts are focused on engineering an antibody with a mutated Fc domain, thus eliminating its effector function and reducing the risk of thrombosis.[231] Another option is to use CD40 antisense oligonucleotides to block CD40L-CD40 signaling.[180,205]

Pateclizumab is a humanized anti-LTα monoclonal antibody that can block both $LT\alpha_3$ and $LT\alpha_1\beta_2$. It has been shown to be safe and effective[232]; however, the effect on RA symptoms after 12 weeks treatment failed to reach statistical significance compared to placebo.[233]

Atacicept is a TACI-Ig fusion protein that prevents binding of BAFF and APRIL to TACI. This has been tested for RA and showed biological activity, but the primary efficacy end point was not achieved.[234] It will continue to be tested in clinical trials for SLE and MS.

An LTβR-Ig fusion protein, baminercept, failed to meet its endpoint in a phase II trial for RA.[235] However, a more recent trial showed that baminercept decreased the IFN signature and increased lymphocyte counts in a subset of RA patients with lymphopenia, but no clinical improvement was observed.[236] Nevertheless, these findings demonstrate the potential for targeting LTβR in a subset of patients with a specific biological signature. LTβR-Ig is currently in a phase II clinical trial for Sjögren's syndrome.

4. Summary

In summary, the TNFSF is a vast family of molecules that are intimately involved in many functions of the immune system, and thus in inflammation. Experimental research, clinical studies, and current therapies have shown that biologics targeting these molecules can successfully ameliorate disease. The path is open, but there is still a long road to pinpoint the specific mechanisms of each TNFSF member in the diversity of human inflammatory disorders.

Acknowledgements

The authors wish to recognize support provided by Perkins Foundation and grants from the National Institutes of Health (5T32AR064194-03, CA164679, AI048073, AI067890 and CA177322).

References

1. Granger GA, Williams TW. (1968). Lymphocyte cytotoxicity in vitro: activation and release of a cytotoxic factor. *Nature*. **218**:1253–1254.
2. Williams TW, Granger GA. (1968). Lymphocyte in vitro cytotoxicity: lymphotoxins of several mammalian species. *Nature*. **219**:1076–1077.
3. Carswell EA, Old LJ, Kassel RL, Green S, Fiore N, Williamson B. (1975). An endotoxin-induced serum factor that causes necrosis of tumors. *Proc Natl Acad Sci USA*. **72**:3666–3670.
4. Gray PW, Aggarwal BB, Benton CV, Bringman TS, Henzel WJ, Jarrett JA *et al.* (1984). Cloning and expression of cDNA for human lymphotoxin, a lymphokine with tumour necrosis activity. *Nature*. **312**:721–724.
5. Gray PW, Chen E, Li CB, Tang WL, Ruddle N. (1987). The murine tumor necrosis factor-beta (lymphotoxin) gene sequence. *Nucleic Acids Res*. **15**:3937.
6. Li CB, Gray PW, Lin PF, McGrath KM, Ruddle FH, Ruddle NH. (1987). Cloning and expression of murine lymphotoxin cDNA. *J Immunol*. **138**:4496–4501.
7. Beutler B, Greenwald D, Hulmes JD, Chang M, Pan YC, Mathison J *et al.* (1985). Identity of tumour necrosis factor and the macrophage-secreted factor cachectin. *Nature*. **316**:552–554.
8. Pennica D, Hayflick JS, Bringman TS, Palladino MA, Goeddel DV. (1985). Cloning and expression in Escherichia coli of the cDNA for murine tumor necrosis factor. *Proc Natl Acad Sci USA*. **82**:6060–6064.
9. Pennica D, Nedwin GE, Hayflick JS, Seeburg PH, Derynck R, Palladino MA *et al.* (1984). Human tumour necrosis factor: precursor structure, expression and homology to lymphotoxin. *Nature*. **312**:724–729.
10. Takeda K, Iwamoto S, Sugimoto H, Takuma T, Kawatani N, Noda M *et al.* (1986). Identity of differentiation inducing factor and tumour necrosis factor. *Nature*. **323**:338–340.
11. Aggarwal BB, Kohr WJ, Hass PE, Moffat B, Spencer SA, Henzel WJ *et al.* (1985). Human tumor necrosis factor. Production, purification, and characterization. *J Biol Chem*. **260**:2345–2354.

12. Aggarwal BB, Eessalu TE, Hass PE. (1985). Characterization of receptors for human tumour necrosis factor and their regulation by gamma-interferon. *Nature.* **318**:665–667.
13. Dembic Z, Loetscher H, Gubler U, Pan YC, Lahm HW, Gentz R *et al.* (1990). Two human TNF receptors have similar extracellular, but distinct intracellular, domain sequences. *Cytokine.* **2**:231–237.
14. Engelmann H, Aderka D, Rubinstein M, Rotman D, Wallach D. (1989). A tumor necrosis factor-binding protein purified to homogeneity from human urine protects cells from tumor necrosis factor toxicity. *J Biol Chem.* **264**:11974–11980.
15. Gray PW, Barrett K, Chantry D, Turner M, Feldmann M. (1990). Cloning of human tumor necrosis factor (TNF) receptor cDNA and expression of recombinant soluble TNF-binding protein. *Proc Natl Acad Sci USA.* **87**:7380–7384.
16. Loetscher H, Pan YC, Lahm HW, Gentz R, Brockhaus M, Tabuchi H *et al.* (1990). Molecular cloning and expression of the human 55 kd tumor necrosis factor receptor. *Cell.* **61**:351–359.
17. Nophar Y, Kemper O, Brakebusch C, Englemann H, Zwang R, Aderka D *et al.* (1990). Soluble forms of tumor necrosis factor receptors (TNF-Rs). The cDNA for the type I TNF-R, cloned using amino acid sequence data of its soluble form, encodes both the cell surface and a soluble form of the receptor. *EMBO.* **9**:3269–3278.
18. Shalaby MR, Aggarwal BB, Rinderknecht E, Svedersky LP, Finkle BS, Palladino MA. (1985). Activation of human polymorphonuclear neutrophil functions by interferon-gamma and tumor necrosis factors. *J Immunol.* **135**:2069–2073.
19. Browning JL, Ngam-ek A, Lawton P, DeMarinis J, Tizard R, Chow EP *et al.* (1993). Lymphotoxin beta, a novel member of the TNF family that forms a heteromeric complex with lymphotoxin on the cell surface. *Cell.* **72**:847–856.
20. Crowe PD, VanArsdale TL, Walter BN, Ware CF, Hession C, Ehrenfels B *et al.* (1994). A lymphotoxin-beta-specific receptor. *Science.* **264**:707–710.
21. Banks TA, Rouse BT, Kerley MK, Blair PJ, Godfrey VL, Kuklin NA *et al.* (1995). Lymphotoxin-alpha-deficient mice. Effects on secondary lymphoid organ development and humoral immune responsiveness. *J Immunol.* **155**:1685–1693.
22. Cupedo T, Mebius RE. (2005). Cellular interactions in lymph node development. *J Immunol.* **174**:21–25.
23. De Togni P, Goellner J, Ruddle NH, Streeter PR, Fick A, Mariathasan S *et al.* (1994). Abnormal development of peripheral lymphoid organs in mice deficient in lymphotoxin. *Science.* **264**:703–707.

24. Camerini D, Walz G, Loenen WA, Borst J, Seed B. (1991). The T cell activation antigen CD27 is a member of the nerve growth factor/tumor necrosis factor receptor gene family. *J Immunol.* **147**:3165–3169.
25. Stamenkovic I, Clark EA, Seed B. (1989). A B-lymphocyte activation molecule related to the nerve growth factor receptor and induced by cytokines in carcinomas. *EMBO.* **8**:1403–1410.
26. Dürkop H, Latza U, Hummel M, Eitelbach F, Seed B, Stein H. (1992). Molecular cloning and expression of a new member of the nerve growth factor receptor family that is characteristic for Hodgkin's disease. *Cell.* **68**:421–427.
27. Mallett S, Fossum S, Barclay AN. (1990). Characterization of the MRC OX40 antigen of activated CD4 positive T lymphocytes--a molecule related to nerve growth factor receptor. *EMBO.* **9**:1063–1068.
28. Kwon BS, Weissman SM. (1989). cDNA sequences of two inducible T-cell genes. *Proc Natl Acad Sci USA.* **86**:1963–1967.
29. Itoh N, Yonehara S, Ishii A, Yonehara M, Mizushima S, Sameshima M *et al.* (1991). The polypeptide encoded by the cDNA for human cell surface antigen Fas can mediate apoptosis. *Cell.* **66**:233–243.
30. Smith CA, Davis T, Wignall JM, Din WS, Farrah T, Upton C *et al.* (1991). T2 open reading frame from the Shope fibroma virus encodes a soluble form of the TNF receptor. *Biochem Biophys Res Commun.* **176**:335–342.
31. Zhai Y, Ni J, Jiang GW, Lu J, Xing L, Lincoln C *et al.* (1999). VEGI, a novel cytokine of the tumor necrosis factor family, is an angiogenesis inhibitor that suppresses the growth of colon carcinomas *in vivo*. *FASEB J.* **13**:181–189.
32. Griffith TS, Brunner T, Fletcher SM, Green DR, Ferguson TA. (1995). Fas ligand-induced apoptosis as a mechanism of immune privilege. *Science.* **270**:1189–1192.
33. Cha SS, Kim MS, Choi YH, Sung BJ, Shin NK, Shin HC *et al.* (1999). 2.8 A resolution crystal structure of human TRAIL, a cytokine with selective antitumor activity. *Immunity.* **11**:253–261.
34. Eck MJ, Ultsch M, Rinderknecht E, de Vos AM, Sprang SR. (1992). The structure of human lymphotoxin (tumor necrosis factor-beta) at 1.9-A resolution. *J Biol Chem.* **267**:2119–2122.
35. Gordon NC, Pan B, Hymowitz SG, Yin J, Kelley RF, Cochran AG *et al.* (2003). BAFF/BLyS receptor 3 comprises a minimal TNF receptor-like module that encodes a highly focused ligand-binding site. *Biochemistry.* **42**:5977–5983.
36. Hymowitz SG, Compaan DM, Yan M, Wallweber HJA, Dixit VM, Starovasnik MA *et al.* (2003). The crystal structures of EDA-A1 and EDA-A2:splice variants with distinct receptor specificity. *Structure.* **11**:1513–1520.

37. Jones EY, Stuart DI, Walker NP. (1992). Crystal structure of TNF. *Immunol Ser.* **56**:93–127.
38. Roschke V, Sosnovtseva S, Ward CD, Hong JS, Smith R, Albert V *et al.* (2002). BLyS and APRIL form biologically active heterotrimers that are expressed in patients with systemic immune-based rheumatic diseases. *J Immunol.* **169**:4314–4321.
39. Pradet-Balade B, Medema JP, López-Fraga M, Lozano JC, Kolfschoten GM, Picard A *et al.* (2002). An endogenous hybrid mRNA encodes TWE-PRIL, a functional cell surface TWEAK-APRIL fusion protein. *EMBO.* **21**:5711–5720.
40. Granger SW, Butrovich KD, Houshmand P, Edwards WR, Ware CF. (2001). Genomic characterization of LIGHT reveals linkage to an immune response locus on chromosome 19p13.3 and distinct isoforms generated by alternate splicing or proteolysis. *J Immunol.* **167**:5122–5128.
41. Bossen C, Ingold K, Tardivel A, Bodmer J-L, Gaide O, Hertig S *et al.* (2006). Interactions of tumor necrosis factor (TNF) and TNF receptor family members in the mouse and human. *J Biol Chem.* **281**:13964–13971.
42. Engelmann H, Holtmann H, Brakebusch C, Avni YS, Sarov I, Nophar Y *et al.* (1990). Antibodies to a soluble form of a tumor necrosis factor (TNF) receptor have TNF-like activity. *J Biol Chem.* **265**:14497–14504.
43. Boldin MP, Mett IL, Varfolomeev EE, Chumakov I, Shemer-Avni Y, Camonis JH *et al.* (1995). Self-association of the "death domains" of the p55 tumor necrosis factor (TNF) receptor and Fas/APO1 prompts signaling for TNF and Fas/APO1 effects. *J Biol Chem.* **270**:387–391.
44. Suda T, Hashimoto H, Tanaka M, Ochi T, Nagata S. (1997). Membrane Fas ligand kills human peripheral blood T lymphocytes, and soluble Fas ligand blocks the killing. *J Exp Med.* **186**:2045–2050.
45. Sata M, Walsh K. (1998). TNFalpha regulation of Fas ligand expression on the vascular endothelium modulates leukocyte extravasation. *Nat Med.* **4**:415–420.
46. Ashkenazi A. (2002). Targeting death and decoy receptors of the tumour-necrosis factor superfamily. *Nat Rev Cancer.* **2**:420–430.
47. Sedy JR, Gavrieli M, Potter KG, Hurchla MA, Lindsley RC, Hildner K *et al.* (2005). B and T lymphocyte attenuator regulates T cell activation through interaction with herpesvirus entry mediator. *Nat Immunol.* **6**:90–98.
48. Cheung TC, Humphreys IR, Potter KG, Norris PS, Shumway HM, Tran BR *et al.* (2005). Evolutionarily divergent herpesviruses modulate T cell activation by targeting the herpesvirus entry mediator cosignaling pathway. *Proc Natl Acad Sci USA.* **102**:13218–13223.
49. Sedy JR, Spear PG, Ware CF. (2008). Cross-regulation between herpesviruses and the TNF superfamily members. *Nat Rev Immunol.* **8**:861–873.

50. Cheung TC, Steinberg MW, Oborne LM, Macauley MG, Fukuyama S, Sanjo H *et al.* (2009). Unconventional ligand activation of herpesvirus entry mediator signals cell survival. *Proc Natl Acad Sci USA.* **106**:6244–6249.
51. Murphy TL, Murphy KM. (2010). Slow down and survive: Enigmatic immunoregulation by BTLA and HVEM. *Annu Rev Immunol.* **28**:389–411.
52. Sedy J, Bekiaris V, Ware CF. (2014). Tumor Necrosis Factor Superfamily in Innate Immunity and Inflammation. *Cold Spring Harb Perspect Biol.*
53. Kollias G. (2005). TNF pathophysiology in murine models of chronic inflammation and autoimmunity. *Semin Arthritis Rheum.* **34**:3–6.
54. McCarthy DD, Summers-Deluca L, Vu F, Chiu S, Gao Y, Gommerman JL. (2006). The lymphotoxin pathway: beyond lymph node development. *Immunol Res.* **35**:41–54.
55. Ware CF. (2005). Network communications: lymphotoxins, LIGHT, and TNF. *Annu Rev Immunol.* **23**:787–819.
56. Sanjo H, Zajonc DM, Braden R, Norris PS, Ware CF. (2010). Allosteric regulation of the ubiquitin:NIK and ubiquitin:TRAF3 E3 ligases by the lymphotoxin-beta receptor. *J Biol Chem.* **285**:17148–17155.
57. Ghosh S, May MJ, Kopp EB. (1998). NF-kappa B and Rel proteins: evolutionarily conserved mediators of immune responses. *Annu Rev Immunol.* **16**:225–260.
58. Karin M, Ben-Neriah Y. (2000). Phosphorylation meets ubiquitination: the control of NF-[kappa]B activity. *Annu Rev Immunol.* **18**:621–663.
59. Schröfelbauer B, Hoffmann A. (2011). How do pleiotropic kinase hubs mediate specific signaling by TNFR superfamily members? *Immunol Rev.* **244**:29–43.
60. Sudhamsu J, Yin J, Chiang EY, Starovasnik MA, Grogan JL, Hymowitz SG. (2013). Dimerization of LTbetaR by LTalpha1beta2 is necessary and sufficient for signal transduction. *Proc Natl Acad Sci USA.* **110**:19896–19901.
61. Eldredge J, Berkowitz S, Corin AF, Day ES, Hayes D, Meier W *et al.* (2006). Stoichiometry of LTbetaR binding to LIGHT. *Biochemistry.* **45**:10117–10128.
62. Coope HJ, Atkinson PG, Huhse B, Belich M, Janzen J, Holman MJ *et al.* (2002). CD40 regulates the processing of NF-kappaB2 p100 to p52. *EMBO J.* **21**:5375–5385.
63. Claudio E, Brown K, Park S, Wang H, Siebenlist U. (2002). BAFF-induced NEMO-independent processing of NF-kappa B2 in maturing B cells. *Nat Immunol.* **3**:958–965.
64. Novack DV, Yin L, Hagen-Stapleton A, Schreiber RD, Goeddel DV, Ross FP *et al.* (2003). The IkappaB function of NF-kappaB2 p100 controls stimulated osteoclastogenesis. *J Exp Med.* **198**:771–781.

65. Saitoh T, Nakayama M, Nakano H, Yagita H, Yamamoto N, Yamaoka S. (2003). TWEAK induces NF-kappaB2 p100 processing and long lasting NF-kappaB activation. *J Biol Chem.* **278**:36005–36012.
66. Ramakrishnan P, Wang W, Wallach D. (2004). Receptor-specific signaling for both the alternative and the canonical NF-kappaB activation pathways by NF-kappaB-inducing kinase. *Immunity.* **21**:477–489.
67. Cavender D, Saegusa Y, Ziff M. (1987). Stimulation of endothelial cell binding of lymphocytes by tumor necrosis factor. *J Immunol.* **139**:1855–1860.
68. Dejana E, Ji-Ming W, Mantovani A. (1987). The recruitment of leukocytes and their interaction with the vessel wall: The role of interleukin-1 and tumor necrosis factor. *Scand J Rheumatol Suppl.* **66**:19–25.
69. Pober JS, Lapierre LA, Stolpen AH, Brock TA, Springer TA, Fiers W *et al.* (1987). Activation of cultured human endothelial cells by recombinant lymphotoxin: comparison with tumor necrosis factor and interleukin 1 species. *J Immunol.* **138**:3319–3324.
70. Cavender DE, Edelbaum D, Ziff M. (1989). Endothelial cell activation induced by tumor necrosis factor and lymphotoxin. *Am J Pathol.* **134**:551–560.
71. Pober JS. (2002). Endothelial activation: intracellular signaling pathways. *Arthritis Res.* **4**(Suppl 3):S109–116.
72. Hollenbaugh D, Mischel-Petty N, Edwards CP, Simon JC, Denfeld RW, Kiener PA *et al.* (1995). Expression of functional CD40 by vascular endothelial cells. *J Exp Med.* **182**:33–40.
73. Karmann K, Hughes CC, Schechner J, Fanslow WC, Pober JS. (1995). CD40 on human endothelial cells: inducibility by cytokines and functional regulation of adhesion molecule expression. *Proc Natl Acad Sci USA.* **92**:4342–4346.
74. Henn V, Slupsky JR, Grafe M, Anagnostopoulos I, Forster R, Muller-Berghaus G *et al.* (1998). CD40 ligand on activated platelets triggers an inflammatory reaction of endothelial cells. *Nature.* **391**:591–594.
75. Chang YH, Hsieh SL, Chao Y, Chou YC, Lin WW. (2005). Proinflammatory effects of LIGHT through HVEM and LTbetaR interactions in cultured human umbilical vein endothelial cells. *J Biomed Sci.* **12**:363–375.
76. Celik S, Langer H, Stellos K, May AE, Shankar V, Kurz K *et al.* (2007). Platelet-associated LIGHT (TNFSF14) mediates adhesion of platelets to human vascular endothelium. *Thromb Haemost.* **98**:798–805.
77. Celik S, Shankar V, Richter A, Hippe HJ, Akhavanpoor M, Bea F *et al.* (2009). Proinflammatory and prothrombotic effects on human vascular endothelial cells of immune-cell-derived LIGHT. *Eur J Med Res.* **14**:147–156.
78. Min JK, Kim YM, Kim SW, Kwon MC, Kong YY, Hwang IK *et al.* (2005). TNF-related activation-induced cytokine enhances leukocyte adhesiveness:

induction of ICAM-1 and VCAM-1 via TNF receptor-associated factor and protein kinase C-dependent NF-kappaB activation in endothelial cells. *J Immunol.* **175**:531–540.
79. Min JK, Cho YL, Choi JH, Kim Y, Kim JH, Yu YS *et al.* (2007). Receptor activator of nuclear factor (NF)-kappaB ligand (RANKL) increases vascular permeability: impaired permeability and angiogenesis in eNOS-deficient mice. *Blood.* **109**:1495–1502.
80. Zauli G, Pandolfi A, Gonelli A, Di Pietro R, Guarnieri S, Ciabattoni G *et al.* (2003). Tumor necrosis factor-related apoptosis-inducing ligand (TRAIL) sequentially upregulates nitric oxide and prostanoid production in primary human endothelial cells. *Circ Res.* **92**:732–740.
81. Secchiero P, Gonelli A, Carnevale E, Milani D, Pandolfi A, Zella D *et al.* (2003). TRAIL promotes the survival and proliferation of primary human vascular endothelial cells by activating the Akt and ERK pathways. *Circulation.* **107**:2250–2256.
82. Chen T, Guo ZP, Li L, Li MM, Wang TT, Jia RZ *et al.* (2013). TWEAK enhances E-selectin and ICAM-1 expression, and may contribute to the development of cutaneous vasculitis. *PLoS One.* **8**:e56830.
83. Yang CR, Hsieh SL, Ho FM, Lin WW. (2005). Decoy receptor 3 increases monocyte adhesion to endothelial cells via NF-kappa B-dependent up-regulation of intercellular adhesion molecule-1, VCAM-1, and IL-8 expression. *J Immunol.* **174**:1647–1656.
84. Madge LA, Kluger MS, Orange JS, May MJ. (2008). Lymphotoxin-alpha 1 beta 2 and LIGHT induce classical and noncanonical NF-kappa B-dependent proinflammatory gene expression in vascular endothelial cells. *J Immunol.* **180**:3467–3477.
85. Sandberg WJ, Yndestad A, Oie E, Smith C, Ueland T, Ovchinnikova O *et al.* (2006). Enhanced T-cell expression of RANK ligand in acute coronary syndrome: possible role in plaque destabilization. *Arterioscler Thromb Vasc Biol.* **26**:857–863.
86. Sato K, Nuki T, Gomita K, Weyand CM, Hagiwara N. (2010). Statins reduce endothelial cell apoptosis via inhibition of TRAIL expression on activated CD4 T cells in acute coronary syndrome. *Atherosclerosis.* **213**:33–39.
87. Suna S, Sakata Y, Shimizu M, Nakatani D, Usami M, Matsumoto S *et al.* (2009). Lymphotoxin-alpha3 mediates monocyte-endothelial interaction by TNFR I/NF-kappaB signaling. *Biochem Biophys Res Commun.* **379**: 374–378.
88. Szmitko PE, Wang CH, Weisel RD, de Almeida JR, Anderson TJ, Verma S. (2003). New markers of inflammation and endothelial cell activation: Part I. *Circulation.* **108**:1917–1923.
89. Zhang H, Park Y, Wu J, Chen X, Lee S, Yang J *et al.* (2009). Role of TNF-alpha in vascular dysfunction. *Clin Sci (Lond).* **116**:219–230.

90. Dupont PJ, Warrens AN. (2007). Fas ligand exerts its pro-inflammatory effects via neutrophil recruitment but not activation. *Immunology*. **120**:133–139.
91. Futosi K, Fodor S, Mocsai A. (2013). Reprint of Neutrophil cell surface receptors and their intracellular signal transduction pathways. *Int Immunopharmacol*. **17**:1185–1197.
92. Klebanoff SJ, Vadas MA, Harlan JM, Sparks LH, Gamble JR, Agosti JM *et al*. (1986). Stimulation of neutrophils by tumor necrosis factor. *J Immunol*. **136**:4220–4225.
93. Shalaby MR, Aggarwal BB, Rinderknecht E, Svedersky LP, Finkle BS, Palladino MA, Jr. (1985). Activation of human polymorphonuclear neutrophil functions by interferon-gamma and tumor necrosis factors. *J Immunol*. **135**:2069–2073.
94. Heo SK, Ju SA, Lee SC, Park SM, Choe SY, Kwon B *et al*. (2006). LIGHT enhances the bactericidal activity of human monocytes and neutrophils via HVEM. *J Leukoc Biol*. **79**:330–338.
95. Murray J, Barbara JA, Dunkley SA, Lopez AF, Van Ostade X, Condliffe AM *et al*. (1997). Regulation of neutrophil apoptosis by tumor necrosis factor-alpha: requirement for TNFR55 and TNFR75 for induction of apoptosis in vitro. *Blood*. **90**:2772–2783.
96. van den Berg JM, Weyer S, Weening JJ, Roos D, Kuijpers TW. (2001). Divergent effects of tumor necrosis factor alpha on apoptosis of human neutrophils. *J Leukoc Biol*. **69**:467–473.
97. Seely AJ, Swartz DE, Giannias B, Christou NV. (1998). Reduction in neutrophil cell surface expression of tumor necrosis factor receptors but not Fas after transmigration: implications for the regulation of neutrophil apoptosis. *Arch Surg*. **133**:1305–1310.
98. Renshaw SA, Timmons SJ, Eaton V, Usher LR, Akil M, Bingle CD *et al*. (2000). Inflammatory neutrophils retain susceptibility to apoptosis mediated via the Fas death receptor. *J Leukoc Biol*. **67**:662–668.
99. Brown SB, Savill J. (1999). Phagocytosis triggers macrophage release of Fas ligand and induces apoptosis of bystander leukocytes. *J Immunol*. **162**:480–485.
100. Kiener PA, Davis PM, Rankin BM, Klebanoff SJ, Ledbetter JA, Starling GC *et al*. (1997). Human monocytic cells contain high levels of intracellular Fas ligand: rapid release following cellular activation. *J Immunol*. **159**:1594–1598.
101. Renshaw SA, Parmar JS, Singleton V, Rowe SJ, Dockrell DH, Dower SK *et al*. (2003). Acceleration of human neutrophil apoptosis by TRAIL. *J Immunol*. **170**:1027–1033.
102. Lum JJ, Bren G, McClure R, Badley AD. (2005). Elimination of senescent neutrophils by TNF-related apoptosis-inducing [corrected] ligand. *J Immunol*. **175**:1232–1238.

103. Hoffmann O, Priller J, Prozorovski T, Schulze-Topphoff U, Baeva N, Lunemann JD *et al.* (2007). TRAIL limits excessive host immune responses in bacterial meningitis. *J Clin Invest.* **117**:2004–2013.
104. McGrath EE, Marriott HM, Lawrie A, Francis SE, Sabroe I, Renshaw SA *et al.* (2011). TNF-related apoptosis-inducing ligand (TRAIL) regulates inflammatory neutrophil apoptosis and enhances resolution of inflammation. *J Leukoc Biol.* **90**:855–865.
105. Zheng SJ, Jiang J, Shen H, Chen YH. (2004). Reduced apoptosis and ameliorated listeriosis in TRAIL-null mice. *J Immunol.* **173**:5652–5658.
106. Baumann R, Yousefi S, Simon D, Russmann S, Mueller C, Simon HU. (2004). Functional expression of CD134 by neutrophils. *Eur J Immunol.* **34**:2268–2275.
107. Dhall S, Do D, Garcia M, Wijesinghe DS, Brandon A, Kim J *et al.* (2014). A novel model of chronic wounds: Importance of redox imbalance and biofilm-forming bacteria for establishment of chronicity. *PLoS One.* **9**:e109848.
108. Petreaca ML, Do D, Dhall S, McLelland D, Serafino A, Lyubovitsky J *et al.* (2012). Deletion of a tumor necrosis superfamily gene in mice leads to impaired healing that mimics chronic wounds in humans. *Wound Repair Regen.* **20**:353–366.
109. Petreaca ML, Yao M, Ware C, Martins-Green MM. (2008). Vascular endothelial growth factor promotes macrophage apoptosis through stimulation of tumor necrosis factor superfamily member 14 (TNFSF14/LIGHT). *Wound Repair Regen.* **16**:602–614.
110. Doherty TA, Soroosh P, Khorram N, Fukuyama S, Rosenthal P, Cho JY *et al.* (2011). The tumor necrosis factor family member LIGHT is a target for asthmatic airway remodeling. *Nat Med.* **17**:596–603.
111. Mana P, Linares D, Silva DG, Fordham S, Scheu S, Pfeffer K *et al.* (2013). LIGHT (TNFSF14/CD258) is a decisive factor for recovery from experimental autoimmune encephalomyelitis. *J Immunol.* **191**:154–163.
112. Krause P, Zahner SP, Kim G, Shaikh RB, Steinberg MW, Kronenberg M. (2014). The tumor necrosis factor family member TNFSF14 (LIGHT) is required for resolution of intestinal inflammation in mice. *Gastroenterology.* **146**:1752–1762.e1754.
113. Pasparakis M, Alexopoulou L, Episkopou V, Kollias G. (1996). Immune and inflammatory responses in TNF alpha-deficient mice: a critical requirement for TNF alpha in the formation of primary B cell follicles, follicular dendritic cell networks and germinal centers, and in the maturation of the humoral immune response. *J Exp Med.* **184**:1397–1411.
114. Zhao L, Chen J, Liu L, Gao J, Guo B, Zhu B. (2015). Essential role of TNF-alpha in development of spleen fibroblastic reticular cells. *Cell Immunol.* **293**:130–136.

115. Furtado GC, Pacer ME, Bongers G, Benezech C, He Z, Chen L *et al.* (2014). TNFalpha-dependent development of lymphoid tissue in the absence of RORgammat(+) lymphoid tissue inducer cells. *Mucosal Immunol.* 7:602–614.
116. Scheu S, Alferink J, Potzel T, Barchet W, Kalinke U, Pfeffer K. (2002). Targeted disruption of LIGHT causes defects in costimulatory T cell activation and reveals cooperation with lymphotoxin beta in mesenteric lymph node genesis. *J Exp Med.* **195**:1613–1624.
117. Wang J, Foster A, Chin R, Yu P, Sun Y, Wang Y *et al.* (2002). The complementation of lymphotoxin deficiency with LIGHT, a newly discovered TNF family member, for the restoration of secondary lymphoid structure and function. *Eur J Immunol.* **32**:1969–1979.
118. Zhu M, Yang Y, Wang Y, Wang Z, Fu YX. (2011). LIGHT regulates inflamed draining lymph node hypertrophy. *J Immunol.* **186**:7156–7163.
119. Shi G, Wu Y, Zhang J, Wu J. (2003). Death decoy receptor TR6/DcR3 inhibits T cell chemotaxis *in vitro* and *in vivo*. *J Immunol.* **171**:3407–3414.
120. Mueller CG, Hess E. (2012). Emerging Functions of RANKL in Lymphoid Tissues. *Front Immunol.* **3**:261.
121. Mebius RE, Streeter PR, Breve J, Duijvestijn AM, Kraal G. (1991). The influence of afferent lymphatic vessel interruption on vascular addressin expression. *J Cell Biol.* **115**:85–95.
122. Browning JL, Allaire N, Ngam-Ek A, Notidis E, Hunt J, Perrin S *et al.* (2005). Lymphotoxin-beta receptor signaling is required for the homeostatic control of HEV differentiation and function. *Immunity.* **23**:539–550.
123. Neyt K, Perros F, GeurtsvanKessel CH, Hammad H, Lambrecht BN. (2012). Tertiary lymphoid organs in infection and autoimmunity. *Trends Immunol.* **33**:297–305.
124. Lee Y, Chin RK, Christiansen P, Sun Y, Tumanov AV, Wang J *et al.* (2006). Recruitment and activation of naive T cells in the islets by lymphotoxin beta receptor-dependent tertiary lymphoid structure. *Immunity.* **25**:499–509.
125. Takemura S, Braun A, Crowson C, Kurtin PJ, Cofield RH, O'Fallon WM *et al.* (2001). Lymphoid neogenesis in rheumatoid synovitis. *J Immunol.* **167**:1072–1080.
126. Columba-Cabezas S, Griguoli M, Rosicarelli B, Magliozzi R, Ria F, Serafini B *et al.* (2006). Suppression of established experimental autoimmune encephalomyelitis and formation of meningeal lymphoid follicles by lymphotoxin beta receptor-Ig fusion protein. *J Neuroimmunol.* **179**:76–86.
127. Kober J, Leitner J, Klauser C, Woitek R, Majdic O, Stockl J *et al.* (2008). The capacity of the TNF family members 4–1.BBL, OX40L, CD70, GITRL, CD30L and LIGHT to costimulate human T cells. *Eur J Immunol.* **38**:2678–2688.

128. Migone TS, Zhang J, Luo X, Zhuang L, Chen C, Hu B *et al.* (2002). TL1A is a TNF-like ligand for DR3 and TR6/DcR3 and functions as a T cell costimulator. *Immunity*. **16**:479–492.
129. Ware CF. (2008). Targeting lymphocyte activation through the lymphotoxin and LIGHT pathways. *Immunol Rev*. **223**:186–201.
130. Watts TH. (2005). TNF/TNFR family members in costimulation of T cell responses. *Annu Rev Immunol*. **23**:23–68.
131. Mahmud SA, Manlove LS, Schmitz HM, Xing Y, Wang Y, Owen DL *et al.* (2014). Costimulation via the tumor-necrosis factor receptor superfamily couples TCR signal strength to the thymic differentiation of regulatory T cells. *Nat Immunol*. **15**:473–481.
132. Chen X, Oppenheim JJ. (2010). TNF-alpha: an activator of CD4+FoxP3+ TNFR2+ regulatory T cells. *Curr Dir Autoimmun*. **11**:119–134.
133. Meylan F, Song YJ, Fuss I, Villarreal S, Kahle E, Malm IJ *et al.* (2011). The TNF-family cytokine TL1A drives IL-13-dependent small intestinal inflammation. *Mucosal Immunol*. **4**:172–185.
134. Taraban VY, Slebioda TJ, Willoughby JE, Buchan SL, James S, Sheth B *et al.* (2011). Sustained TL1A expression modulates effector and regulatory T-cell responses and drives intestinal goblet cell hyperplasia. *Mucosal Immunol*. **4**:186–196.
135. Cella M, Scheidegger D, Palmer-Lehmann K, Lane P, Lanzavecchia A, Alber G. (1996). Ligation of CD40 on dendritic cells triggers production of high levels of interleukin-12 and enhances T cell stimulatory capacity: T-T help via APC activation. *J Exp Med*. **184**:747–752.
136. Morel Y, Truneh A, Sweet RW, Olive D, Costello RT. (2001). The TNF superfamily members LIGHT and CD154 (CD40 ligand) costimulate induction of dendritic cell maturation and elicit specific CTL activity. *J Immunol*. **167**:2479–2486.
137. He B, Santamaria R, Xu W, Cols M, Chen K, Puga I *et al.* (2010). The transmembrane activator TACI triggers immunoglobulin class switching by activating B cells through the adaptor MyD88. *Nat Immunol*. **11**:836–845.
138. Zan H, Casali P. (2013). Regulation of Aicda expression and AID activity. *Autoimmunity*. **46**:83–101.
139. Ding BB, Bi E, Chen H, Yu JJ, Ye BH. (2013). IL-21 and CD40L synergistically promote plasma cell differentiation through upregulation of Blimp-1 in human B cells. *J Immunol*. **190**:1827–1836.
140. Duhen T, Pasero C, Mallet F, Barbarat B, Olive D, Costello RT. (2004). LIGHT costimulates CD40 triggering and induces immunoglobulin secretion; a novel key partner in T cell-dependent B cell terminal differentiation. *Eur J Immunol*. **34**:3534–3541.
141. Wang J, Anders RA, Wu Q, Peng D, Cho JH, Sun Y *et al.* (2004). Dysregulated LIGHT expression on T cells mediates intestinal inflammation and contributes to IgA nephropathy. *J Clin Invest*. **113**:826–835.

142. Kang HS, Chin RK, Wang Y, Yu P, Wang J, Newell KA *et al.* (2002). Signaling via LTbetaR on the lamina propria stromal cells of the gut is required for IgA production. *Nat Immunol.* **3**:576–582.
143. Kruglov AA, Grivennikov SI, Kuprash DV, Winsauer C, Prepens S, Seleznik GM *et al.* (2013). Nonredundant function of soluble LTalpha3 produced by innate lymphoid cells in intestinal homeostasis. *Science.* **342**:1243–1246.
144. Ware CF. (2013). Protein therapeutics targeted at the TNF superfamily. *Adv Pharmacol.* **66**:51–80.
145. Feldmann M, Brennan FM, Elliott M, Katsikis P, Maini RN. (1994). TNF alpha as a therapeutic target in rheumatoid arthritis. *Circ Shock.* **43**:179–184.
146. Calmon-Hamaty F, Audo R, Combe B, Morel J, Hahne M. (2014). Targeting the Fas/FasL system in Rheumatoid Arthritis therapy: Promising or risky? *Cytokine.* **75**:228–233.
147. Vinay DS, Kwon BS. (2012). Targeting TNF superfamily members for therapeutic intervention in rheumatoid arthritis. *Cytokine.* **57**:305–312.
148. Tang R, Sinnwell JP, Li J, Rider DN, de Andrade M, Biernacka JM. (2009). Identification of genes and haplotypes that predict rheumatoid arthritis using random forests. *BMC Proc.* **3**(Suppl 7):S68.
149. Lee YH, Ji JD, Song GG. (2007). Tumor necrosis factor-alpha promoter -308 A/G polymorphism and rheumatoid arthritis susceptibility: a metaanalysis. *J Rheumatol.* **34**:43–49.
150. Coenen MJ, Trynka G, Heskamp S, Franke B, van Diemen CC, Smolonska J *et al.* (2009). Common and different genetic background for rheumatoid arthritis and coeliac disease. *Hum Mol Genet.* **18**:4195–4203.
151. El-Gabalawy HS, Robinson DB, Daha NA, Oen KG, Smolik I, Elias B *et al.* (2011). Non-HLA genes modulate the risk of rheumatoid arthritis associated with HLA-DRB1 in a susceptible North American Native population. *Genes Immun.* **12**:568–574.
152. Okada Y, Wu D, Trynka G, Raj T, Terao C, Ikari K *et al.* (2014). Genetics of rheumatoid arthritis contributes to biology and drug discovery. *Nature.* **506**:376–381.
153. Raychaudhuri S, Remmers EF, Lee AT, Hackett R, Guiducci C, Burtt NP *et al.* (2008). Common variants at CD40 and other loci confer risk of rheumatoid arthritis. *Nat Genet.* **40**:1216–1223.
154. Murch SH, Lamkin VA, Savage MO, Walker-Smith JA, MacDonald TT. (1991). Serum concentrations of tumour necrosis factor alpha in childhood chronic inflammatory bowel disease. *Gut.* **32**:913–917.
155. Slebioda TJ, Kmiec Z. (2014). Tumour necrosis factor superfamily members in the pathogenesis of inflammatory bowel disease. *Mediators Inflamm.* **2014**:325129.

156. Shih DQ, Michelsen KS, Barrett RJ, Biener-Ramanujan E, Gonsky R, Zhang X *et al.* (2011). Insights into TL1A and IBD pathogenesis. *Adv Exp Med Biol.* **691**:279–288.
157. Cohavy O, Zhou J, Ware CF, Targan SR. (2005). LIGHT is constitutively expressed on T and NK cells in the human gut and can be induced by CD2-mediated signaling. *J Immunol.* **174**:646–653.
158. Wang J, Anders RA, Wang Y, Turner JR, Abraham C, Pfeffer K *et al.* (2005). The critical role of LIGHT in promoting intestinal inflammation and Crohn's disease. *J Immunol.* **174**:8173–8182.
159. Bamias G, Jia LG, Cominelli F. (2013). The tumor necrosis factor-like cytokine 1A/death receptor 3 cytokine system in intestinal inflammation. *Curr Opin Gastroenterol.* **29**:597–602.
160. Funke B, Autschbach F, Kim S, Lasitschka F, Strauch U, Rogler G *et al.* (2009). Functional characterisation of decoy receptor 3 in Crohn's disease. *Gut.* **58**:483–491.
161. Brost S, Koschny R, Sykora J, Stremmel W, Lasitschka F, Walczak H *et al.* (2010). Differential expression of the TRAIL/TRAIL-receptor system in patients with inflammatory bowel disease. *Pathol Res Pract.* **206**:43–50.
162. Reenaers C, Franchimont N, Oury C, Belaiche J, Malaise M, Bours V *et al.* (2008). Sensitivity of intestinal fibroblasts to TNF-related apoptosis-inducing ligand-mediated apoptosis in Crohn's disease. *Scand J Gastroenterol.* **43**:1334–1345.
163. Kawashima R, Kawamura YI, Oshio T, Son A, Yamazaki M, Hagiwara T *et al.* (2011). Interleukin-13 damages intestinal mucosa via TWEAK and Fn14 in mice-a pathway associated with ulcerative colitis. *Gastroenterology.* **141**:2119–2129.e2118.
164. Liu Z, Colpaert S, D'Haens GR, Kasran A, de Boer M, Rutgeerts P *et al.* (1999). Hyperexpression of CD40 ligand (CD154) in inflammatory bowel disease and its contribution to pathogenic cytokine production. *J Immunol.* **163**:4049–4057.
165. Lopez-Hernandez R, Valdes M, Campillo JA, Martinez-Garcia P, Salama H, Salgado G *et al.* (2014). Genetic polymorphisms of tumour necrosis factor alpha (TNF-alpha) promoter gene and response to TNF-alpha inhibitors in Spanish patients with inflammatory bowel disease. *Int J Immunogenet.* **41**:63–68.
166. Jostins L, Ripke S, Weersma RK, Duerr RH, McGovern DP, Hui KY *et al.* (2012). Host-microbe interactions have shaped the genetic architecture of inflammatory bowel disease. *Nature.* **491**:119–124.
167. Tello-Ruiz MK, Curley C, DelMonte T, Giallourakis C, Kirby A, Miller K *et al.* (2006). Haplotype-based association analysis of 56 functional candidate genes in the IBD6 locus on chromosome 19. *Eur J Hum Genet.* **14**:780–790.

168. Douni E, Akassoglou K, Alexopoulou L, Georgopoulos S, Haralambous S, Hill S *et al.* (1995). Transgenic and knockout analyses of the role of TNF in immune regulation and disease pathogenesis. *J Inflamm.* **47**:27–38.
169. Kontoyiannis D, Pasparakis M, Pizarro TT, Cominelli F, Kollias G. (1999). Impaired on/off regulation of TNF biosynthesis in mice lacking TNF AU-rich elements: implications for joint and gut-associated immunopathologies. *Immunity.* **10**:387–398.
170. Croft M, Duan W, Choi H, Eun SY, Madireddi S, Mehta A. (2012). TNF superfamily in inflammatory disease: Translating basic insights. *Trends Immunol.* **33**:144–152.
171. Murata K, Nose M, Ndhlovu LC, Sato T, Sugamura K, Ishii N. (2002). Constitutive OX40/OX40 ligand interaction induces autoimmune-like diseases. *J Immunol.* **169**:4628–4636.
172. Mori L, Iselin S, De Libero G, Lesslauer W. (1996). Attenuation of collagen-induced arthritis in 55-kDa TNF receptor type 1 (TNFR1)-IgG1-treated and TNFR1-deficient mice. *J Immunol.* **157**:3178–3182.
173. Drutskaya MS, Efimov GA, Zvartsev RV, Chashchina AA, Chudakov DM, Tillib SV *et al.* (2014). Experimental models of arthritis in which pathogenesis is dependent on TNF expression. *Biochemistry (Mosc).* **79**:1349–1357.
174. Chiang EY, Kolumam GA, Yu X, Francesco M, Ivelja S, Peng I *et al.* (2009). Targeted depletion of lymphotoxin-alpha-expressing TH1 and TH17 cells inhibits autoimmune disease. *Nat Med.* **15**:766–773.
175. Fava RA, Notidis E, Hunt J, Szanya V, Ratcliffe N, Ngam-Ek A *et al.* (2003). A role for the lymphotoxin/LIGHT axis in the pathogenesis of murine collagen-induced arthritis. *J Immunol.* **171**:115–126.
176. Oflazoglu E, Boursalian TE, Zeng W, Edwards AC, Duniho S, McEarchern JA *et al.* (2009). Blocking of CD27-CD70 pathway by anti-CD70 antibody ameliorates joint disease in murine collagen-induced arthritis. *J Immunol.* **183**:3770–3777.
177. Yoshioka T, Nakajima A, Akiba H, Ishiwata T, Asano G, Yoshino S *et al.* (2000). Contribution of OX40/OX40 ligand interaction to the pathogenesis of rheumatoid arthritis. *Eur J Immunol.* **30**:2815–2823.
178. Seo SK, Choi JH, Kim YH, Kang WJ, Park HY, Suh JH *et al.* (2004). 4–1BB-mediated immunotherapy of rheumatoid arthritis. *Nat Med.* **10**:1088–1094.
179. Durie FH, Fava RA, Foy TM, Aruffo A, Ledbetter JA, Noelle RJ. (1993). Prevention of collagen-induced arthritis with an antibody to gp39, the ligand for CD40. *Science.* **261**:1328–1330.
180. Andreakos E, Rauchhaus U, Stavropoulos A, Endert G, Wendisch V, Benahmed AS *et al.* (2009). Amphoteric liposomes enable systemic antigen-presenting cell-directed delivery of CD40 antisense and are therapeutically effective in experimental arthritis. *Arthritis Rheum.* **60**:994–1005.

181. Bull MJ, Williams AS, Mecklenburgh Z, Calder CJ, Twohig JP, Elford C *et al.* (2008). The Death Receptor 3-TNF-like protein 1A pathway drives adverse bone pathology in inflammatory arthritis. *J Exp Med.* **205**:2457–2464.
182. Lai Kwan Lam Q, King Hung Ko O, Zheng BJ, Lu L. (2008). Local BAFF gene silencing suppresses Th17-cell generation and ameliorates autoimmune arthritis. *Proc Natl Acad Sci USA.* **105**:14993–14998.
183. Zhang H, Yang Y, Horton JL, Samoilova EB, Judge TA, Turka LA *et al.* (1997). Amelioration of collagen-induced arthritis by CD95 (Apo-1/Fas)-ligand gene transfer. *J Clin Invest.* **100**:1951–1957.
184. Song K, Chen Y, Goke R, Wilmen A, Seidel C, Goke A *et al.* (2000). Tumor necrosis factor-related apoptosis-inducing ligand (TRAIL) is an inhibitor of autoimmune inflammation and cell cycle progression. *J Exp Med.* **191**:1095–1104.
185. Yao Q, Wang S, Gambotto A, Glorioso JC, Evans CH, Robbins PD *et al.* (2003). Intra-articular adenoviral-mediated gene transfer of trail induces apoptosis of arthritic rabbit synovium. *Gene Ther.* **10**:1055–1060.
186. Yao Q, Seol DW, Mi Z, Robbins PD. (2006). Intra-articular injection of recombinant TRAIL induces synovial apoptosis and reduces inflammation in a rabbit knee model of arthritis. *Arthritis Res Ther.* **8**:R16.
187. Odani-Kawabata N, Takai-Imamura M, Katsuta O, Nakamura H, Nishioka K, Funahashi K *et al.* (2010). ARG098, a novel anti-human Fas antibody, suppresses synovial hyperplasia and prevents cartilage destruction in a severe combined immunodeficient-HuRAg mouse model. *BMC Musculoskelet Disord.* **11**:221.
188. Scheinin T, Butler DM, Salway F, Scallon B, Feldmann M. (2003). Validation of the interleukin-10 knockout mouse model of colitis: Antitumour necrosis factor-antibodies suppress the progression of colitis. *Clin Exp Immunol.* **133**:38–43.
189. Kojouharoff G, Hans W, Obermeier F, Mannel DN, Andus T, Scholmerich J *et al.* (1997). Neutralization of tumour necrosis factor (TNF) but not of IL-1 reduces inflammation in chronic dextran sulphate sodium-induced colitis in mice. *Clin Exp Immunol.* **107**:353–358.
190. Lindebo Holm T, Poulsen SS, Markholst H, Reedtz-Runge S. (2012). Pharmacological Evaluation of the SCID T Cell Transfer Model of Colitis: As a Model of Crohn's Disease. *Int J Inflam.* **2012**:412178.
191. Takedatsu H, Michelsen KS, Wei B, Landers CJ, Thomas LS, Dhall D *et al.* (2008). TL1A (TNFSF15) regulates the development of chronic colitis by modulating both T-helper 1 and T-helper 17 activation. *Gastroenterology.* **135**:552–567.
192. Obermeier F, Schwarz H, Dunger N, Strauch UG, Grunwald N, Scholmerich J *et al.* (2003). OX40/OX40L interaction induces the expression of CXCR5 and contributes to chronic colitis induced by dextran sulfate sodium in mice. *Eur J Immunol.* **33**:3265–3274.

193. Dohi T, Rennert PD, Fujihashi K, Kiyono H, Shirai Y, Kawamura YI *et al.* (2001). Elimination of colonic patches with lymphotoxin beta receptor-Ig prevents Th2 cell-type colitis. *J Immunol.* **167**:2781–2790.
194. Manocha M, Rietdijk S, Laouar A, Liao G, Bhan A, Borst J *et al.* (2009). Blocking CD27-CD70 costimulatory pathway suppresses experimental colitis. *J Immunol.* **183**:270–276.
195. Higgins LM, McDonald SA, Whittle N, Crockett N, Shields JG, MacDonald TT. (1999). Regulation of T cell activation *in vitro* and *in vivo* by targeting the OX40-OX40 ligand interaction: amelioration of ongoing inflammatory bowel disease with an OX40-IgG fusion protein, but not with an OX40 ligand-IgG fusion protein. *J Immunol.* **162**:486–493.
196. Sun X, Yamada H, Shibata K, Muta H, Tani K, Podack ER *et al.* (2010). CD30 ligand is a target for a novel biological therapy against colitis associated with Th17 responses. *J Immunol.* **185**:7671–7680.
197. Somada S, Muta H, Nakamura K, Sun X, Honda K, Ihara E *et al.* (2012). CD30 ligand/CD30 interaction is involved in pathogenesis of inflammatory bowel disease. *Dig Dis Sci.* **57**:2031–2037.
198. McNamee EN, Masterson JC, Jedlicka P, Collins CB, Williams IR, Rivera-Nieves J. (2013). Ectopic lymphoid tissue alters the chemokine gradient, increases lymphocyte retention and exacerbates murine ileitis. *Gut.* **62**:53–62.
199. Mackay F, Browning JL, Lawton P, Shah SA, Comiskey M, Bhan AK *et al.* (1998). Both the lymphotoxin and tumor necrosis factor pathways are involved in experimental murine models of colitis. *Gastroenterology.* **115**:1464–1475.
200. Malmstrom V, Shipton D, Singh B, Al-Shamkhani A, Puklavec MJ, Barclay AN *et al.* (2001). CD134L expression on dendritic cells in the mesenteric lymph nodes drives colitis in T cell-restored SCID mice. *J Immunol.* **166**:6972–6981.
201. Totsuka T, Kanai T, Uraushihara K, Iiyama R, Yamazaki M, Akiba H *et al.* (2003). Therapeutic effect of anti-OX40L and anti-TNF-alpha MAbs in a murine model of chronic colitis. *Am J Physiol Gastrointest Liver Physiol.* **284**:G595–603.
202. De Jong YP, Comiskey M, Kalled SL, Mizoguchi E, Flavell RA, Bhan AK *et al.* (2000). Chronic murine colitis is dependent on the CD154/CD40 pathway and can be attenuated by anti-CD154 administration. *Gastroenterology.* **119**:715–723.
203. Liu Z, Geboes K, Colpaert S, Overbergh L, Mathieu C, Heremans H *et al.* (2000). Prevention of experimental colitis in SCID mice reconstituted with CD45RBhigh CD4+ T cells by blocking the CD40-CD154 interactions. *J Immunol.* **164**:6005–6014.
204. Lee J, Lee EN, Kim EY, Park HJ, Chang CY, Jung DY *et al.* (2005). Administration of agonistic anti-4–1BB monoclonal antibody leads to the

amelioration of inflammatory bowel disease. *Immunol Lett.* **101**:210–216.
205. Arranz A, Reinsch C, Papadakis KA, Dieckmann A, Rauchhaus U, Androulidaki A *et al.* (2013). Treatment of experimental murine colitis with CD40 antisense oligonucleotides delivered in amphoteric liposomes. *J Control Release.* **165**:163–172.
206. Blumberg RS, Saubermann LJ, Strober W. (1999). Animal models of mucosal inflammation and their relation to human inflammatory bowel disease. *Curr Opin Immunol.* **11**:648–656.
207. Wehrens EJ, Prakken BJ, van Wijk F. (2013). T cells out of control--impaired immune regulation in the inflamed joint. *Nat Rev Rheumatol.* **9**:34–42.
208. Bhol KC, Tracey DE, Lemos BR, Lyng GD, Erlich EC, Keane DM *et al.* (2013). AVX-470:a novel oral anti-TNF antibody with therapeutic potential in inflammatory bowel disease. *Inflamm Bowel Dis.* **19**:2273–2281.
209. Huang Z, Gan J, Jia L, Guo G, Wang C, Zang Y *et al.* (2015). An orally administrated nucleotide-delivery vehicle targeting colonic macrophages for the treatment of inflammatory bowel disease. *Biomaterials.* **48**:26–36.
210. Vandenbroucke K, de Haard H, Beirnaert E, Dreier T, Lauwereys M, Huyck L *et al.* (2010). Orally administered L. lactis secreting an anti-TNF Nanobody demonstrate efficacy in chronic colitis. *Mucosal Immunol.* **3**:49–56.
211. Elliott MJ, Maini RN, Feldmann M, Kalden JR, Antoni C, Smolen JS *et al.* (1994). Randomised double-blind comparison of chimeric monoclonal antibody to tumour necrosis factor alpha (cA2) versus placebo in rheumatoid arthritis. *Lancet.* **344**:1105–1110.
212. Li J, Hsu HC, Mountz JD. (2012). Managing macrophages in rheumatoid arthritis by reform or removal. *Curr Rheumatol Rep.* **14**:445–454.
213. Kabat EA. (1988). Antibody complementarity and antibody structure. *J Immunol.* **141**:S25–36.
214. Papp K. (2010). Clinical development of onercept, a tumor necrosis factor binding protein, in psoriasis. *Curr Med Res Opin.* **26**:2287–2300.
215. Horiuchi T, Mitoma H, Harashima S, Tsukamoto H, Shimoda T. (2010). Transmembrane TNF-alpha: structure, function and interaction with anti-TNF agents. *Rheumatology (Oxford).* **49**:1215–1228.
216. Nesbitt A, Fossati G, Bergin M, Stephens P, Stephens S, Foulkes R *et al.* (2007). Mechanism of action of certolizumab pegol (CDP870): *In vitro* comparison with other anti-tumor necrosis factor alpha agents. *Inflammatory Bowel Diseases.* **13**:1323–1332.1310.1002/ibd.20225.
217. Van den Brande JM, Braat H, van den Brink GR, Versteeg HH, Bauer CA, Hoedemaeker I *et al.* (2003). Infliximab but not etanercept induces apoptosis in lamina propria T-lymphocytes from patients with Crohn's disease. *Gastroenterology.* **124**:1774–1785.

218. Gregory AP, Dendrou CA, Attfield KE, Haghikia A, Xifara DK, Butter F *et al.* (2012). TNF receptor 1 genetic risk mirrors outcome of anti-TNF therapy in multiple sclerosis. *Nature*. **488**:508–511.
219. Scallon B, Cai A, Solowski N, Rosenberg A, Song XY, Shealy D *et al.* (2002). Binding and functional comparisons of two types of tumor necrosis factor antagonists. *J Pharmacol Exp Ther*. **301**:418–426.
220. Palm NW, de Zoete MR, Cullen TW, Barry NA, Stefanowski J, Hao L *et al.* (2014). Immunoglobulin A coating identifies colitogenic bacteria in inflammatory bowel disease. *Cell*. **158**:1000–1010.
221. Fallahi-Sichani M, Flynn JL, Linderman JJ, Kirschner DE. (2012). Differential risk of tuberculosis reactivation among anti-TNF therapies is due to drug binding kinetics and permeability. *J Immunol*. **188**:3169–3178.
222. Wallis RS. (2011). Biologics and infections: lessons from tumor necrosis factor blocking agents. *Infect Dis Clin North Am*. **25**:895–910.
223. Katsanos AH, Katsanos KH. (2014). Inflammatory bowel disease and demyelination: more than just a coincidence? *Expert Review of Clinical Immunology*. **10**:363–373.
224. Solomon AJ, Spain RI, Kruer MC, Bourdette D. (2011). Inflammatory neurological disease in patients treated with tumor necrosis factor alpha inhibitors. *Mult Scler*. **17**:1472–1487.
225. Desroches M, Louis G, Gleizes A, Krzysiek R, Emilie D. (2010). Treatment failure with antagonists of TNF-alpha: Mechanisms and implications for the care of patients. *Eur Cytokine Netw*. **21**:226–231.
226. Bartelds GM, Krieckaert CL, Nurmohamed MT, van Schouwenburg PA, Lems WF, Twisk JW *et al.* (2011). Development of antidrug antibodies against adalimumab and association with disease activity and treatment failure during long-term follow-up. *JAMA*. **305**:1460–1468.
227. Sandborn WJ. (2010). State-of-the-art: Immunosuppression and biologic therapy. *Dig Dis*. **28**:536–542.
228. Martyn-Simmons CL, Green L, Ash G, Groves RW, Smith CH, Barker JN. (2009). Adalimumab for psoriasis patients who are non-responders to etanercept: open-label prospective evaluation. *J Eur Acad Dermatol Venereol*. **23**:1394–1397.
229. Croft M, Benedict CA, Ware CF. (2013). Clinical targeting of the TNF and TNFR superfamilies. *Nat Rev Drug Discov*. **12**:147–168.
230. Kawai T, Andrews D, Colvin RB, Sachs DH, Cosimi AB. (2000). Thromboembolic complications after treatment with monoclonal antibody against CD40 ligand. *Nat Med*. **6**:114.
231. Xie JH, Yamniuk AP, Borowski V, Kuhn R, Susulic V, Rex-Rabe S *et al.* (2014). Engineering of a novel anti-CD40L domain antibody for treatment of autoimmune diseases. *J Immunol*. **192**:4083–4092.

232. Emu B, Luca D, Offutt C, Grogan JL, Rojkovich B, Williams MB *et al.* (2012). Safety, pharmacokinetics, and biologic activity of pateclizumab, a novel monoclonal antibody targeting lymphotoxin alpha: results of a phase I randomized, placebo-controlled trial. *Arthritis Res Ther.* **14**:R6.
233. Kennedy WP, Simon JA, Offutt C, Horn P, Herman A, Townsend MJ *et al.* (2014). Efficacy and safety of pateclizumab (anti-lymphotoxin-alpha) compared to adalimumab in rheumatoid arthritis: a head-to-head phase 2 randomized controlled study (The ALTARA Study). *Arthritis Res Ther.* **16**:467.
234. Genovese MC, Kinnman N, de La Bourdonnaye G, Pena Rossi C, Tak PP. (2011). Atacicept in patients with rheumatoid arthritis and an inadequate response to tumor necrosis factor antagonist therapy: results of a phase II, randomized, placebo-controlled, dose-finding trial. *Arthritis Rheum.* **63**:1793–1803.
235. Browning JL. (2008). Inhibition of the lymphotoxin pathway as a therapy for autoimmune disease. *Immunol Rev.* **223**:202–220.
236. Bienkowska J, Allaire N, Thai A, Goyal J, Plavina T, Nirula A *et al.* (2014). Lymphotoxin-LIGHT pathway regulates the interferon signature in rheumatoid arthritis. *PLoS One.* **9**:e112545.

Chapter 2

Complement as a Mediator of Inflammation

B. Paul Morgan*

1. Introduction to the complement system

1.1. *What is complement?*

Complement comprises a network of proteins present in plasma and on cells that interact to provide defense against infection, efficient clearance of debris, and a myriad of other important physiological activities, all delivered by the activation products generated when the system is triggered. As befits its destructive nature, complement is rigidly controlled in health, with multiple intrinsic regulating features and an array of complement regulators that outnumber the complement system proteins. As a consequence, complement does not normally damage self-cells but remains primed ready to respond instantly and in a focused manner to pathogen or other trigger. When this homeostatic balance is disturbed in disease, control of complement activation is lost leading to dysregulation and injury to

*Division of Infection and Immunity, School of Medicine, Cardiff University, Cardiff CF144XN, UK.

self that exacerbates the pathology. As a consequence, complement is a contributing factor in many diseases where inflammation is a driver, and anti-complement therapies can be of benefit in these many contexts.

1.2. *Initiation of complement activation*

At the core of the complement network sit the activation pathways that initiate, amplify, and propagate the response to an initial stimulus. Initiation involves a pattern recognition event whereby an activating surface binds a complement protein. In the *Classical* activation pathway (CP) the activating surface usually comprises antibody (IgG or IgM) bound to antigen; multi-point binding of the large and complex C1q molecule to specific sites in the antibody Fc begins the process. On non-self surfaces, initiation does not necessarily require antibody; instead, the pattern recognition event involves the recognition of pathogen-specific sugars by one of several C1q-like collectin molecules (mannan binding lectin (MBL), ficolins), termed the *Lectin* activation pathway (LP). Non-self surfaces may also be recognized based on their lack of complement regulators; intrinsic tick-over activation in plasma showers all surfaces with activation products that are mopped up by regulators on self-cells but survive and amplify on pathogens, the *Alternative* activation pathway (AP), synonymous with the amplification loop.

1.3. *Amplification in the activation pathways*

Once initiated, complement activation proceeds to the amplification stage where a small initial stimulus can translate rapidly into a large response (Fig. 1). The pattern recognition molecules C1q and MBL each carry with them proenzymes that are activated upon binding ligand. In the CP, C1q carries the enzymes C1r and C1s in a $C1qr_2s_2$ complex; binding triggers conformational change in C1q that causes auto-activation of C1r that in turn cleaves and activates C1s. In the LP, MBL carries MBL-associated proteases (MASPs)-1 and -2; ligand binding triggers cleavage and activation of these enzymes.

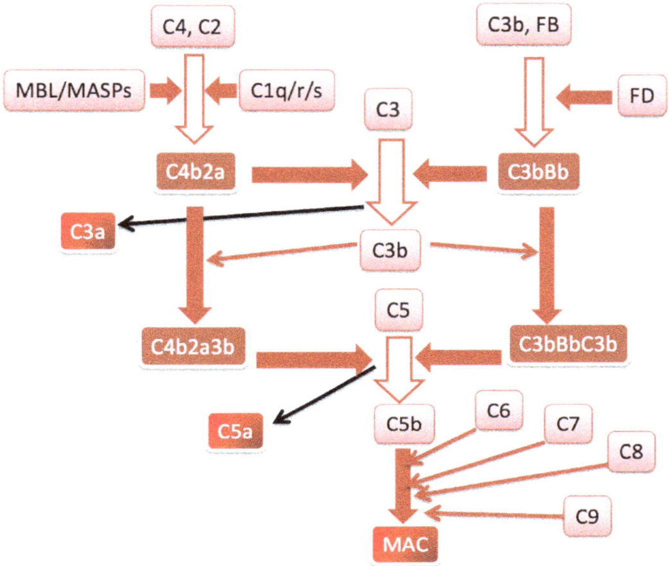

Fig. 1. The complement system. The figure summarizes the critical pathways in the complement system, beginning with an initiation step, proceeding through several layers of amplification, and converging on a common terminal pathway. The enzymatic cleavages are represented by empty arrows and show the responsible enzymes alongside. Further explanation is found in the text.

The substrates of C1s in the C1q r_2s_2 and MASP-2 in the MBL/MASP complex are identical — the plasma proteins C4 and C2. First, C4 is cleaved at a single site, releasing a small fragment C4a and exposing a reactive thioester on the large fragment C4b that binds covalently to adjacent surfaces. Each enzyme cleaves many C4 molecules so the activating surface rapidly becomes coated in C4b, the first amplification step. C4b binds C2 and presents it for cleavage by an adjacent enzyme (C1s or MASP-2), releasing a fragment, C2b, and leaving the enzymatically active C2a fragment tightly bound to C4b. C2a in the C4b2a complex is the second amplifying enzyme with the abundant plasma protein C3 as substrate; cleavage releases a small biologically active fragment C3a and exposes a reactive thioester on the large fragment C3b that binds covalently to adjacent surfaces. Each C4b2a enzyme cleaves many C3 molecules so the activating surface rapidly becomes coated in C3b, the second amplification step.

1.4. *The amplification loop of the alternative pathway*

Although amplification in the CP and LP described above are important, they are limited by endogenous and exogenous factors; the former including the lability of the thioester and the dependence on proximity to an activating enzyme, the latter a battery of regulatory proteins described below. The AP provides an additional, strong and less spatially restricted means of activation; indeed, the AP is better described as an amplification loop. C3b (or hydrolyzed C3), generated in the activation pathways or by tickover, is the initiator. Once formed, C3b, whether covalently bound to a surface or in the fluid phase, binds the plasma protein factor B (FB; a structural homolog of C2), altering its conformation to allow cleavage at a single site by the plasma protease factor D (FD). The Ba fragment is released and the enzymatically active Bb fragment remains attached to C3b; Bb in the C3bBb complex cleaves more C3 to generate more C3b on adjacent surfaces and in the fluid phase, each of which can bind FB and repeat the cycle. Left unregulated, the AP amplification loop cycles to consume all available C3.

1.5. *Amplification at the stage of C5 cleavage*

The final amplification step involves cleavage of the plasma protein C5, a close structural homolog of C4 and C3 but without a thioester. The C5- cleaving enzyme comprises either C4b2a or C3bBb with an additional C3b molecule attached through its thioester to the complex (i.e., C4b2aC3b or C3bBbC3b); the role of the additional C3b is to capture C5 and present it for cleavage by the enzyme (C2a or Bb) in the complex. The small biologically active fragment C5a is released and the C5b fragment remains associated with the enzyme complex. Once C5b is released as described below, the tri-molecular enzyme can cleave more C5, thus further amplifying the response.

1.6. *Assembly of the membrane attack complex*

Cleavage of C5 is the final amplification step and last enzymatic event in the complement pathway; it is also the first step in the terminal pathway. C5b binds the plasma proteins C6 and C7 and alters conformation to release the tri-molecular C5b67 complex and create in the complex a hydrophobic membrane binding site. Those C5b67 complexes that encounter membrane during the brief life of this site bind tightly and sequentially recruit the plasma proteins C8 and C9 to create the membrane attack complex (MAC), a transmembrane pore containing one molecule each of C5b, C6, C7, and C8 with as many as eighteen C9 molecules, these elongating and aggregating to form the walls of the pore.

1.7. *Active products of complement activation*

The nature and properties of complement activation products will be discussed in more detail in later sections; here, I provide a simplified overview. Three sorts of activation products are generated during complement activation: *opsonins*, *anaphylatoxins*, and *cytotoxins* (Fig. 2(a)). The first group comprise those complement proteins and fragments that coat target surfaces and label them for recognition by phagocytes or other effector cells. C3b and its breakdown products iC3b and C3d are foremost in this group, although C4d and its breakdown products and the pattern recognition molecules C1q and MBL also have opsonic roles in some contexts. The second group comprises those complement fragments that attract (chemotactic) and activate (anaphylactic) phagocytes and other effectors. C5a is the critical product in this group and is a key pro-inflammatory molecule; C3a has had a checkered history and appears to have a complex palate of activities,

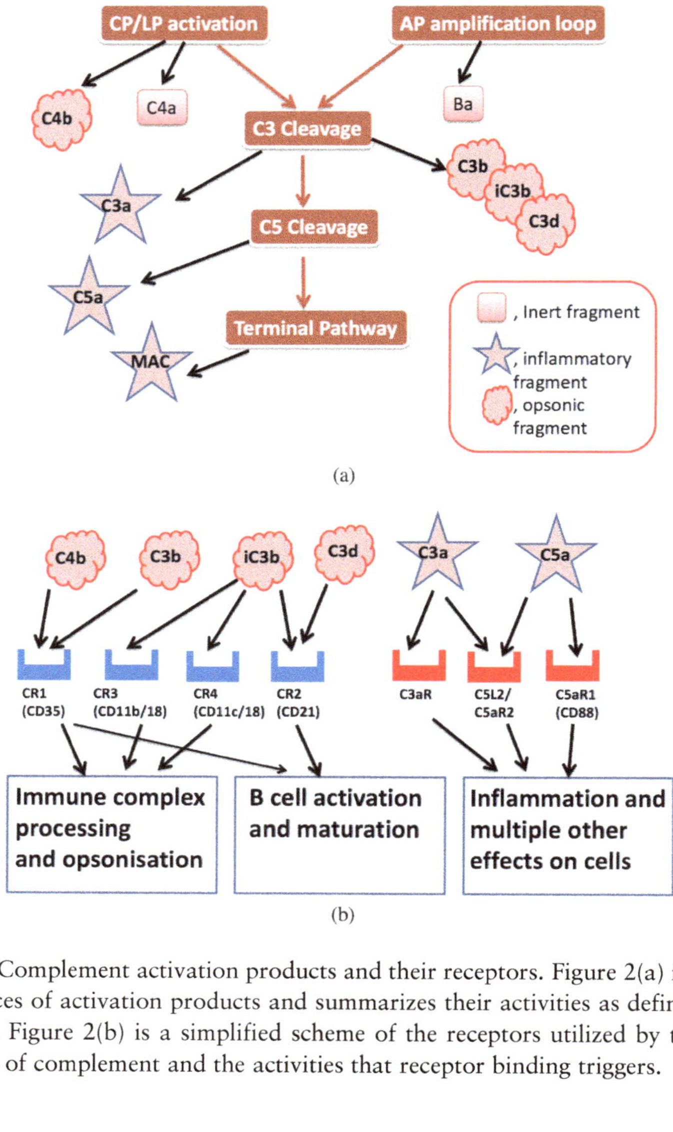

Fig. 2. Complement activation products and their receptors. Figure 2(a) illustrates the sources of activation products and summarizes their activities as defined in the key box. Figure 2(b) is a simplified scheme of the receptors utilized by the active products of complement and the activities that receptor binding triggers.

some pro-inflammatory and others anti-inflammatory depending on the target cell. The third group has a single member, the MAC, which can cause lysis of inert cell targets and some pathogens by disrupting osmotic barriers.

1.8. Complement regulation

It is obvious that an auto-activating, self-amplifying cascade requires rigid control to avoid a catastrophic forest fire. Control is provided by in-built inefficiencies and exogenous regulators. Many of the key intermediates and enzymes are transient: the thioester groups in nascent C4b and C3b are inactivated by hydrolysis within a few milliseconds of exposure; the multi-molecular enzyme complexes of the activation pathways break up (decay) spontaneously within minutes of formation; the membrane-binding site on the MAC precursor C5b67 complex exists for only a fraction of a second. On top of this endogenous control, exogenous regulators act at almost every step in the pathway. The initiating C1q r_2s_2 and MBL–MASP complexes are regulated by the plasma protein C1-inhibitor (C1INH) which strips the enzyme components from the recognition moiety. The C3/C5 cleaving enzymes are controlled by proteins in plasma (Factor H [FH], C4b binding protein [C4BP], factor I [FI]) and on membranes (CD46, CD55, CR1 [CD35]) that either accelerate the natural decay of the enzyme complex (FH, C4BP, CD55), or collaborate to cause irreversible inactivation of the enzyme (FH/FI, C4BP/FI, CD46/FI). The anaphylactic peptides C3a and C5a are inactivated by plasma carboxypeptidase-N. MAC assembly is inhibited by plasma proteins that bind C5b67 and prevent its association with membrane (vitronectin, clusterin) and by membrane proteins that lock into the forming MAC to prevent pore formation (CD59).

1.9. Complement receptors

The majority of the effects of complement and its activation products require receptor engagement. Several C1q receptors have been described, binding either the globular head (gC1qR) or collagenous tail (cC1qR) region; none are specific for C1q but nevertheless may provide an explanation for observed opsonic effects of C1q in clearance of apoptotic cells and other targets. Receptors for C3 activation products are numerous and biologically important (Fig. 2(b)). Complement receptor 1 (CR1; CD35) binds C3b and C4b and has key roles in the processing of opsonized particles and pathogens, described below. CR2 (CD21) binds the C3b degradation products iC3b and C3d. CR3 (CD11b/CD18) and CR4 (CD11c/CD18) both bind iC3b and play roles in handling of opsonized particles. Two receptors for C3a are described, C3aR and C5L2; both are heptaspan receptors but only the former is G- protein coupled. C5a also binds two receptors, C5aR1 (CD88) and C5L2 (also termed C5aR2); the latter binds C3a, C5a, and the inactivated (desArg) forms of these molecules and was originally described as a decoy receptor.

2. Complement roles in health

2.1. *Protection against infection*

The principal contribution of complement to health is its role in prevention of bacterial infections. Complement is activated on bacterial surfaces through the LP, AP, or (in the presence of antibacterial antibody) CP, leading to opsonization with C3b/iC3b. Phagocytes, attracted to the site of infection and activated by locally generated C3a and/or C5a, bind, predominantly via CR3, and phagocytose the bacterium for intracellular destruction. For the majority of bacteria, opsonization and phagocyte uptake is the most important innate immune defense; the exception is provided by pathogenic Gram-negative bacteria of the genus *Neisseria*, *N. meningitidis* and *N. gonorrhoeae*: these agents are relatively resistant to opsonization but sensitive to lytic killing by the MAC.

2.2. *Immune complex solubilisation*

Immune complexes (ICs), comprising conglomerates of antibody and particulate antigen, tend to grow by aggregation and accretion, eventually precipitating in capillary beds to cause pathology. ICs activate complement via the CP and become coated with C3b/iC3b; this masks antigen, restricting further growth, and enables IC to hitch a lift on erythrocytes by C3b binding to CR1. CR1 is a cofactor for FI-mediated cleavage of C3b to iC3b and CR1 does not bind the latter; hence, no sooner has a C3b-coated IC bound erythrocyte CR1 than it is released as the C3b is cleaved, only to bind again through another of the abundant C3b molecules on the IC. Dynamic binding and C3b cleavage are critical factors in the final disposal of ICs. Tissue macrophages in the spleen and other reticuloendothelial components express CR3 that binds iC3b on the IC and initiates phagocytosis; ICs are stripped off the transporter erythrocyte without damaging the erythrocyte, engulfed, and destroyed.

2.3. *Priming adaptive immunity*

The adaptive immune response involves both cellular (effector T cells) and humoral (antibody) components. Over the past 20 years, an important contribution of complement to the humoral immune response has emerged.[1,2] ICs bind cells expressing the cognate B cell receptor (BCR) and trigger B cell activation and maturation into antibody-secreting plasma cells; simultaneous binding of C3d on the IC to B cell CR2 (CD21) engages a second signaling pathway that lowers the threshold for B cell activation and increases the amplitude of the final response. B cells also express CR1 in the same signaling complexes, and it is likely that CR1 plays important roles in the initial capture by binding C3b on ICs, and in processing down to iC3b, C3dg, and C3d, all ligands for CR2. CR2 is also expressed on follicular dendritic cells, APCs present in lymph nodes; these can capture ICs by C3d binding to CR2 and present antigen in the IC to the BCR of an adjacent B cell. Indeed, this provides an efficient system for uptake of opsonized ICs from the lymphatics and delivery to FDCs and B cells in the lymphoid follicles.[3] Roles for complement in regulation of T cell activation have also emerged with C3 activation products signaling T cell activation through engagement of CD46.[4,5] Local production and activation of C3 may be the primary factor in these emerging roles in adaptive immunity.

2.4. *Regulating lipid metabolism*

The first evidence implicating complement in control of lipid metabolism came from an unexpected finding. Adipsin, a serine protease made exclusively in adipose tissue and implicated in lipid metabolism, was shown by gene sequencing to be identical to FD, the key enzyme of complement AP amplification.[6,7] Around the same time, acylation stimulating protein (ASP), an autocrine stimulator of triglyceride synthesis in adipose tissue, was shown to be C3adesArg.[8,9] From these observations arose the concept of an adipsin-ASP pathway as an important regulator of lipid handling in adipose tissue. Adipocytes are the major source of FD/adipsin and also produce C3 and FB, the raw materials for AP activation. Locally generated C3adesArg/ASP binds receptors (C5L2/C5aR2) to signal increased triglyceride synthesis.[10]

3. Complement roles in disease

3.1. *Complement and autoimmunity*

Whenever and wherever an autoantibody binds its antigen on tissues, cells, or in immune complexes, then complement will be activated and, in many autoimmune diseases, is the main driver of pathology. The list of autoimmune conditions, organ-specific and non-organ-specific, in which complement has been implicated is very long, and I will provide just a few examples in the different categories. In most cases of *myasthenia gravis* (MG), autoantibodies target the acetylcholine receptor (AChR) at the neuromuscular junction (NMJ) and activate complement, which in turn effects the destruction of the NMJ. MG patients suffer episodes of profound muscle weakness and fatigue.[11] Proof of the critical role for complement has been provided by the dramatic efficacy of anti-complement drugs in many animal models of MG and, more recently, in human AChR antibody-positive MG.[12,13] *Neuromyelitis optica* (NMO) is a rare autoimmune demyelinating disease characterized by progressive weakness and vision loss. Autoantibodies against the aquaporin-4 water channel bind astrocytes, activate complement and drive cell damage and inflammation. Again, evidence from animal models and human trials demonstrate the central role of complement.[14,15] *Systemic lupus erythematosus* (SLE) is an autoimmune disease in which autoantibodies against common cell constituents such as double-stranded DNA are produced that bind in many different tissues, including skin, kidney, nerves, and brain; activate complement; and drive inflammation.[16] It is now clear that a major aspect of the disease is failure of systems for clearing apoptotic cells and other debris in tissues, and here too complement plays roles.[17]

3.2. *Complement deficiencies*

Deficiencies of each of the components of complement, most of the regulators, and some of the receptors have been described; most are rare but clinical consequences can be devastating and early detection life-saving.[18] Deficiencies arise from mutations that either prevent protein synthesis or cause loss of function, the former characterized by absence of protein the latter by presence of inactive protein. As might be anticipated from the discussion above, the most common consequences of complement component deficiencies are infections and IC-mediated disease. The clinical picture is dictated by the stage in the system that the deficiency impacts. Deficiencies of CP components (C1q, C1r, C1s, C4, C2) uniquely predispose to IC disease, graphically illustrating the key role of the CP in IC processing.[19] Frequency and severity of disease is highest in those deficient in C1 proteins, almost all of whom develop a severe SLE-like illness in childhood, and lowest in C2 deficient individuals, the majority remaining symptom-free. Total C4 deficiency is very rare because the gene is duplicated (*C4A* and *C4B*), with the majority of individuals carrying a total of 4 copies; however, partial deficiencies are common and predispose to IC disease in the expected risk order (1 copy>2 copies>3 copies). C3 is the most abundant and important of the complement proteins, source of the majority of active products, and a choke-point for downstream activation. Individuals deficient in C3 suffer frequent, recurrent, and severe infections with a diverse spectrum of bacteria, often resulting in death in infancy. Early diagnosis and prophylactic use of broad-spectrum antibiotics can be life- saving. Deficiency of MBL is extremely common, present in up to 5% of Caucasians; most are symptom-free though statistically they are at increased risk of bacterial infections.[20] MASP-2 deficiency is very rare and the clinical consequences are unclear. Deficiencies of components of the AP amplification loop (FB, FD) are very rare and predispose to *Neisseria* infections.

Individuals deficient in components of the MAC (C5, C6, C7, C8α, C8β and C9) are at risk of infections with *Neisseria*, confirming its specific role in controlling this group of bacteria. C5 deficiency not only ablates MAC but also causes loss of capacity to generate C5a; the consequences appear to be additional risk of infection and IC disease.[21] MAC component deficiencies are rare in Caucasians; however, C9 deficiency is very common in Japan (1:1000 of the population) and to a lesser extent in Korea and China.[22]

Deficiencies of complement regulators lead to dysregulation in the system and disease. C1INH is the sole plasma regulator of the initiation stages of the classical and lectin pathways and also regulates the kinin system, an important source of bradykinin and other vasoactive peptides. Individuals deficient in C1INH suffer episodes of soft tissue swelling, a condition termed hereditary angioedema (HAE).[23] Attacks can be frequent or infrequent, localized or widespread; critically, attacks can cause laryngeal oedema leading to respiratory distress or gut mucosal swelling that may lead to gut obstruction. Individuals with HAE are usually heterozygotes for C1INH deficiency so have reduced but not absent plasma levels of C1INH. Insults such as minor trauma or even stress can trigger low-grade complement and kinin system activation in the tissues that is initially controlled by C1INH, but in HAE the regulator is rapidly consumed, control is lost, and the resultant burst of inflammatory mediators causes swelling. Because heterozygous deficiency causes disease, HAE is relatively common and is the most frequent complement deficiency disease in Caucasians affecting perhaps 1:10,000.

Deficiencies of either FI or FH, both very rare, cause loss of control of the AP amplification loop and complete consumption of C3; the consequences are the same as those of primary C3 deficiency — severe, recurrent bacterial infections. The regulators

CD55 and CD59 are attached to the membrane via a glycosylphosphatidyl inositol (GPI) anchor. Defects in the machinery of GPI anchor synthesis can arise spontaneously in hemopoietic cells resulting in a clone of blood cells that have little or no GPI anchored proteins, including CD55 and CD59; the GPI-negative clone can remain small or expand to dominate.[24] The resultant disease, paroxysmal nocturnal hemoglobinuria (PNH) is characterized by hemolytic crises, anemia, and thrombosis. PNH erythrocytes are extremely susceptible to spontaneous complement hemolysis because they have no membrane regulators — unlike most cells, erythrocytes do not express CD46.

3.3. *Complement mutations and polymorphisms*

Mutations in complement genes can cause changes that stop short of complete absence or complete loss of function but instead cause reduced expression or altered function. Common polymorphisms can similarly alter expression level or function of a complement protein, and these changes, though often subtle, can markedly impact disease susceptibility. Mutations and polymorphisms can either reduce (loss-of-function) or enhance (gain-of-function) activities, and examples of both are numerous in complement proteins. The impact of complement mutations and polymorphisms on structure and function and the lessons taught by these experiments of nature have been well-reviewed recently;[26] here, I will focus on just a few disease exemplars.

Atypical hemolytic uremic syndrome (aHUS) is characterized by the triad of intravascular hemolysis, thrombocytopenia, and renal failure. It is a rare disease, distinguished from the more common diarrhoeal form of HUS (an epidemic disease the result of food-borne exposure to some strains of *E. coli*) by its chronic course and lack of a diarrhoeal prodrome. aHUS is a disease of complement dysregulation caused by polymorphisms and mutations in genes encoding complement proteins, most commonly in FH.[27] Scores of different mutations have been described, most clustering in the carboxy-terminus, that disrupt the capacity of FH to bind endothelia and other surfaces rendering them susceptible to complement-mediated injury. Mutations in other AP protein genes have also been found in aHUS; gain-of function mutations in C3 and FB were shown to increase the efficiency of C3 convertase formation, thus predisposing to dysregulation. Common polymorphisms in FH, the FH-related proteins (FHRs), and the membrane regulator CD46 all affect risk of developing aHUS. Indeed, for most of the aHUS-associated mutations, penetrance is incomplete, and within families co-existing risk polymorphisms dictate whether or not disease occurs.

Age-related macular degeneration (AMD), the commonest cause of blindness in the western world, is caused by a build-up of debris (drusen) in the retina that drives inflammation and retinal damage. Complement was first implicated because drusen deposits contain complement fragments and regulators; however, the demonstration that a common polymorphism in FH (FH_{Y402H}) is an important risk factor for AMD brought complement center stage.[28,29] Several other complement polymorphisms are strongly associated with AMD, including in C3, FB, and FI, another in FH, and several in the FH-related proteins.[30] The functional basis of the association has been ascertained for several of these; in summary, each confers a small increase in complement activity, thus increasing the propensity for inflammation.[31]

4. Complement as a driver of inflammation

4.1. *General principles*

Many of the physiological and most of the pathological effects of complement activation involve inflammation. Complement is a very potent pro-inflammatory cascade that responds to pathogens, damaged tissue, and other triggers to generate local inflammation and recruit inflammatory cells. The mediators of these effects are the activation products generated during activation.

4.2. Complement anaphylatoxins

Activation of each of the homologous complement proteins C4, C3, and C5 involves a proteolytic cleavage that releases a small peptide termed, respectively, C4a, C3a, and C5a. After much debate, the consensus is that C4a is biologically inert; however, the C3a and C5a fragments are very active, binding specific receptors on diverse cell targets to mediate their effects (Fig. 2). C3a and C5a were considered to be very similar in terms of their biological effects, differing only in relative activity; however, recent evidence suggests that they display quite different and often antagonist effects in some targets.[32]

For simplicity, I will first focus on C5a, a 74 amino acid pro-inflammatory peptide.[33] The principal receptor for C5a, termed C5aR1 (CD88), is a classical 7-transmembrane domain G-protein coupled receptor expressed on many cell types but in high abundance on innate (neutrophils, macrophages, mast cells) and adaptive (T cells) immune cells. For the purposes of this review I will focus on innate immune cell expression. C5a, generated at a site of infection or injury, binds its receptor on adjacent neutrophils and macrophages and triggers a signaling cascade ending in cell degranulation with release of multiple inflammatory mediators. In all expressing cells, C5aR1 is G-protein coupled (predominantly $G\alpha i2$) and binding of ligand begins a cascade of activation events; receptor engagement by ligand activates the G-protein receptor kinases, other associated kinases, and phospholipase C; these in turn activate multiple signaling pathways, including the Akt, MAPK/ERK kinase (MEK), and phosphatidylinositol 3-kinase (PI3K) pathways (Fig. 3). Downstream consequences of these events are in general pro-inflammatory but are cell type-dependent. In neutrophils, downstream effects include delayed apoptosis, chemotaxis, reactive oxygen species production, and packaging and reorientation of secretory machinery in the cell. Neutrophils and macrophages traffic along the chemotactic gradient toward the source, all the time becoming more prepared to respond, arriving at the source fully primed and ready to degranulate. Tissue mast cells also express C5aR1 and are induced to degranulate upon binding C5a, further exacerbating local inflammation.

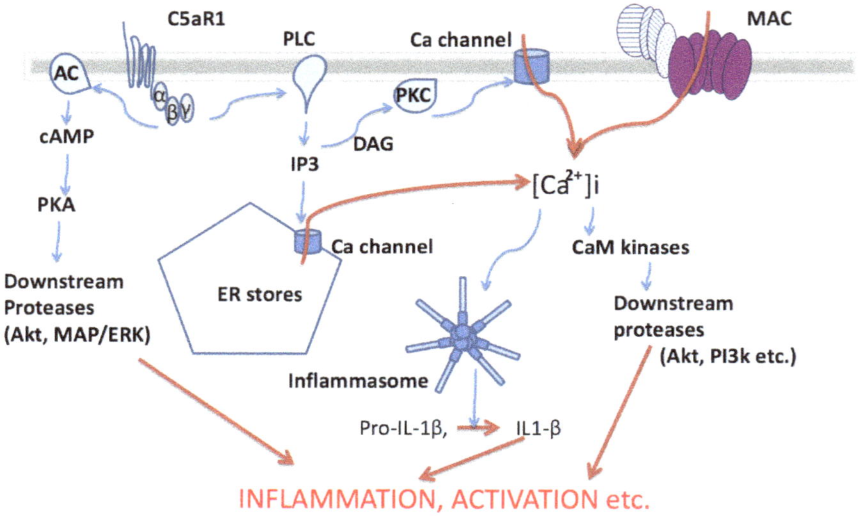

Fig. 3. Cell activation by C5a and the membrane attack complex. C5a binds its GPCR, C5aR1, to trigger multiple signaling pathways in the cell; receptor-associated G proteins directly activate phospholipase C in the membrane to produce inositol triphosphate (IP3) and diacylglycerol (DAG), second messengers that trigger opening of Ca^{2+} channels in the membrane and the endoplasmic reticulum to increase intracellular Ca^{2+} concentration ($[Ca^{2+}]i$). Receptor-associated G proteins can also activate adenylate cyclase (AC) to produce the second messenger cyclic adenosine monophosphate (cAMP) that causes opening of membrane ion channels and activation of protein kinase A (PKA); this in turn activates multiple downstream proteases. The MAC causes rapid influx of Ca^{2+}; when the increased $[Ca^{2+}]i$ exceeds the activating threshold, calmodulin is activated through conformational change caused by binding multiple Ca^{2+} ions, triggering the downstream activation of numerous calmodulin-dependent proteases. Increased $[Ca^{2+}]i$ and likely other complement-derived signals triggers inflammasome activation in some cell types leading to the production of pro-IL-1β and pro-IL-18 and their processing through caspase cleavage to the active inflammatory cytokines.

Effects of C5a are localized because carboxypeptidases in plasma and on cell surfaces efficiently cleave the carboxy-terminal arginine residue, the resultant C5adesArg still binds C5aR1 but its affinity for the receptor and activating capacity is reduced by more than 90%. C5adesArg is stable, and its residual activity is important in attracting cells toward the source. Of note, clinical assays that purport to measure C5a in plasma are in fact measuring C5adesArg.

A second receptor for C5a, termed C5L2 or C5aR2, first described in 2000, is also a seven-transmembrane domain receptor expressed widely and in a similar distribution to C5aR1.[34] One difference in expression patterns is that C5aR2 is abundantly expressed on adipose tissue and plays key roles in lipid metabolism outside the scope of this chapter's review. Importantly, C5aR2 binds both C5a and C5adesArg with high affinity, the latter with much higher affinity than C5R1. C5aR2 lacks the motif that effects G-protein coupling, so it has no obvious link to signaling systems leading to the suggestion that it was a decoy receptor, acting to mop up C5a and C5adesArg and modulate inflammation. More recently, studies using cell or whole animal knockouts or specific blockers of the two receptors have revealed a much more complicated situation that remains a subject of hot debate. In different studies and on different cell types, the presence of C5aR2 has been shown to either enhance or inhibit C5aR1 response to ligand.[35,36] The data suggest that C5aR2 engagement can be strongly pro-inflammatory in some contexts and profoundly anti-inflammatory in others. Precisely how C5aR2 mediates signaling also remains to be demonstrated, although it has been shown to interact with C5aR1, β-arrestin, TLRs, and other signaling molecules in the membrane.[37,38] In support of this, TLR4 ligands markedly increased leukocyte response to C5a; this effect was absolutely dependent on the presence of C5aR2, suggesting that it mediated cross-talk between the signaling receptors.

C3a is a 77-amino acid peptide, long considered to be a pro-inflammatory functional analogue of C5a. The principal receptor for C3a is C3aR, a classical 7-transmembrane domain G-protein coupled receptor that likely engages the same signaling pathways as C5aR1. Its distribution is not well documented, but it is expressed in many tissues and cell types, including innate immune cells. Like C5a and its receptor, C3a binds C3aR on innate immune cells to trigger activation and inflammation. Like C5a, C3a is efficiently cleaved by carboxypeptidases to form C3adesArg; however, this metabolite has a very low affinity for C3aR and essentially no activating capacity.

Yet more controversy surrounds the role of C5aR2 (or C5L2) as a receptor for C3a and C3adesArg; data from different groups and in different cell types are starkly contradictory, with some claiming no binding and others binding and important biological effects. There is no consensus on whether C3a and/or C3adesArg bind C5aR2 on immune cells to modulate signaling through C3aR (and maybe C5aR1?). In adipose tissue, it is clear that C5aR2 binds locally generated C3adesArg to signal triglyceride uptake — although even here the signaling pathways remain undefined.[39]

T cells, B cells, and antigen-presenting cells all express C3aR and C5aR1, and a growing body of evidence suggests that both C3a and C5a play important roles in regulating the adaptive immune response. This evolving field has been well reviewed recently,[40] and will not be revisited here. C4a is a structural analog of the anaphylactic peptides C3a and C5a and was originally considered an anaphylatoxin; however, there is no specific receptor for C4a and no evidence that C4a binds the C3a or C5a receptors.[41] It is therefore unlikely that it has any biological effect. The activation fragments C2b and Ba have also been ascribed biological activities, but the lack of candidate receptors make this unlikely.

4.3. *Membrane attack complex*

The MAC has evolved to bring about lytic killing of pathogens. When complement is activated on self-cells, defense mechanisms and regulators described above protect from lytic killing in all but the most extreme circumstances. Nevertheless, assembly of numerous large protein-walled channels in the cell membrane is not without consequence. The first consequence is calcium ion (Ca^{2+}) influx through the pore that in turn triggers Ca^{2+}-activated Ca^{2+} store release; intracellular Ca^{2+} concentration increases from low nM resting levels into the micromolar range within seconds.[42] Increased intracellular Ca^{2+} concentration translates into cell responses by binding multiple cytoplasmic Ca^{2+}-binding proteins, notably calmodulin, that in turn activate downstream calmodulin-dependent kinases to drive events in the cell (Fig. 3). Although Ca^{2+} is the principle mediator of MAC effects, cell activation occurs even when Ca^{2+} influx is prevented by removal of extracellular Ca^{2+} and/or intracellular Ca^{2+} chelation. A direct interaction of the MAC with the Giα-subunit, classically linked to G-protein-coupled receptor family members, has been described, providing a route to regulation of cyclic AMP (cAMP) production. Precisely how MAC intercalates with the Giα-subunit and other signal transducers in the membrane is unresolved; however, the growing body of evidence that MAC interacts with toll receptors, GPCRs, and other signaling receptors in the membrane provides a possible explanation — although no structure/function explanation has yet emerged for these MAC interactions.

The literature on downstream signalling pathways triggered by MAC is complicated by the hotch-potch of different cell types, tissues, complement sources, definition of non-lytic attack, and outcome measures. Nevertheless, common pathways do emerge from multiple studies, notably the PI3kinase, Akt/FOX01, and ERK1 pathways.[43–45] We recently undertook an unbiased comparison of gene expression in MAC-attacked and control tumor cells; ERK1 emerged as a central signaling node, supporting its central role in MAC signaling. MAC-dependent activation of the cyclin-dependent kinases (CDKs) 2 and 4 has been described, leading to cell activation and proliferation.[46] MAC triggering of apoptotic pathways through BCP-2-associated death receptor (Bad) phosphorylation leading to caspase activation has been described in multiple cell types.

Proinflammatory consequences of non-lytic MAC have been reported in numerous cell types. Neutrophils (and macrophages) are triggered to degranulate, releasing their arsenal of inflammatory mediators and induced to secrete inflammatory cytokines. Non-lytic MAC causes T cell triggering of inflammatory cytokine release.[47] Retinal epithelial cells exposed to non-lytic MAC were stimulated to release IL-6, IL-8, MCP-1, and VEGF.[48] MAC-triggered platelet activation has been described in many reports with effects including release of microparticles and surface changes that enhance stickiness.[49]

4.4. Complement and inflammasome activation

Inflammasomes are oligomeric signaling platforms present in diverse cell types that integrate multiple signals from pathogen recognition molecules and other "danger" detectors to deliver an appropriately targeted inflammatory response. The NLRP3 inflammasome has been most studied in the context of inflammation because of its broad distribution and capacity to respond to numerous triggers. NLRP3 inflammasome triggering causes activation of caspase-1 that in turn leads to the maturation and secretion of IL-1β and IL-18. In innate immune cells, this pathway plays a central role in switching on both inflammation and apoptotic cell death.[50] Increased intracellular Ca^{2+} and resultant mitochondrial injury have been implicated as mediators of inflammasome activation. This key role of Ca^{2+} led us to investigate whether non-lytic MAC could trigger inflammasome activation. Sub-lytic MAC triggered NLRP3 inflammasome assembly and activation in lung epithelial cells, resulting in co-localization of the component proteins and markedly increased IL-1β production.[51] Increased intracellular Ca^{2+}, both through influx via the pore and release of stores, was an early and key event that also triggered mitochondrial damage and apoptotic pathways. In a separate study, exposure of murine dendritic cells to sub-lytic MAC triggered NLRP3 inflammasome activation and production of IL-1β and IL-18.[52] These findings were recapitulated *in vivo* where inflammasome activation in LPS-treated mice, assessed by measuring plasma IL-1β and IL-18, was markedly reduced in C6-deficient mice (unable to make MAC) and in wild-type mice given MAC-blocking antibodies. The authors proposed that their findings showed that MAC triggered inflammation primarily through inflammasome activation; by extension, they argued that drugs targeting IL-1β would be effective in MAC-driven pathologies.

Both C3a and C5a have also been implicated in inflammasome activation. C3a was required for LPS-triggered NLRP3 inflammasome activation, assessed by measuring IL-1β production, in human macrophages and DCs, and enhanced activation in monocytes.[53] Although the pathway to activation was not fully elucidated, it involved C3aR engagement of ERK signaling pathways and regulation of ATP levels.

Critically, these events increased the induction of pro-inflammatory Th17 cells. Cholesterol crystals, a hallmark of atherosclerosis, are among many particulate triggers of inflammasome activation.[54] A role for C5a in this process was recently proposed based on the observation that cholesterol crystals spontaneously activated complement and elimination of complement activation removed their capacity to activate the inflammasome.[55] C5-depleted serum was inactive, focusing attention on C5a (although not eliminating MAC as a trigger). Regardless, the data suggest that cholesterol crystal-induced inflammation in atherosclerosis requires complement triggers and may be treatable with anti-complement drugs.

5. Complement inhibitors as anti-inflammatory drugs

The recent explosion in research and pharmaceutical interest in anti-complement drugs has been matched by an explosion of similar proportions in the number of reviews of the area. I do not seek here to add to this long list but will instead provide a brief summary. By definition, any drug that inhibits complement activation will be anti-inflammatory because complement is such a pro-inflammatory system. Nevertheless, the effects of such drugs will depend on the steps in the cascade that they impact, among many other variables. The first anti-complement drugs on the market were targeted to niche applications, for example, C1INH replacement therapy in hereditary angioedema (HAE; a rare inflammatory disease caused by deficiency of this regulator). Newer agents are targeting more common diseases or disease groups, and choice of agent is a complicated balance of immunological, clinical, and financial considerations.

5.1. *Pathway blockers as anti-inflammatory drugs*

Drugs that block one or more of the activation pathways or the terminal pathway can have profound anti-inflammatory effects by reducing the supply of the pro-inflammatory active products described above. C1INH blocks the classical and lectin pathways (and several other pro-inflammatory cascades), and deficiency leads to loss of control in all these pathways and generation of multiple pro-inflammatory molecules.[56] Replacement therapy is very effective as an emergency for acute attacks in HAE and increasingly as maintenance therapy. Despite the fact that C1INH has been in clinical use in HAE for over 25 years, only recently has it come to the fore as a potent anti-inflammatory that may be of benefit in many different diseases.[57] Cost is one major obstacle to its wider use. A large number of other activation pathway blockers, small molecules to biological, are in development and near the clinic, many targeted to treat acute and chronic inflammation.

The amplification loop of the alternative pathway is an attractive target, and many blocking drugs are in the pipeline.[58] C3, the chokepoint of complement activation and most abundant protein, is the target of a small peptide inhibitor compstatin that is, after a very long gestation, finally entering clinical trials.[59] A concern with blockers of the activation pathways is that they reduce or eliminate complement opsonization, an important defense against bacterial infection.

The terminal pathway is the source of the two most inflammatory products of complement, C5a and the MAC. The anti-C5 mAb eculizumab burst on the scene in 2002 and rapidly became a blockbuster drug. Eculizumab binds C5 and prevents its cleavage by complement C5 convertase. Initially developed for treatment of the rare hemolytic disorder paroxysmal nocturnal hemoglobinuria,[60] eculizumab is now in or near the clinic for numerous and diverse inflammatory diseases.[61] A flood of similar agents either targeting C5 or other MAC components are heading for the clinic. An advantage of terminal pathway blockade is that opsonization is unaffected and infection risk is restricted to *Neisseria*, uniquely requiring MAC for killing.

5.2. *Blocking C3a and C5a to inhibit inflammation*

Although the pathway blockers are effective anti-inflammatories, they carry risk of infection and other side effects. Targeting the anaphylactic fragments in diseases where these are the major drivers is attractive. C5a is a major pro-inflammatory molecule in many diseases involving complement activation and a prime target for drugs.[62] Drugs might target the receptor or the ligand. Numerous C5a receptor blockers have been developed ranging from large mAb or mAb fragments to small molecule or peptide blockers. These target C5aR1, the broadly expressed G-protein coupled receptor that mediates the pro-inflammatory effects of C5a. Some of these agents likely also target C5aR2, and the consequences of this are less clear. Ligand blockers targeting C5a and C5adesArg are also in development, the majority of these are mAb, mAb fragments, or related binding proteins. Several C5a/C5aR blockers are in clinical trials in a broad range of inflammatory diseases from psoriasis to rheumatoid arthritis, and some will likely enter the clinic soon.

C3a/C3adesArg as a drug target presents a conundrum in that it has a complex set of activities some of which are pro-inflammatory but others anti-inflammatory or homeostatic; for example, its role in lipid handling. A few drugs targeting the C3a/C3aR axis are in development as anti-inflammatories, but their safety and efficacy remains to be proven.

6. Summary and future prospects

This chapter serves as a reminder, should it be needed, that the complement system is a major driver of physiological and pathological inflammation. The former involves its capacity to signal danger, attract, and activate immune cells to respond; the latter involves dysregulation and activation to excess, causing damage to self-cells and tissues. New is the recent realization that complement acts in concert with other danger signals better to respond to the threat,[63] and that complement products directly trigger the inflammatory machinery embedded in many cell types. Coupled with the revolution in anti-complement drugs to target inflammatory diseases,[64] it seems that the time is ripe for complement to regain its historical place as the cornerstone of inflammation.

References

1. Fearon DT. (1998). The complement system and adaptive immunity. *Semin Immunol.* **10**:355–361.
2. Fearon DT, Carroll MC. (2000). Regulation of B lymphocyte responses to foreign and self- antigens by the CD19/CD21 complex. *Annu Rev Immunol.* **18**:393–422.
3. Carroll MC, Isenman DE. (2012). Regulation of humoral immunity by complement. *Immunity.* **37**:199–207.
4. Kemper C, Verbsky JW, Price JD, Atkinson JP. (2005). T-cell stimulation and regulation: with complements from CD46. *Immunol Res.* **32**:31–43.
5. Heeger PS, Kemper C. (2012). Novel roles of complement in T effector cell regulation. *Immunobiology.* **217**:216–224.
6. Cook KS, Min HY, Johnson D, Chaplinsky RJ, Flier JS, Hunt CR, Spiegelman BM. (1987). Adipsin: a circulating serine protease homolog secreted by adipose tissue and sciatic nerve. *Science.* **237**(4813): 402–405.
7. Rosen BS, Cook KS, Yaglom J, Groves DL, Volanakis JE, Damm D, White T, Spiegelman BM. (1989). Adipsin and complement factor D activity: an immune-related defect in obesity. *Science.* **244**(4911): 1483–1487.
8. Cianflone KM, Sniderman AD, Walsh MJ, Vu HT, Gagnon J, Rodriguez MA. (1989). Purification and characterization of acylation stimulating protein. *J Biol Chem.* **264**:426–430.
9. Sniderman AD, Cianflone K. (1994). The adipsin-ASP pathway and regulation of adipocyte function. *Ann Med.* **26**:388–393.
10. MacLaren R, Cui W, Cianflone K. (2008). Adipokines and the immune system: an adipocentric view. *Adv Exp Med Biol.* **632**:1–21.
11. Verschuuren JJ, Huijbers MG, Plomp JJ, Niks EH, Molenaar PC, Martinez-Martinez P, Gomez AM, De Baets MH, Losen M. (2013). Pathophysiology of myasthenia gravis with antibodies to the acetylcholine receptor, muscle-specific kinase and low-density lipoprotein receptor-related protein 4. *Autoimmun Rev.* **12**:918–923.
12. Hepburn NJ, Chamberlain-Banoub JL, Williams AS, Morgan BP, Harris CL. (2008). Prevention of experimental autoimmune myasthenia gravis by rat Crry-Ig: A model agent for long-term complement inhibition in vivo. *Mol Immunol.* **45**:395–405.
13. Howard JF Jr, Barohn RJ, Cutter GR, Freimer M, Juel VC, Mozaffar T, Mellion ML, Benatar MG, Farrugia ME, Wang JJ, Malhotra SS, Kissel JT. (2013). MG Study Group. A randomized, double-blind, placebo-controlled phase II study of eculizumab in patients with refractory generalized myasthenia gravis. *Muscle Nerve.* **48**:76–84.
14. Pittock SJ, Lennon VA, McKeon A, Mandrekar J, Weinshenker BG, Lucchinetti CF, O'Toole O, Wingerchuk DM. (2013). Eculizumab in

AQP4-IgG-positive relapsing neuromyelitis optica spectrum disorders: an open-label pilot study. *Lancet Neurol.* **12**:554–562.
15. Zhang H, Verkman AS. (2014). Longitudinally extensive NMO spinal cord pathology produced by passive transfer of NMO-IgG in mice lacking complement inhibitor CD59. *J Autoimmun.* **53(9)**: 67–77.
16. Manderson AP, Botto M, Walport MJ. (2004). The role of complement in the development of systemic lupus erythematosus. *Annu Rev Immunol.* **22**:431–456.
17. Poon IK, Lucas CD, Rossi AG, Ravichandran KS. (2014). Apoptotic cell clearance: basic biology and therapeutic potential. *Nat Rev Immunol.* **14**:166–180.
18. Morgan BP, Walport MJ. (1991). Complement deficiency and disease. *Immunol Today.* **12**:301–306.
19. Truedsson L, Bengtsson AA, Sturfelt G. (2007). Complement deficiencies and systemic lupus erythematosus. *Autoimmunity.* **40**:560–566.
20. Heitzeneder S, Seidel M, Förster-Waldl E, Heitger A. (2012). Mannan-binding lectin deficiency — Good news, bad news, doesn't matter? *Clin Immunol.* **143**:22–38.
21. Skattum L, van Deuren M, van der Poll T, Truedsson L. (2011). Complement deficiency states and associated infections. *Mol Immunol.* **48**:1643–1655.
22. Grumach AS, Kirschfink M. (2014). Are complement deficiencies really rare? Overview on prevalence, clinical importance and modern diagnostic approach. *Mol Immunol.* **61**:110–117.
23. Cicardi M, Zanichelli A. (2010). Replacement therapy with C1 esterase inhibitors for hereditary angioedema. *Drugs Today (Barc).* **46**:867–874.
24. Hall C, Richards SJ, Hillmen P. (2002). The glycosylphosphatidylinositol anchor and paroxysmal nocturnal haemoglobinuria/aplasia model. *Acta Haematol.* **108**:219–230.
25. Harris CL, Heurich M, Rodriguez de Cordoba S, Morgan BP. (2012). The complotype: dictating risk for inflammation and infection. *Trends Immunol.* **33**:513–521.
26. de Cordoba SR, Tortajada A, Harris CL, Morgan BP. (2012). Complement dysregulation and disease: from genes and proteins to diagnostics and drugs. *Immunobiology.* **217**:1034–1046.
27. Le Quintrec M, Roumenina L, Noris M, Frémeaux-Bacchi V. (2010). A typical hemolytic uremic syndrome associated with mutations in complement regulator genes. *Semin Thromb Hemost.* **36**:641–652.
28. Donoso LA, Kim D, Frost A, Callahan A, Hageman G. (2006). The role of inflammation in the pathogenesis of age-related macular degeneration. *Surv Ophthalmol.* **51**:137–152.
29. Thakkinstian A, Han P, McEvoy M, Smith W, Hoh J, Magnusson K, Zhang K, Attia J. (2006). Systematic review and meta-analysis of the association

between complement factor H Y402H polymorphisms and age-related macular degeneration. *Hum Mol Genet.* **15**:2784–2790.
30. Zipfel PF, Lauer N, Skerka C. (2010). The role of complement in AMD. *Adv Exp Med Biol.* **703**:9–24.
31. Heurich M, Martínez-Barricarte R, Francis NJ, Roberts DL, Rodríguez de Córdoba S, Morgan BP, Harris CL. (2011). Common polymorphisms in C3, factor B, and factor H collaborate to determine systemic complement activity and disease risk. *Proc Natl Acad Sci USA.* **108**:8761–8766.
32. Engelke C, Wiese AV, Schmudde I, Ender F, Ströver HA, Vollbrandt T, König P, Laumonnier Y, Köhl J. (2014). Distinct roles of the anaphylatoxins C3a and C5a in dendritic cell-mediated allergic asthma. *J Immunol.* **193**:5387–5401.
33. Manthey HD, Woodruff TM, Taylor SM, Monk PN. (2009). Complement component 5a (C5a). *Int J Biochem Cell Biol.* **41**:2114–2117.
34. Li R, Coulthard LG, Wu MC, Taylor SM, Woodruff TM. (2013). C5L2:a controversial receptor of complement anaphylatoxin, C5a. *FASEB J.* **27**:855–864.
35. Chen NJ, Mirtsos C, Suh D, Lu YC, Lin WJ, McKerlie C, Lee T, Baribault H, Tian H, Yeh WC. (2007). C5L2 is critical for the biological activities of the anaphylatoxins C5a and C3a. *Nature.* **446**:203–207.
36. Hao J, Wang C, Yuan J, Chen M, Zhao MH. (2013). A pro-inflammatory role of C5L2 in C5a-primed neutrophils for ANCA-induced activation. *PLoS One.* 8(6):e66305.
37. Bamberg CE, Mackay CR, Lee H, Zahra D, Jackson J, Lim YS, Whitfeld PL, Craig S, Corsini E, Lu B, Gerard C, Gerard NP. (2010). The C5a receptor (C5aR) C5L2 is a modulator of C5aR-mediated signal transduction. *J Biol Chem.* **285**:7633–7644.
38. Tang H, Amara U, Tang D, Barnes MA, McDonald C, Nagy LE. (2013). Synergistic interaction between C5a and NOD2 signaling in the regulation of chemokine expression in RAW 264.7 macrophages. *Adv Biosci Biotechnol.* 4(8C): 30–37.
39. Cui W, Lapointe M, Gauvreau D, Kalant D, Cianflone K. (2009). Recombinant C3adesArg/acylation stimulating protein (ASP) is highly bioactive: a critical evaluation of C5L2 binding and 3T3-L1 adipocyte activation. *Mol Immunol.* **46**:3207–3217.
40. Sacks SH. (2010). Complement fragments C3a and C5a: the salt and pepper of the immune response. *Eur J Immunol.* **40**:668–670.
41. Klos A, Wende E, Wareham KJ, Monk PN. (2013). International Union of Basic and Clinical Pharmacology. LXXXVII. Complement peptide C5a, C4a, and C3a receptors. *Pharmacol Rev.* **65**:500–543.
42. Morgan BP. (1989). Complement membrane attack on nucleated cells: resistance, recovery and non-lethal effects. *Biochem J.* **264**:1–14.

43. Fosbrink M, Niculescu F, Rus V, Shin ML, Rus H. (2006). C5b-9-induced endothelial cell proliferation and migration are dependent on Akt inactivation of forkhead transcription factor FOXO1. *J Biol Chem.* **281**:19009–19018.
44. Ren G, Huynh C, Bijian K, Cybulsky AV. (2008). Role of apoptosis signal-regulating kinase 1 in complement-mediated glomerular epithelial cell injury. *Mol Immunol.* **45**:2236–2246.
45. Qiu W, Zhang Y, Liu X, Zhou J, Li Y, Zhou Y, Shan K, Xia M, Che N, Feng X, Zhao D, Wang Y. (2012). Sublytic C5b-9 complexes induce proliferative changes of glomerular mesangial cells in rat Thy-1 nephritis through TRAF6-mediated PI3K-dependent Akt1 activation. *J Pathol.* **226**:619–632.
46. Tegla CA, Cudrici C, Patel S, Trippe R 3rd, Rus V, Niculescu F, Rus H. (2011). Membrane attack by complement: the assembly and biology of terminal complement complexes. *Immunol Res.* **51**:45–60.
47. Chauhan AK, Moore TL. (2011). T cell activation by terminal complex of complement and immune complexes. *J Biol Chem.* **286**:38627–38637.
48. Lueck K, Wasmuth S, Williams J, Hughes TR, Morgan BP, Lommatzsch A, Greenwood J, Moss SE, Pauleikhoff D. (2011). Sub-lytic C5b-9 induces functional changes in retinal pigment epithelial cells consistent with age-related macular degeneration. *Eye (Lond).* **25**:1074–1082.
49. Martel C, Cointe S, Maurice P, Matar S, Ghitescu M, Théroux P, Bonnefoy A. (2011). Requirements for membrane attack complex formation and anaphylatoxins binding to collagen-activated platelets. *PLoS One.* **6**(4):e18812.
50. Horng T. (2014). Calcium signaling and mitochondrial destabilization in the triggering of the NLRP3 inflammasome. *Trends Immunol.* **35**:253–261.
51. Triantafilou K, Hughes TR, Triantafilou M, Morgan BP. (2013). The complement membrane attack complex triggers intracellular Ca2+ fluxes leading to NLRP3 inflammasome activation. *J Cell Sci.* **126**:2903–2913.
52. Laudisi F, Spreafico R, Evrard M, Hughes TR, Mandriani B, Kandasamy M, Morgan BP, Sivasankar B, Mortellaro A. (2013). Cutting edge: the NLRP3 inflammasome links complement-mediated inflammation and IL-1β release. *J Immunol.* **191**:1006–1010.
53. Asgari E, Le Friec G, Yamamoto H, Perucha E, Sacks SS, Köhl J, Cook HT, Kemper C. (2013). C3a modulates IL-1β secretion in human monocytes by regulating ATP efflux and subsequent NLRP3 inflammasome activation. *Blood.* **122**:3473–3481.
54. Rajamäki K, Lappalainen J, Oörni K, Välimäki E, Matikainen S, Kovanen PT, Eklund KK. (2010). Cholesterol crystals activate the NLRP3 inflammasome in human macrophages: a novel link between cholesterol metabolism and inflammation. *PLoS One.* **5**(7):e11765.
55. Samstad EO, Niyonzima N, Nymo S, Aune MH, Ryan L, Bakke SS, Lappegård KT, Brekke OL, Lambris JD, Damås JK, Latz E, Mollnes TE, Espevik T.

(2014). Cholesterol crystals induce complement-dependent inflammasome activation and cytokine release. *J Immunol.* **192**:2837–2845.
56. Davis AE 3rd, Lu F, Mejia P. (2010). C1 inhibitor, a multi-functional serine protease inhibitor. *Thromb Haemost.* **104**:886–893.
57. Caliezi C, Wuillemin WA, Zeerleder S, Redondo M, Eisele B, Hack CE. (2000). C1-Esterase inhibitor: an anti-inflammatory agent and its potential use in the treatment of diseases other than hereditary angioedema. *Pharmacol Rev.* **52**:91–112.
58. Holers VM. (2008). The spectrum of complement alternative pathway-mediated diseases. *Immunol Rev.* **223**:300–316.
59. Ricklin D, Lambris JD. (2008). Compstatin: a complement inhibitor on its way to clinical application. *Adv Exp Med Biol.* **632**:273–292.
60. Schrezenmeier H, Höchsmann B. (2009). Eculizumab opens a new era of treatment for paroxysmal nocturnal hemoglobinuria. *Expert Rev Hematol.* **2**:7–16.
61. Wong EK, Kavanagh D. (2015). Anticomplement C5 therapy with eculizumab for the treatment of paroxysmal nocturnal hemoglobinuria and atypical hemolytic uremic syndrome. *Transl Res.* **165**:306–320.
62. Woodruff TM, Nandakumar KS, Tedesco F. (2011). Inhibiting the C5-C5a receptor axis. *Mol Immunol.* **48**:1631–1642.
63. Raby AC, Holst B, Davies J, Colmont C, Laumonnier Y, Coles B, Shah S, Hall J, Topley N, Köhl J, Morgan BP, Labéta MO. (2011). TLR activation enhances C5a-induced pro-inflammatory responses by negatively modulating the second C5a receptor, C5L2. *Eur J Immunol.* **41**:2741–2752.
64. Morgan BP, Harris CL. (2015). Complement, a target for therapy in inflammatory and degenerative diseases. *Nat Rev Drug Discov.* **14**:857–877.

Chapter 3

Lipids and Inflammation

Valerie B. O'Donnell*, Robert C. Murphy† and Garret A. FitzGerald‡

1. Introduction

Lipids (or fats) play essential roles in all cellular processes. They are structural, provide an important energy source, and act as key signaling mediators in cell differentiation, development, and inflammation. However, excess lipid deposition (obesity) is a major pro-inflammatory risk factor for chronic disease and death and is a public health problem worldwide. In this chapter, we will discuss lipids at a whole-body level, including what is currently known about their participation in inflammatory diseases. Following this, our current knowledge on the role of lipids as specific signaling mediators in inflammation will be summarized.

* Systems Immunity Research Institute and Institute of Infection and Immunity, School of Medicine, Cardiff University, Cardiff, CF14 4XN, UK. E-mail: o-donnellvb@cardifff.ac.uk

† Department of Pharmacology, University of Colorado Denver, Aurora, CO 80045, USA.

‡ Institute for Translational Medicine and Therapeutics, 3400 Civic Center Boulevard, Building 421, 10th Floor, Room 122, Philadelphia, PA 19104-5158, USA.

Most lipids reside in hydrophobic compartments, including the cell membrane and lipid bodies, or circulate in plasma bound with lipoproteins. During acute inflammation, rapid alterations in lipid pools take place, mediated by the action of numerous phospholipases, acyltransferases, and kinases. The results in the generation of a complex and still not fully characterized myriad of potent signaling mediators. Some, including eicosanoids, are soluble and can be secreted to act on neighboring cells via paracrine activation of G protein-coupled receptors (GPCRs). Others, including phosphoinositides, are retained in the cell membrane and interact with local proteins to alter conformational structure and enzymatic activities in the cytoplasm.

In the last 10–15 years, our ability to analyze and quantify lipids that signal in inflammation has been revolutionized by the introduction of new-generation liquid chromatography–mass spectrometry instruments, in particular tandem and high-resolution mass spectrometers, and the emergence of Lipidomics as a sub-discipline of Metabolomics. Lipid imaging using matrix-assisted laser desorption ionization (MALDI) can now define the location of specific lipids within tissues. The increasing availability of these new analytical modalities is rapidly changing our ability to identify, quantify, and map lipids of inflammation, leading to novel discoveries and broader insights into their key roles in inflammation.

2. Lipids and inflammation in obesity

In the Western world, obesity, characterized by excess body lipid deposition in adipose tissue, has reached epidemic proportions and is a major risk factor for global fatalities. WHO stated that 3.4 million adults a year die because of an obesity-associated complication (WHO, Obesity and overweight, Fact sheet No. 311, updated August 2014). This is caused by a combination of factors that include increased caloric intake, with higher proportion of lipids and refined carbohydrates, coupled with lower levels of exercise. There is also an emerging role for a specific gut microbiota composition in promoting lipid deposition, although as yet the mechanisms linking microbes and body lipid deposition are poorly understood.[1,2]

Adipose tissue is either subcutaneous or visceral, with white adipocytes containing a single large lipid droplet, and can represent up to 60% of total body weight.[3] However, the number of adipocytes is static in humans, with visceral fat considered the most important in terms of inflammatory signaling. In this regard, it is now widely accepted that adipose tissue is not an inert organ, or merely a store for excess lipids, but that it is metabolically active, generating over 600 hormones termed adipokines, that include leptin, estrogen, and pro-inflammatory cytokines.[4] Adipose tissue is also a major source of circulating fatty acids and their metabolites.[5,6] These not only act locally, but are also secreted into the circulation leading to a chronic low-grade pro-inflammatory state, and they also act centrally to influence feeding behavior.[7] Such circulating mediators are considered to be of major importance in the link between obesity and numerous diseases including cardiovascular disease, diabetes, asthma, arthritis, autoimmune disease, non-alcoholic fatty liver disease, and neuropsychiatric disorders.[8–12]

Inflammation in adipose tissue is considered centrally to involve adipose tissue macrophages (ATMs), which generate either pro- or anti-inflammatory adipokines, at least in part depending on the level of adiposity and their phenotype. Recent studies have shown that lipolysis or short-term low-calorie diets in humans can lead to accumulation of M2 (anti-inflammatory) ATMs, while conversely, in obesity, white fat tissue contains more M1 (pro-inflammatory ATMs).[13–15] How this is controlled is currently unclear but may relate to lipid-dependent signaling initiated by the adipocytes themselves. Indeed, these cells are known sources of many immunomodulatory lipid mediators, including prostaglandins, leukotrienes, and mono- and di-hydroxy unsaturated fatty acids (see Ref. 3 for a recent review). White adipose tissue expresses numerous enzymes that generate lipid mediators, including cyclooxygenases (COXs)-1 and -2, and several prostaglandin synthase enzymes including PGD synthase and thromboxane synthase.[16–18] Cultured adipocytes also express membrane receptors for several prostaglandins and appear to modulate lipolysis via the PGE_2 receptor, EP3.[19] Finally, adipose tissue expresses all enzymes necessary for leukotriene generation and signaling, including 5-lipoxygenase (LOX), 5-LOX activating protein (FLAP), leukotriene A4 hydrolase, leukotriene C4 synthase, and the receptors BLT1 and 2 and CysLT1 and 2.[20] These mediators may play a central role in controlling inflammatory activation by ATM, but the mechanistic links between these and adipocytes are not yet fully clarified.

3. Circulating plasma lipids and inflammation

Atherosclerosis is a chronic low-grade inflammation of the vascular wall characterized by lipid deposition and oxidation and by infiltration of innate and adaptive immune cells, resulting from an inappropriate response to injury. Elevated levels of circulating lipids, in particular cholesteryl esters (CEs) present in circulating low-density lipoproteins (LDLs), are classic risk and causal factors for development of atherosclerosis and for prediction of secondary vascular events.[21–23] LDL is a major source of circulating cholesterol and cholesteryl esters, with LDL-C being a common measure for total LDL levels used clinically. Lowering LDL using statins is a key strategy for reducing risk of vascular events and has been developed following strong evidence from both primary and secondary trials.[21–24] However, there is clear evidence that statins also act directly via reducing inflammation associated with elevated lipids. In this way, they exert an anti-inflammatory action on the vessel wall through influencing a variety of pathways in the innate and adaptive immune systems, and via regulating isoprenoid formation.[25] As an inhibitor of HMG-CoA reductase (the first rate-limiting step of cholesterol biosynthesis), statins prevent formation of intermediates required for protein isoprenylation. This is required for effective functioning of a number of important GTP-binding proteins, including Ras, Rho, and Rac. These are involved in expression of pro-inflammatory cytokines, generation of oxidative intermediates, and proliferation, adhesion and apoptosis, and their inhibition is a key aspect of the anti-atherogenic properties of these drugs (see Ref. 25 and references therein).

Triglycerides (TGs) are the second major lipid component of circulating lipoproteins and are principally contained in TG-rich lipoproteins (TGRLs), either chylomicrons (dietary) or very-low-density lipoprotein (VLDL, hepatic). They consist of at least 200 individual molecular species, differing in fatty acid composition.[26] Chylomicron elevation is associated with pancreatic inflammation, while VLDL increases endothelial inflammation, promoting cell migration into the vessel wall. TG lipolysis by lipoprotein lipases (LPL) on the vessel wall releases products that are known to induce inflammation and apoptosis, with known involvement of the transcription factor ATF-3 and kinases such as p38, c-Jun N-terminal kinases, mitogen-activated protein kinases (MAPK), and cytokines that include interleukins (IL)-1α, -6, and -8 and vascular endothelial growth factor (VEGF).[27–30] Following a high fat meal, patients with hypertriglyceridemia produce high levels of TGRLs, with a defined pro-inflammatory fatty acid composition that can upregulate TNF and VCAM-1 expression on endothelial cells. In contrast, TGRLs with low TG content are anti-inflammatory.[31–33]

CEs and TGs are families of lipids that contain hundreds of different molecular species, some of which may be considerably more important than others in terms of inflammatory bioactivities within the vasculature.[26] One interesting feature is that circulating CE molecular species within plasma lipoproteins contain high levels of polyunsaturated fatty acids such as linoleic acid and arachidonic acid, CE(18:2) and CE(20:4), respectively. This is likely a major conduit providing these essential fatty acids to cells throughout the body. With the advent of ever more sensitive and specific high-resolution and quantitative lipidomic profiling methodologies, significant opportunities now exist to map the plasma lipidome in terms of CE and TG molecular composition in different forms of dyslipidemias, in order to identify which molecular species are more relevant in terms of promoting disease in patients with different genetic backgrounds. This information could potentially be used clinically to (i) uncover novel disease mechanisms and (ii) guide lipid-lowering treatment strategies.

4. Specific lipid classes in inflammation

4.1. *Eicosanoids and related lipids*

Acute activation of innate immune cells switches on phospholipase A_2 (PLA_2) enzymes, of which there are three main families: cytosolic (calcium-dependent, $cPLA_2$, *PLA2G4A*), calcium-independent ($iPLA_2$, *PLA2G6*), and secretory ($sPLA_2$, *PLA2G2A*). These hydrolyze phospholipids releasing fatty acids, most importantly arachidonate, that act as substrates for eicosanoid biosynthesis. Eicosanoids are formally defined as oxidized metabolites of fatty acids with a 20-carbon hydrophobic chain, most commonly arachidonate (AA). They include prostaglandins (PG), thromboxanes (TX) — both of which contain unique ring structures — and other mediators, including mono-, di-, and tri-hydroxy-fatty acids. Longer and shorter chain analogs are also generated via 18- or 22-carbon fatty acid oxidation, e.g. docosanoids from docosahexaenoic acid (DHA, 22:6, n3).

In the context of inflammation, there are three main pathways for formation of eicosanoids and related mediators, COX, LOX, and cytochrome P450 (CYP), with constitutive or inducible isoforms of each, as follows.

4.1.1. *COX enzymes, products, and their receptors*

There are two isoforms of COX: constitutive (COX-1, *PTGS1*) and inducible (COX-2, *PTGS2*). COX-1 is expressed in platelets and the gastric system constitutively, where it is considered homeostatic. However, platelet COX-1 is important in the innate immune response, facilitating platelet aggregation via synthesis of thromboxane A_2 (TXA_2) to promote hemostasis and prevent bacterial invasion following wounding. COX-2 is inducible, via exogenous bacterial/fungal signals or endogenous cytokines, and generates higher levels of eicosanoids than COX-1 in both acute and chronic inflammation. COX isoforms have two catalytic activities, cyclooxygenase and peroxidase, and their final product is always PGH_2.[34] This gets transformed either enzymatically or non-enzymatically to a variety of

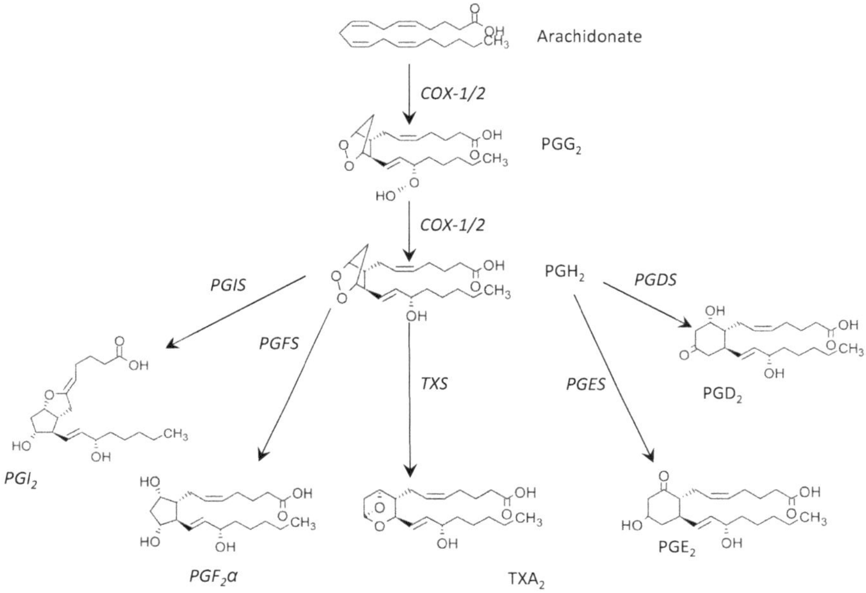

Fig. 1. Cyclooxygenase metabolism of arachidonate to form bioactive mediators. COX enzymes oxidize arachidonate (AA) to form PGG_2 which is reduced by the COX heme peroxidase to form PGH_2. Following this, PGH_2 can be metabolized by several other enzymes, depending on the cell type, to form secondary products as shown. PGIS; PGI synthase, PGFS; PGF synthase, TXS; thromboxane synthase, PGES; PGE synthase, PGDS; PGD synthase.

secondary mediators, including PGE_2, PGD_2, and $PGF_2\alpha$ (Fig. 1).[35] In general, COX-1-derived PGH_2 is utilized by thromboxane synthase (*TBXAS1*), PGF synthase, or cytosolic PGE synthase (PGES, *PTGES3*), while COX-2 derived PGH_2 is metabolized by prostacyclin synthase (PGIS, *PTGIS*) and microsomal PGES (*PTGES*).[36] The profile of eicosanoid formation from COX is thus determined by the cellular profile of enzymes that further metabolize PGH_2. Thus, platelets generate primarily TXA_2, with small amounts of PGE_2 and D_2 generated non-enzymatically, while rodent macrophages generate large amounts of primarily PGD_2, with some PGE_2 following induction of COX-2 by lipopolysaccharide. Platelets also generate significant amounts of 12-hydroxyheptadecatrienoic acid (12-HHTrE) via TX synthase. This has recently been recognized as an activator of the BLT1 receptor.[37] It is generally thought that COX enzymes are catalytically active when expressed, but that their turnover is governed by substrate supply and thus by PLA_2 activity.

COX products are predominantly secreted and act in a paracrine manner via activation of G protein-coupled receptors. There are eight members of the prostanoid receptor family: E prostanoid receptor (EP) 1, EP2, EP3, and EP4; PGD receptor (DP1); PGF receptor (FP); PGI receptor (IP); and thromboxane receptor (TP). Several isoforms, including TPα, TPβ, FP_A, FP_B, and eight EP3s form via alternative splicing.[38,39] Prostanoid receptors activate a series of intracellular signaling pathways including adenylyl cyclase (increasing cAMP), phosphoinositide metabolism (forming IP3), phospholipase C (PLC), and guanine nucleotide exchange factors of the small G protein, Rho.[35] Several G proteins are involved, including G_s, G_h, G_i, G_q, and G_{13} families.

COX enzymes generate PGG_2 via the COX domain, which uses a tyrosyl radical to abstract hydrogen from arachidonate, in the first stage of oxygenation. PGG_2 is then converted to the final product, PGH_2, via a heme peroxidase cycle. The reducing substrates for this activity in mammalian cells are not totally clear, but likely include glutathione present in the cytosol at millimolar concentrations. COXs exist as homodimers, with one protein monomer acting as the catalytic site and the other as an allosteric regulator.[40]

COX-2 is considered the primary source of eicosanoids in inflammation; however, COX-1 can also generate these lipids during acute stages, at least in part since it is already expressed by innate immune cells that have not been exposed to infectious or damage stimuli.[36] Indeed, a role for both enzymes as amplifiers in inflammatory responses has been revealed using knockout mice.[41–43] The role of COX-2 in various diseases has been reported as either pro- or anti-inflammatory, and in mouse models of vascular disease to either prevent, promote, or have no effect.[35] This may reflect differences in effects or the enzymes in acute or chronic settings (where there is evidence of a pro-resolving role through uncharacterized mechanisms) or inherent changes in mice genetically lacking these pathways.[44,45]

4.1.2. *Inhibition of COXs*

COXs are inhibited by a series of compounds, called non-steroidal anti-inflammatory drugs (NSAIDs) that include the newer COX-2 selective inhibitors, which were originally developed to avoid the gastrointestinal bleeding side effects associated with NSAIDs. Generally, these act via competitive transient inhibition at the COX active site.[35] Blocking COX-2 thus prevents pro-inflammatory PG generation, alleviating pain and edema. In contrast, aspirin acts instead as a covalent irreversible inhibitor, and at lower doses selectively blocks platelet TX generation in humans, while higher doses inhibit both COX isoforms. Examples of NSAIDs include those that block both isoforms with comparable potency (ibuprofen, ketoprofen), intermediate COX-2-selective inhibitors (nimesulide, meloxicam, diclofenac, celecoxib), and highly selective COX-2 inhibitors (rofecoxib, etoricoxib, lumiracoxib).[46] Acidic NSAIDs have been shown to concentrate at inflammatory sites (diclofenac, ibuprofen, ketoprofen), leading to a sustained therapeutic effect.[47] While aspirin is clearly cardioprotective, other NSAIDs are associated with increased cardiovascular risk, due primarily to PGI_2 blockade in the vasculature.[48] The cardiovascular effects of NSAIDs are also complex, for example, NSAIDs targeting COX-1 can prevent acetylation of platelet COX-1 by aspirin, thus decreasing its cardioprotective effects.[47] NSAIDs remain a major treatment strategy for acute and chronic inflammation. Knowledge of factors affecting their safety and tolerability, including their selectivity, and pharmacokinetics needs to be used clinically to guide their use. These have been recently summarized in Ref. 49.

4.1.3. *COX metabolites in inflammation*

PGE_2 is an important biologically active lipid that plays numerous roles in health as well as in immune/inflammatory disease. In inflammation, it is centrally involved in mediating pain and edema through acting on peripheral and central neurons, and causing vasodilation.[50] It is generated either via cPGES, mPGES-1 or -2. Mice deficient in mPGES-1 show marked alterations in inflammation and demonstrate a role for PGE_2 in promoting arthritis, subcutaneous inflammation and atherogenesis.[51,52] PGE_2 signals primarily via EP3 and EP4 in promoting arthritis *in vivo*, through stimulating IL-6 and IL-1 generation.[35] It can also stimulate Th1/IL-23-dependent Th17 cell differentiation, and induce migration of dendritic cells to draining lymph nodes.[53,54] However, PGE_2 can also be anti-inflammatory, for example in both neuroinflammation and atherosclerosis, there is evidence of both pro- and anti-inflammatory actions, all mediated by EP2 and EP4.[35] Thus, the biology of PGE_2 is complex, and largely results from differences in receptor expression at target sites of inflammation.

PGI_2 is a major regulator of vascular tone generated by endothelial cells to mediate vasodilation and prevent adhesion of platelets and white cells.[55] Mice deficient in IP show enhanced vascular responses to injury, accelerated atherogenesis, and elevated hypertension.[35] Due to its vasoactive effects, PGI_2 is a key mediator of edema and pain in acute inflammation. It is generated in high amounts in human arthritic synovial fluid as well as in the inflamed murine peritoneal cavity.[56,57] It also contributes to pain via triggering of IP in spinal cord and dorsal root ganglions. In support, IP antagonists reduce pain in a number of animal inflammatory models.[58,59]

PGD_2 regulates both homeostasis and inflammation and is generated by mast cells, dendritic cells, and Th2 cells.[60–62] It is a major mediator in allergy and asthma, and elicits bronchoconstriction and eosinophil infiltration. Its pro-inflammatory actions are elicited by both DP1 and DP2/CRTH2 receptors expressed on bronchial epithelium and circulating immune cells, respectively. However, in some models of airway inflammation, PGD_2 also elicits anti-inflammatory actions. For example, acting via DP1, PGD_2 blocks migration of dendritic cells and eosinophils to lung in mouse allergy models.[63,64] PGD_2 has been suggested to modulate inflammation via its degradation to form 15d-PGJ_2, which then acts via PPARγ or NFκB. However, definitive evidence that this lipid forms in amounts sufficient to be bioactive *in vivo* are currently lacking.

$PGF_2\alpha$ is primarily formed from PGH_2 via PGF synthase, but can also form via metabolism of other PGs, as a minor product. It plays a major role in brain injury and pain.[65,66] It has been reported to be elevated in several forms of arthritis, diabetes, obesity, and smoking, although in acute models, its generation may coincide with isoprostane formation (see below) and thus be at least partly non-enzymatic.[35]

TX is mainly generated via COX-1 and TX synthase in platelets, but can also form in lower amounts via COX-2 in macrophages. It stimulates platelet adhesion/aggregation, smooth muscle contraction, and endothelial inflammation.[67] A major role for TX in inflammation is not currently known, although its receptor, TP, can be activated by a number of other PGs generated during disease, including PGH_2, isoprostanes, and hydroxyeicosatetraenoic acids (HETEs).[68,69] Mice deficient in TP show less platelet activation and are protected against hypertension, atherosclerosis, and cardiac hypertrophy.[70–72]

4.1.4. *LOX enzymes, products, and their receptors*

Mammalian cells express LOXs that include immune cell and epidermal isoforms. The immune cell LOXs are named by the position of oxygen insertion into AA, specifically 12-LOX (platelets, *ALOX12*), 5-LOX (neutrophils, mast cells, *ALOX5*), 15-LOX1 (human, IL-4 cultured monocytes, eosinophils, airway epithelia, *ALOX15*), and its murine homolog 12/15-LOX which is highly expressed in naïve peritoneal macrophages.[73] LOXs contain a non-sulfur-bound non-heme iron. Substrate specificity is isoform dependent with 12/15- and 15-LOXs able to oxidize not only AA but also linoleate, and other fatty acids, and complex lipids where fatty acids are attached to larger functional groups including phospholipids and cholesteryl esters. In contrast, 5- and 12-LOXs only oxidize free acid substrates, primarily AA[73] (Fig. 2) While several isoforms can modulate inflammatory disease *in vivo*, it is likely that their physiologic roles instead relate to promoting innate immunity and wound healing responses under healthy conditions.

12/15-LOXs can regulate the outcome of acute and chronic inflammatory disease in several mouse models including cardiovascular disease, diabetes, hypertension, and allergic asthma.[74–77] In human cells, 15-LOX1 is strongly induced by Th2 cytokines (IL-4 and -13) via STAT6, that polarize macrophages to an M2 phenotype.[78] This correlates with elevated levels of its lipids in allergic and autoimmune diseases, including asthma.[79] Macrophages lacking this enzyme show numerous functional defects in Toll-like receptor 4 signaling, PPARγ activation, and defective membrane processing during autophagy and phagocytosis.[80,81] The primary products of this enzyme are 13S-hydroperoxyoctadecadienoic acid (HpODE) or 12S/15S-hydroperoxyeicosatetraenoic acids (HpETE), which are rapidly reduced to the corresponding 13S-HODEs or 12/15S-HETEs (Fig. 2).

The 5-LOX is cytosolic in resting cells, but on calcium mobilization it translocates to either the nuclear or plasma membrane. It has three phosphorylation sites, for MAP-KAP, ERK2, and PKA, which

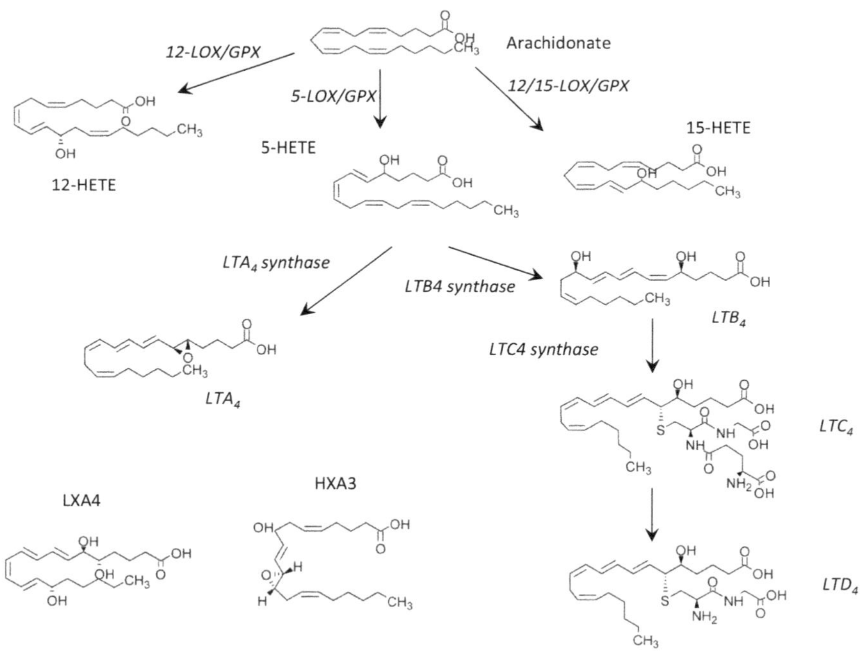

Fig. 2. Lipoxygenase metabolism of arachidonate to form bioactive mediators. LOXs oxidize AA to form hydroperoxyeicosatetraenoic acids, which are rapidly reduced by cellular GPX to hydroxyeicosatetraenoic acids (HETEs). These can be further metabolized to leukotrienes in neutrophils. An example of a hepoxilin (HX) and a lipoxin (LX) is also shown.

can either activate or suppress catalytic turnover. It also requires the presence of an accessory protein, 5-LOX activating protein (FLAP), which predominantly localizes at the nuclear membrane. For a detailed review of 5-LOX enzymatic regulation see Ref. 82. 5-LOX products are important mediators of allergic responses in airway disease.[83] Although expressed in foam cells of atheroma, there is limited evidence for its participation in causing disease.[84] Evidence also exists for leukotrienes involved in traumatic brain injury and FLAP inhibitors improving outcomes in rats when administered after traumatic brain injury.[85,86] Several studies have suggested that 5-LOX can participate in the pathogenesis of Alzheimer's disease (AD) as another example of the role of this pathway in mediating neuroinflammatory events. For example, 5-LOX can modulate levels of amyloid-β and tau phosphorylation in cultured cells, and a pilot study linked 5-LOX gene polymorphisms with early and late onset disease. Finally, mice lacking 5-LOX are protected against age-dependent AD learning and memory insults in transgenic disease models (Tg2576, 3xTg).[87] These studies in the brain suggest an emerging understanding of 5-LOX activity in neuroinflammation. Currently, the 5-LOX pathway is targeted indirectly by montelukast, a cysteinyl leukotriene receptor antagonist, used in asthma.[88]

4.1.5. *LOX metabolites in inflammation*

The primary product of LOX catalysis are HpETEs, which are rapidly reduced in cells via glutathione peroxidases (GPx) to HETEs. H(p)ETEs are considered to act biologically primarily through their cellular metabolism to secondary lipid mediators (Fig. 2). In particular, 5-HpETEs are converted by further LOX activities to hepoxilins or lipoxins or by 5-LOX and leukotriene (LT) synthases to cystenyl leukotrienes (CysLTs). Mice deficient in LTs display reduced inflammation, e.g. in zymosan peritonitis. LTB_4 is a potent neutrophil chemotactic agent that acts via two GPCRs, BLT_1 (high affinity), and BLT_2 (low affinity). BLT_1 is primarily expressed by immune cells and plays a major role in allergic asthma, dermatitis, and conjunctivitis.[89] The CysLTs, LTC_4, D_4, and E_4 are major mediators of asthma and allergic rhinitis and are generated by eosinophils, mast cells, and macrophages. They act via $CysLT_1$ and $CysLT_2$, which mediate their effects in asthma and also promote airway remodeling and mucus edema *in vivo*.[89]

Hepoxilins contain epoxy hydroxy groups and form via metabolism of 12-HpETE by either eLOX3 or 12/15-LOX (Fig. 2). These lipids are chemically and biologically unstable, forming tri-hydroxy metabolites *in vivo*. They elevate calcium in neutrophils, promote chemotaxis, and elevate skin permeability, and have been found during several forms of acute inflammation and infection.[90]

4.1.6. *Transcellular generation of eicosanoids*

Early studies showed that *in vitro*, primary LOX- and COX-derived lipids could move from their cell of origin and be metabolized to additional products in other cell types. Specifically, incubation of indomethacin-treated aortic rings with platelet-rich plasma showed generation of PGI_2, where the COX-derived PGH_2 from platelets was metabolized by endothelial PGI2 synthase.[91] Similarly, PGH_2 from endothelium was shown to be metabolized to TXA_2 by platelet TXS.[92] LTs have also been shown to form via transcellular mechanisms, with over 50% of neutrophil LTA_4 being released from neutrophils, and at least some being further metabolized in red cells to form LTB_4, or to LTC_4 by endothelial cells.[93]

Evidence that transcellular biosynthesis could occur *in vivo* has been provided using chimeric mice. Leukocytes in these mice lack the complete machinery to generate LTB_4 or LTC_4. However, during inflammatory challenge, significant amounts of both lipids were formed, indicating that interactions between bone marrow and stromal cells together contribute toward bioactive mediator generation.[94,95]

Lipoxins (LX, lipoxygenase interaction products), which are tri-hydroxytetraene eicosanoids) have been shown to form *in vitro* via several different mechanisms that include (i) 5- and 12-LOX, (ii) 15- and 5-LOX, (iii) acetylated COX-2, and 5-LOX[93] (structure shown in Fig. 2). Thus, co-operation among several cell types including platelets, eosinophils, neutrophils, monocytes, epithelial cells, and endothelial cells could potentially be involved in their *in vivo* generation. However, they may also form via non-enzymatic further oxidation of primary LOX products. In this case, multiple isobaric isomeric species would be expected, which would be visible on LC-MS/MS analysis. However, many investigators use ELISAs to measure these lipids from clinical or animal model systems. While several studies have shown that LXs can prevent neutrophil infiltration and promote monocyte and NK cell activation, functional studies using the proposed receptor, ALX/FPR2, have been contradictory.[96,97] Currently, exactly how LXs are formed *in vivo* and their definitive signaling actions are not fully understood.[93]

In addition to AA, both EPA and DHA can be metabolized by LOXs to generate lipids that have been proposed to act as specialized pro-resolving mediators (SPM), including resolvins, maresins, or protectins.[98,99] These are anti-inflammatory when added exogenously in a variety of *in vivo* and *in vitro* models. This has led to development of mimetics as pro-resolving mediators for therapeutic use.[100] However, questions remain regarding their *in vivo* generation and ability to act as endogenous mediators. Some studies measuring these lipids in biological samples have used ELISAs, which can overestimate due to lack of antibody specificity. Additionally, cells can generate higher amounts of lipid mediators when supplied with exogenous substrates than are often seen when using receptor-dependent agonists, highlighting the difference between capacity and actual biosynthesis. A recent study of serum generated *in vitro* showed that this contains an array of eicosanoids not present in plasma, including SPMs.[101] Even the use of plasma is not without sampling artifacts, since blood taking can result in artefactual generation of eicosanoids; thus, urinary metabolites should be always considered the gold standard for systemic eicosanoid estimations, if assays for these are available.[102] Last, given the close structural relationship between many of these lipid mediators, chiral chromatography coupled with LC-MS/MS has been suggested as a way to greatly improve unequivocal identification of their generation *in vivo*.[103]

4.1.7. *Endocannabinoids and inflammation*

Endocannabinoids are esterified forms of AA that include N-arachidonylethanolamide (AEA) and 2-arachidonoylglycerol (2-AG) that signal in appetite, pain, and memory. Recently, they were found to be substrates for COX isoforms, generating esterified PGs that signal differently to the free acid PG forms and may play novel roles in inflammation. Both LOXs and COXs can oxidize AEA and 2-AG (Fig. 3). 15-LOX, but not platelet 12- or 5-LOX, can form HpETE-EA or -AG, with roughly the same efficiency as free AA, and with the same regio- and stereoselectivity.[104] LOXs also oxidize lipo-amino acids, and other fatty acids (e.g. DHA)

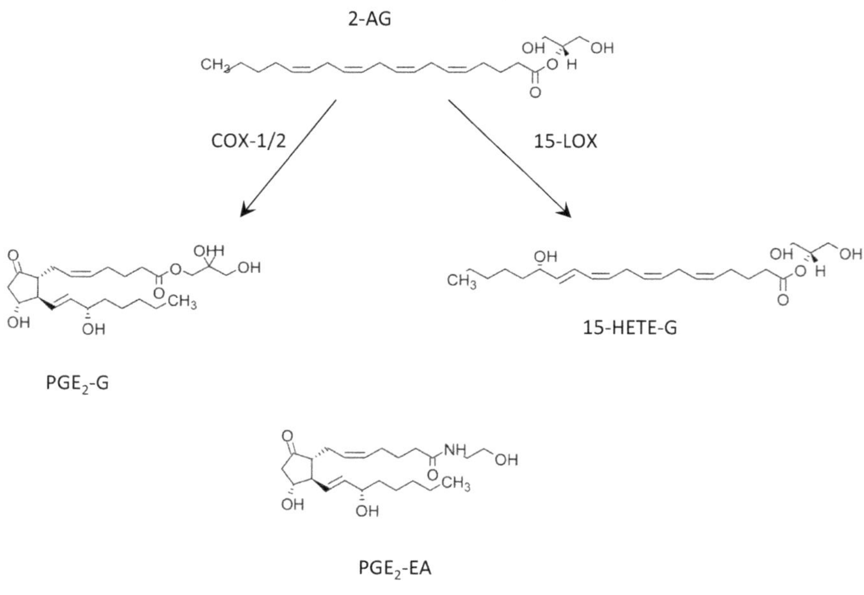

Fig. 3. Metabolism of endocannabinoids by oxidative enzymes. 2-arachidonoyl-glycerol (2-AG) or arachidonyl-ethanolamide (AEA) are oxidized directly by COX or LOX to form esterified eicosanoids.

attached to EA in a similar manner, generating esterified products that may signal in inflammation. Indeed, 17-hydroxy-DHEA has been found in mouse brain homogenate, suggesting a physiological role for these lipids.[104]

COXs, in particular COX-2, can oxidize esterified fatty acids with small functional groups, including AEA and 2-AG (but not phospholipids or diglycerides). Unlike LOXs, the efficiency of oxidation of AEA is lower, for COX-2 it is only about 27% that of AA.[105] In contrast, COX-2 oxidation of 2-AG is comparable to AA. For AEA, the product is an esterified PGE_2 derivative, while for 2-AG, a mix of products including glyceryl esters of PGE_2, D_2, 11-HETE, 15-HETE, and 12-HHT are formed.[106] Similar to LOX isoforms, COX-2 can also oxidize lipo-amino acids. Finally, cytochrome P450 enzymes, in particular the 4F2 (kidney) and 34A (liver), can form epoxyeicosatetraenoic acid-EA (EET-EA) from AEA. In contrast, there is little evidence for P450-mediated oxidation of 2-AG.[104]

Several of these unique lipids have been reported as being generated by immune cells, suggesting they may play a role in inflammation, although *in vivo* levels are generally extremely low and require exogenous administration of substrates (e.g. AEA) to stimulate their formation. *In vitro*, these include: 15S-HETE-EA (neutrophils), 12-HETE-taurine (resident peritoneal macrophages), PGD_2-EA and –G (LPS/IFNγ-treated RAW264.7 cells).[104] COX-derived oxygenated endocannabinoids are not active at known PG or endocannabinoid receptors. In contrast, several HETE-EAs are effective CB1 receptor ligands, and 6-EET-EA is a higher affinity ligand for CB2 than AEA.[107,108]

PG-Gs or -EAs possess biological activities that are different from their free acid analogs. $PGF_2\alpha$-EA and its analog bimatoprost are beneficial in glaucoma, but this action is independent of FP, and appears to be a result of expression of a splice variant of FP, altFP4. In RAW264.7 cells, PGE_2-G, but not PGD_2-G, or PGF_2 cause calcium mobilization, along with an increase in inositol triphosphate, activation of protein kinase C, and phosphorylation of mitogen-activated protein kinases (MAPK). The receptors involved in this process are unknown. Interestingly, replacing the ester linkage of the glycerol with a thioester, or changing to the EA derivative, abolished activity. This suggests the presence of a specific receptor for PGE_2-G in immune cell signaling.[104]

Extensive literature around the enzymatic oxidation of endocannabinoids has developed, along with measurements of very low levels *in vivo*. What is less certain as yet is under which circumstances, if any, these lipids play a role in modulation of inflammation *in vivo*.

4.1.8. *Isoprostanes and inflammation*

Isoprostanes are regioisomers and enantiomers of prostaglandins, generated through non-enzymatic oxidation of AA. Hundreds of potential structures exist, with several having been found *in vivo*. One of the best characterized are F2 isoprostanes, for which there are four families, the 5-, 8-, 12-, and 15-series. One of these is 8-iso-$PGF_2\alpha$, an isomer of $PGF_2\alpha$ and a member of the 15-series lipids.[109] This is a widely used biomarker of free radical-mediated "oxidative stress" in human disease, being elevated in both tissue and urine during atherosclerosis, type 2 diabetes, and obesity.[109] However, while this lipid is not formed directly by any known catalytic activity, this may not rule out a role for enzymes in its generation *in vivo*. For example, secondary oxidation reactions initially triggered by enzymes that include LOXs, COXs, and other oxidative pathways in inflammatory cells may be involved. Currently, the detailed pathways that initiate formation of isoprostanes *in vivo* are not known.

4.2. *Phospholipids in inflammation*

Phospholipids (PLs) are the primary structural component of cell membranes. There are five main classes: phosphatidylcholine (PC), phosphatidylethanolamine (PE), phosphatidylserine (PS), phosphatidylglycerol (PG), and phosphatidylinositol (PI). Phospholipids can also be divided into acyl (ester), plasmalogen (vinyl ether), and ether (alkyl ether). Both plasmalogens and ethers are found with PC or PE headgroups, and in some tissues (brain, immune, and vascular system), plasmalogens comprise up to 30–70% of total PC.

4.2.1. *Aminophospholipid translocation in inflammation*

Under resting conditions, PC is the most prominent PL on the cell surface, while the aminophospholipids (aPLs) PE and PS are mainly face the cytosol of the lipid bilayer. When immune cells become activated (e.g. by bacterial products or when platelets are aggregating), or during cell ageing and apoptosis, PE and PS translocate to the cell surface where they support coagulation and facilitate opsonization and clearance by the reticuloendothelial system. This is mediated by calcium-dependent activation of scramblase. aPL externalization is an important process required for effective inflammation both in the acute and resolving stages. This is routinely measured by fluorescent annexin V binding; however, a lipidomic method was recently developed that allows mapping and quantitation of aPL molecular species on the surface of cells. This showed that lipids with 18–20 carbon fatty acids are optimum for supporting coagulation, and are the most abundant on the platelet surface following activation by thrombin, and induction of apoptosis.[110,111]

4.2.2. *Oxidized phospholipids in inflammation*

Oxidized PL (oxPL) are well known as biomarkers in a variety of diseases, including atherosclerosis, lung injury, ischemia, and multiple sclerosis.[112] In the 1990s, they were identified as a component of minimally modified low density lipoprotein, able to activate monocyte inflammatory signaling.[113,114] At that time, air oxidation of PC was used as an *in vitro* model system in order to characterize how these lipids can signal in inflammation. However, this contains >100s of species. Thus, in many experiments the specific structures and mechanisms that mediate their bioactivities were not clarified. Later on, fractionation of air oxidized lipid mixtures led to identification of molecules responsible for specific activities. Examples of PCs identified in this way include both non-fragmented (e.g. isofurans, epoxyisoprostane, endoperoxides) and fragmented forms (oxovaleryl, glutaryl, furan).[112] These lipids can signal through multiple mechanisms, including acting as antigens, ligands for scavenging receptors, and other receptors including those for RAGE, PAF, PG, VEGF, and also TLR receptors and PPARs. They can promote platelet activation, are angiogenic, and modulate cytoskeleton, adhesion, and endothelial permeability. Finally, they have been found to play a role in adaptive immunity, through modulating dendritic cells and T cell anergy. A comprehensive review has recently been published.[112]

Up to 2007, oxPL were all presumed to form non-enzymatically. However, since then, 40–50 individual molecular species of oxPL generated acutely in innate immune cells on agonist activation have been identified. The most prominent are enantiomeric HETE-PE and PCs, generated via LOX oxidation of membrane PLs in platelets, neutrophils, and monocytes following activation by thrombin, collagen, fMLP, or calcium ionophore.[115–120] There are also corresponding analogs of PGE_2 and PGD_2-PEs formed by platelets via COX-1, but in much lower quantities.[121] 15-HETE-PLs generated by 15-LOX or 12/15-LOX form via direct membrane oxidation; however, those from platelet 12-LOX, 5-LOX, or COX-1 require $cPLA_2$-dependent AA hydrolysis from the membrane prior to enzymatic oxidation, followed by fast re-esterification into the membrane (Fig. 4).

HETE-PE/PCs are thrombogenic, promoting plasma coagulation factor activities (in particular prothrombin and other gla-domain proteins). They dampen TLR4 activity in monocytes, act as low affinity PPARγ ligands, and modulate neutrophil antibacterial actions, notably IL-8, superoxide generation, and neutrophil extracellular trap (NET) release.[115,117–120] HETE-PE/PCs and their keto-eicosatetraenoic acid (KETE)-PE analogs, formed via prostaglandin dehydrogenase, have been detected during *in vivo* inflammation and infection, in both human and murine bacterial peritonitis, and in lung allergy and cystic fibrosis.[115,116,118]

Given their known bioactivities, it is likely that enzymatically generated oxidized PLs play a central role in mediating acute wound responses *in vivo*, as part of the innate immune system. On the other hand, their uncontrolled generation in terms of amounts, location, and myriad molecular species results in inappropriate inflammation in the vessel wall, contributing to promotion and progression of atherosclerosis and other vascular diseases in humans.

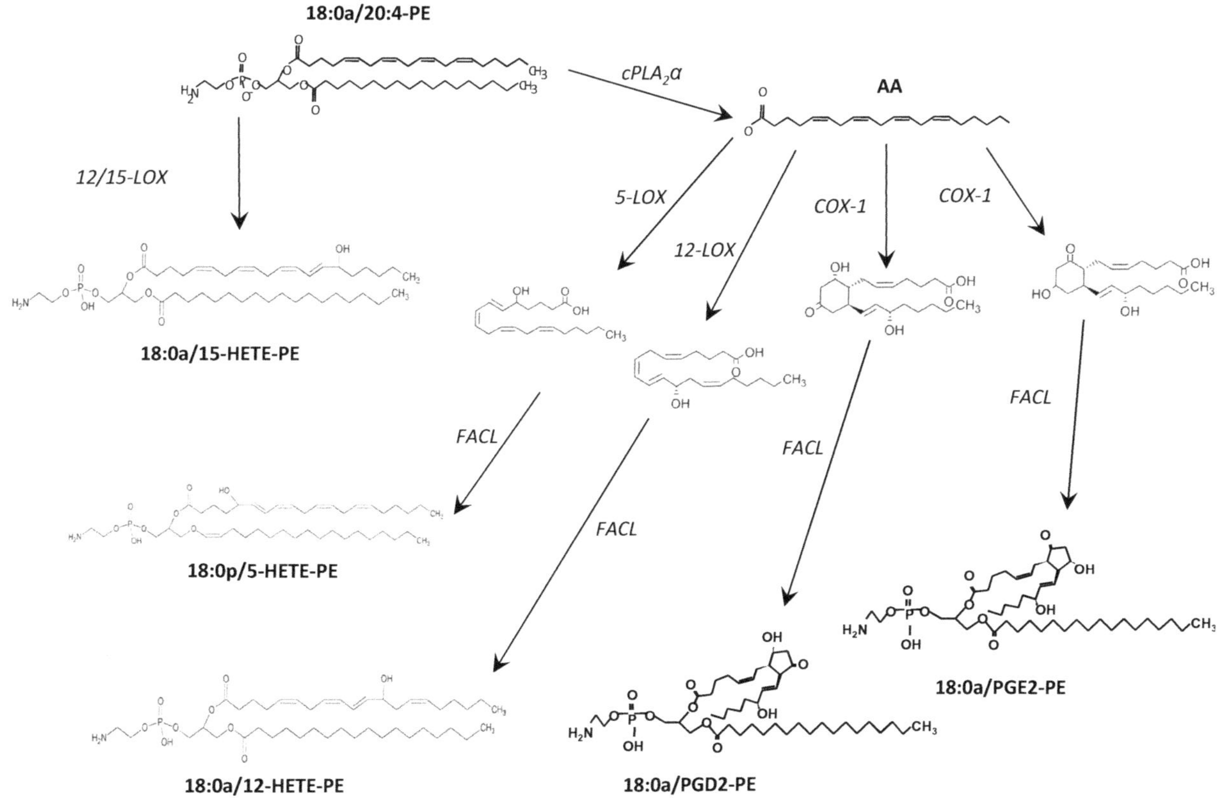

Fig. 4. Formation of esterified eicosanoids by COX or LOX enzymes. AA is hydrolyzed from phospholipids by PLA$_2$. Following its oxidation by COX or LOXs, it can then be re-esterified back into phospholipids, primarily PE. In contrast, PE can be directly oxidized by 12/15- or 15-LOXs in monocytes/macrophages. In all cases, the primary products will be the hydroperoxides that are reduced by GPX (not shown).

4.2.3. *Lysophospholipids (LP) and phosphatidic acid (PA)*

Phospholipids are metabolized by PLA_2 or PLA_1, and PLD to generate LPs and lysophosphatidic acid (LPA) (Fig. 5). These can also be generated via phosphorylation of monoglycerides (MGs) or diacylglycerides (DAGs), e.g. by DAG kinase. PA is generated by removal of the PL headgroup, by PLD, or by acylation of LPA by LPA-acyltransferases (LPAAT). LPs are a complex mix of species, which formally include LPA and sphingosine-1-phosphate (S1P), that have a phosphate head group and single fatty acid attached to a glycerol backbone. Many species can be formed depending on the fatty acid composition at *sn1* and *sn2*, although whether different molecular species possess distinct biological actions is not yet known. LPs bind to GPCRs, with there being six known for LPA (LPA_{1-5}). These play multiple roles in development, homeostasis, pain, and immunity.[122,123] For example, LPA_3 regulates chemotaxis of dendritic cells

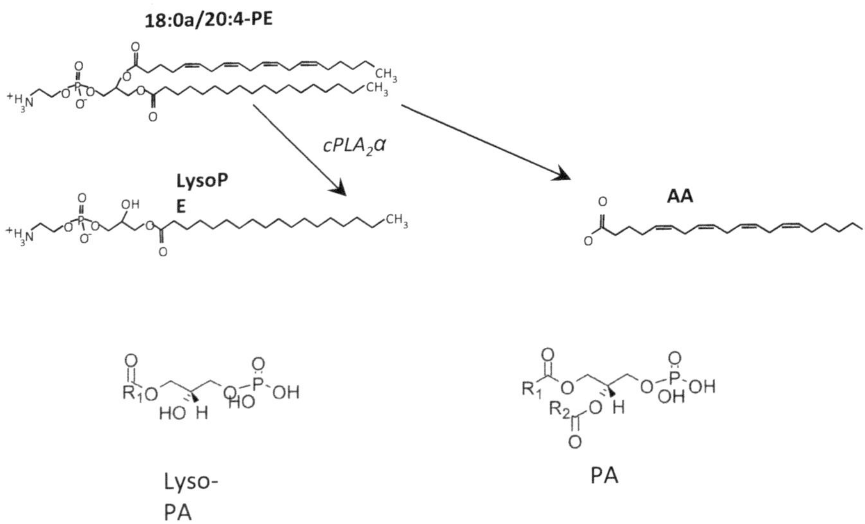

Fig. 5. Formation of lysophospholipids and phosphatidic acid. A phospholipid is hydrolyzed by PLA_2 to form a lyso-PE and AA. Examples of a lysophosphatidic acid (lyso-PA) and phosphatidic acid (PA) are also shown.

and pain.[122,123] Furthermore, antagonists of LPA_1 are currently in clinical development for LPA_1 for fibrosis. LPA is generated by thrombin-stimulated platelets and is itself prothrombogenic.[124] Plasma contains micromolar amounts of LPAs that are proposed to be formed via autotaxin, a plasma lysophospholipase D.[125]

LPs, including lyso-PI and -PS, have also been shown to activate specific GPCRs. Lyso-PS has several functions of relevance to immunity, including stimulation of mast cell histamine release and subsequent anaphylactic shock in rodents.[132,133] It also suppresses T-cell proliferation, and can activate TLR2 during parasite infection.[134,135] It signals via several GPCRs including GPR34, P2Y10, and GPR174.[136] In neutrophils, lyso-PI activates GPR55 to form filamentous actin, via RhoA.[137] At this time, the detailed biological roles of lyso-PS and -PI are not known, although lyso-PS has been shown recently to be generated in a mouse wound model *in vivo*.[138] Whether they form in sufficient amounts to mediate significant bioactivity has not yet been determined.

4.2.4. *Phosphoinositides*

Phosphoinositides are a large family of related lipids containing an inositol (Fig. 6). Reversible phosphorylation of the headgroup is mediated by several related families of tightly regulated PI-kinase enzymes. In addition, phospholipase C cleavage of PI(4,5,)P2 leads to formation of two potent signaling mediators, the protein kinase C (PKC) activator, diacylglycerol (DAG), and a potent activator of intracellular calcium mobilization, I(1,4,5)P3 (IP3). DAG and IP3 are key mediators of the acute activation of immune cells, including platelets, neutrophils, T-cells, and monocytes. PIP3, formed by phosphorylation of PI(4,5)P2 by PI3-kinases (PI3K), binds to a domain of 120 amino acids, termed a pleckstrin homology (PH) domain. These are present in several signaling and cytoskeleton proteins, along with SH2 and SH3 domains. This binding leads to both membrane association and conformational changes, further transducing cell signaling during inflammation and immune regulation.

PI3Ks are major players in inflammatory disorders, cell proliferation, cancer, differentiation, and apoptosis. They are highly

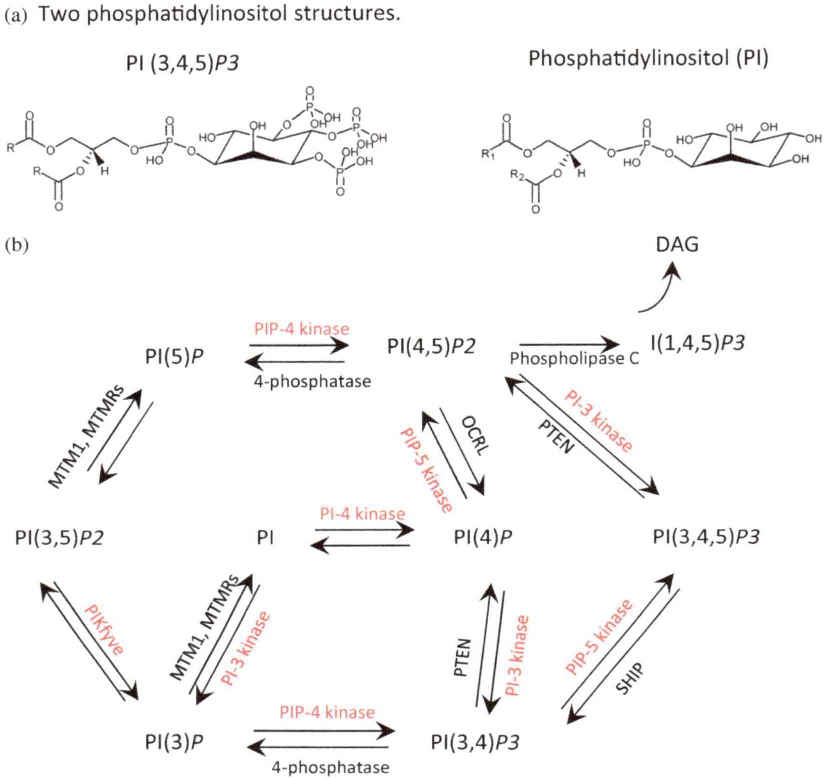

Fig. 6. Phosphoinositide metabolism pathways. (a) Examples of 2 polyphosphorylated forms of PI. (b) The complex metabolic interconversion of phosphoinositides. Kinases are shown in red. Adapted from Ref. 135.

expressed in leukocytes where they regulate chemokine-mediated recruitment of innate immune cells. They also play a central role in antigen receptor-stimulated development, differentiation, and function of lymphocytes.[139] For example, through regulating immunoreceptor tyrosine-based activation motif (ITAM) receptors, they can influence hemostasis and platelet activation.[140] Targeting PI3K decreases viral infection in chronic obstructive pulmonary disease (COPD).[141] They also regulate vesicle trafficking and induction of autophagy, pathogen killing, and immune cell survival.

For detailed reviews of the role of PI3K in inflammation, see Refs. 139 and 142.

One of the most important phosphoinositides is PI(3,4,5)P3. This unique lipid interacts with many proteins through specific binding domains and regulates a large variety of cellular functions including survival, proliferation, cytoskeletal rearrangement, and gene expression. Altered generation of PI(3,4,5)P3 contributes to cancer, diabetes, inflammation, and vascular disease.[143]

There are multiple isoforms of all enzymes involved in PI metabolism, making signaling via this pathway extremely complex. For example, platelets alone express five variants of PLC (PLC-β (β1, β2, β3, β4) and PLC-γ) and all four class I isoforms of PI3K. Murine studies have enabled determination of roles of individual isoforms of these proteins, showing multiple and often overlapping functions and revealing important new targets for therapeutic development in hemostasis.[144]

4.3. *Ceramides/sphingolipids*

Sphingolipids are a ubiquitous class of lipids that include ceramide, sphingomyelin, and many different glycosphingolipids that contain a sphingoid base backbone. The simplest of these is ceramide, which contains a sphingosine and fatty acid (Fig. 7). Sphingosine or ceramide can be phosphorylated, e.g. sphingosine by sphingosine kinases 1 and 2, forming sphingosine-1-phosphate (S1P). The three key lipids from this pathway in terms of inflammatory and immune signaling are ceramide, ceramide-1-phosphate (C1P), and S1P. These play important roles in responses to infection/injury; however, their unregulated generation is implicated in numerous diseases, including edema, asthma, bowel disease, cancer, multiple sclerosis, and arthritis.[145] Thus, these lipids are important bioactive metabolites of relevance to cell growth, survival, immune cell migration, vascular integrity, inflammation, and cancer.[126,146] For recent reviews of this topic, see Refs. 126, 145, 147 and 148. In the last 10 years, our knowledge of this class of lipids has rapidly advanced. This was driven by the cloning of sphingolipid regulatory proteins and

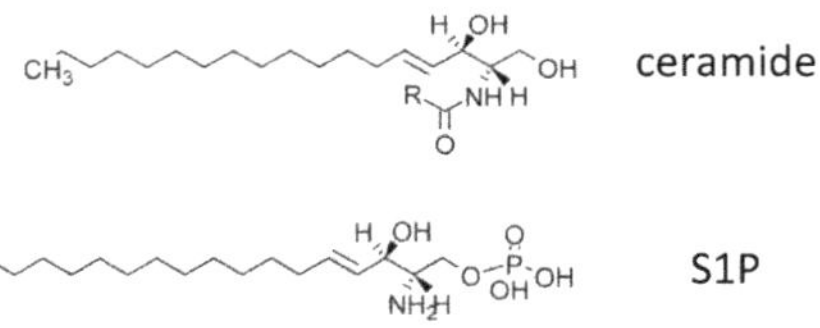

Fig. 7. Structures of ceramide and sphingosine-1-phosphate.

enzymes, coupled with the generation of synthesis/response protein-deficient mice, and the advent of new-generation high-sensitive mass spectrometry. New antagonists and agonists have been developed, in particular, fingolimod, a sphingosine analog now used clinically for multiple sclerosis.[145]

Five receptors are known for S1P ($S1P_{1–5}$).[126,127] In general, these mediate intracellular signaling including inhibition of cAMP generation, cytosolic calcium elevation, and activation of MAPK and small GTPase Rac.[128] Several have known functions of relevance for inflammation and immunity. For example, $S1P_1$ activates cell migration and lymphocyte trafficking, leading to B and T cell retention in lymphoid germinal centers.[126] $S1P_4$ is involved in thrombopoiesis, leukocyte migration, and T_H17 differentiation.[129] S1P is abundant in blood and lymph, and plays important homeostatic roles in vascular integrity and immune cell trafficking. S1P also enhances vascular endothelial (VE)-cadherin expression, maintaining integrity of high endothelial venules during immune responses.[130,131] Thus, it attenuates increased endothelial permeability induced by inflammatory cytokine signaling.

Ceramide has been reported to exist in specialized microdomains which have been implicated in B cell activation, pathogen responses, and cytokine release.[131] Its levels increase in endothelial cells in response to cytokines and injury, are linked with vascular permeability, and result from acid/neutral sphingomyelinase activation. Ceramide triggers caspase activation and increases mitochondrial permeability, and it is responsible for damage associated with emphysema, sepsis, and ARDS. Finally, ceramide-1-phosphate (C1P) inhibits ADAM17 (tumor necrosis factor (TNF)-converting enzymes, TACE), the major protease that cleaves pro-TNF to TNF.[149]

5. Lipid receptors in inflammation: PPAR and LXR

Bioactive lipids transduce their signaling through several mechanisms, but in particular via binding and activation of receptors and transcription factors. In many cases, these bioactive lipids are steroids and steroid hormones but also include lipid vitamins such as retinoic acid and vitamin D.[150–152] Earlier sections described lipid GPCRs that primarily interact with free acid mediators to regulate acute inflammatory cell signaling. Here, we focus on a series of important receptors that act as lipid-sensing transcription factors, responding to dynamic changes in lipid levels through regulating gene expression and metabolism: peroxisome proliferator-activated receptors (PPARs), retinoic acid receptors (RXRs), and liver X receptor (LXR).

5.1. *Peroxisome proliferator-activated receptors (PPAR)*

PPARs are a family of nuclear receptors that act as transcription factors and respond to a diverse range of fatty acids and their metabolites.[153] They are involved in differentiation, development, and metabolism and are considered to be major therapeutic targets in inflammatory disease, in particular type 2 diabetes. There are three PPAR isoforms, α, δ, and γ, with having three alternatively spliced forms γ .[153] PPARs heterodimerize with the retinoid X receptor (RXR) to induce gene expression, in response to multiple agonists, and via recruitment of coactivator proteins.

PPARγ (*PPARG*) is a major regulator of adipocyte differentiation, insulin sensitivity, lipogenesis, and adipocyte survival.[154,155] While its isoforms are major targets for diabetes treatment, agonists have been of limited use due to major side effects caused by activation of PPARγ in non-target organs. Genome-wide profiling has recently demonstrated that PPARγ:RXR bind to thousands of sites in adipocytes.[156,157] Sequence analysis has identified a degenerate direct repeat 1 (DR1) element as the primary binding site. These are strongly enriched near genes induced during differentiation, in particular related to fatty acid and glucose metabolism, indicating a direct role in activating these pathways during adipogenesis.[154] Many lipids bind to PPARγ and act as low-affinity ligands (e.g. with activation in the high nanomolar to low micromolar range). These include polyunsaturated fatty acids, oxidized phospholipids, nitrolipids, eicosanoids, and the prostaglandin 15-deoxy-Δ12, 14-prostaglandin J_2 (15d-PGJ_2), many of which are present at levels *in vivo* that would be too low to individually activate this pathway.[116,158,159] To date, no high-affinity ligands have been identified, suggesting that lipid sensing by PPARγ relates more to sensing global levels of multiple related lipids, via binding to a large and rather open binding site, as opposed to a high-affinity response to a single or small number of specific molecular species.

PPARα (*PPARA*) is a receptor for a similarly diverse range of lipid species, including phospholipids such as 1-palmitoyl-2-oleoyl-sn-glycerol-3-phosphocholine (16:0/18:1-GPC), generated by fatty acid synthase.[160] It also binds a variety of unsaturated fatty acids at physiological concentrations, which act (as before) as low-affinity ligands. Dietary unsaturated fatty acids have a diverse range of effects, including insulin, cardiovascular, and immune regulation, and these are at least in part mediated via activation of this transcription factor.[161,162] This isoform is a major sensor of dietary and liver lipids, responding rapidly in fasting and starvation. It is also important in modulating genes during inflammation, in particular relating to lipotoxicity, inflammation, endothelial dysfunction, and thrombogenesis.[163–165] A recent review has been published regarding this.[166]

Similar to other PPARs, PPARδ heterodimerizes with RXR to induce gene transcription. However, this isoform also can transrepress transcription and also act in a non-genomic manner. Transrepression occurs via interaction with other transcription factors, including Bcl6, to prevent cell proliferation. Thus, PPARδ can act in either pro- or anti-inflammatory manner depending on whether it is unbound or ligand bound.[167] Finally, it can act non-genomically, e.g. via binding to PKCα in platelets to block adhesion, or by opening of calcium-operated potassium channels.[168] Similar to other PPARs, this isoform also binds saturated and unsaturated fatty acids, including prostacyclin and 15d-PGJ_2. Several analogs were developed for clinical use, in particular for hypercholesterolemia and dyslipidemia; however, these failed due to accelerated tumor development in humans.[169,170] Currently, agonists are being evaluated for pulmonary hypertension, septic shock, atherosclerosis, and liver disease.[171]

5.2. *Liver X receptor (LXR)*

Liver X receptors (LXRs) exist as α and β isoforms and are transcription factors regulated by cholesterol derivatives, including oxysterols and desmosterol.[172,173] Similar to PPARs, LXRs bind with RXR in order to mediate their transcriptional activities. Binding of ligand induces removal of the heterodimer from its promoter region, enabling release of nuclear receptor coactivators and allowing gene expression.[174–176] LXRα (*NR1H3*) is expressed in liver, intestine, macrophages, and adipose tissue, while LXRβ (*NR1H2*) is more generally expressed.[177] These proteins play a major role in regulation of genes required for cholesterol uptake, transport, and excretion.[178] This includes control of reverse cholesterol transport, where excess cholesterol is returned to the liver from peripheral tissues by high-density lipoprotein (HDL).[179] This has made them important targets for atherosclerosis, through development of agonists that prevent foam cell formation. Several agonists have progressed to clinical trials, and these are summarized in Ref. 179. Proteins targeted for transcriptional repression by LXR include members of the ABC family of membrane transporters, e.g. ABCA1, ABCG1, ABCG5, and ABCG8.[179] As a result of their effects on lipogenesis, LXRs also can regulate glucose homeostasis, thus making them targets for treatment of type 2 diabetes as well.

6. Lipidomics of inflammation: Analysis of bioactive lipids

Lipidomics refers to the application of new-generation mass spectrometry (MS) profiling methodologies to the analysis of lipids. Over the last 10 years, these instruments have revolutionized our ability to discover and quantify lipid mediators of inflammation. Several configurations are now in routine use, for example tandem/triple quadrupole instruments for high-sensitivity quantitation, time-of-flight or Orbitrap/Fourier transform mass spectrometry for high-resolution analysis, suited for structural elucidation, and MALDI for tissue lipid imaging. One new approach, termed ion mobility, measures movement of lipids in a carrier gas and can distinguish isobaric lipids (with the same mass) and, in some cases, enantiomers. Lipidomics is broadly divided into two approaches, (i) shotgun, where lipids are not separated prior to introduction into the mass spectrometer, and (ii) liquid chromatography MS/MS.[180,181] The latter is generally required for analysis of lipid signaling mediators of relevance to inflammation since these are often present at low concentrations and not amenable to shotgun methodologies.

Signaling lipids can be isolated using several methods including organic solvent extraction or with solid phase columns. For liquid/liquid methods, the traditional Bligh and Dyer (chloroform/methanol) or a hexane/isopropanol mixture is often used, although where investigators are interested in a single lipid or series of related structures, careful optimization of extraction parameters is recommended.[117,182] Antibody-based ELISA kits are available for several lipids and can be attractive due to cost and ease of use. However, these should not be employed for complex biological mixtures due to lack of specificity. If used, they should always be carefully validated by comparison with MS methods before application to experimental samples.

A wide variety of tissues can be used for measurement of lipids of inflammation. For cohort studies, serum should always be avoided since it is generated through *in vitro* clotting of blood, a process that induces significant activation of white cells and platelets. Thus, eicosanoids measured in serum will always be artifactually generated during sample acquisition. While the use of plasma avoids this problem, sampling artifacts (e.g. activation of platelets or white cells at a low level during bloodletting) can also lead to generation of cell-derived lipid mediators that would not have been present *in vivo*. To minimize this, slow blood drawing combined with a wide bore needle is recommended, and vacutainers must be avoided. The use of fasted samples, especially if tri-glycerides and cholesterol esters are being determined, is always recommended for plasma lipid determination. The gold standard for systemic measurement of circulating eicosanoid metabolites is urinary metabolites. Several are available, e.g. for PGI_2, TXA_2, $PGF_2\alpha$, and PGE_2.[183–186] Older methods used gas chromatography for these, but LC-MS/MS methods are now in wide use.

7. Summary

Lipids play multiple and complex roles in both acute and chronic inflammatory processes in all organs. In this chapter, we have summarized the current knowledge of the state-of-the-art of lipid signaling in this context both at a cellular and whole-body level. Given the complexity of this area, several comprehensive reviews are cited in individual sections so that the reader can delve into particular topics in more detail where desired.

References

1. Kotzampassi K, Giamarellos-Bourboulis EJ, Stavrou G. (2014). Obesity as a consequence of gut bacteria and diet interactions. *ISRN Obesity*. **2014**:651895.
2. Burcelin R, Serino M, Chabo C, Garidou L, Pomie C, Courtney M, Amar J, Bouloumie A. (2013). Metagenome and metabolism: The tissue microbiota hypothesis. *Diabetes, Obesity Metabolism*. **15**(Suppl 3): 61–70.
3. Masoodi M, Kuda O, Rossmeisl M, Flachs P, Kopecky J. (2015). Lipid signaling in adipose tissue: Connecting inflammation & metabolism. *Biochimica et biophysica acta*. **1851**:503–518.
4. Trayhurn P, Wood IS. (2004). Adipokines: Inflammation and the pleiotropic role of white adipose tissue. *The Brit J Nutr*. **92**:347–55.
5. Lehr S, Hartwig S, Lamers D, Famulla S, Muller S, Hanisch FG, Cuvelier C, Ruige J, Eckardt K, Ouwens DM, Sell H, Eckel J. (2012). Identification and validation of novel adipokines released from primary human adipocytes. *Molecular Cellular Proteomics: MCP*. **11**:M111 010504.
6. Lehr S, Hartwig S, Sell H. (2012). Adipokines: A treasure trove for the discovery of biomarkers for metabolic disorders. *Proteomics Clin appl*. **6**:91–101.
7. Paschos GK, Ibrahim S, Song WL, Kunieda T, Grant G, Reyes TM, Bradfield CA, Vaughan CH, Eiden M, Masoodi M, Griffin JL, Wang F, Lawson JA,

Fitzgerald GA. (2012). Obesity in mice with adipocyte-specific deletion of clock component Arntl. *Nat Med.* **18**:1768–77.

8. Aguilar-Valles A, Inoue W, Rummel C, Luheshi GN. (2015). Obesity, adipokines and neuroinflammation. *Neuropharmacology.* **96**(A): 124–34.
9. Thijssen E, van Caam A, van der Kraan PM. (2015). Obesity and osteoarthritis, more than just wear and tear: Pivotal roles for inflamed adipose tissue and dyslipidaemia in obesity-induced osteoarthritis. *Rheumatology.* **54**:588–600.
10. Leiria LO, Martins MA, Saad MJ. (2015). Obesity and asthma: Beyond T(H)2 inflammation. *Metabolism: Clin Expe.* **64**:172–81.
11. Versini M, Jeandel PY, Rosenthal E, Shoenfeld Y. (2014). Obesity in autoimmune diseases: Not a passive bystander. *Autoimmun Revi.* **13**:981–1000.
12. Gruben N, Shiri-Sverdlov R, Koonen DP, Hofker MH. (2014). Nonalcoholic fatty liver disease: A main driver of insulin resistance or a dangerous liaison? *Biochimica et biophysica acta.* **1842**:2329–2343.
13. Capel F, Klimcakova E, Viguerie N, Roussel B, Vitkova M, Kovacikova M, Polak J, Kovacova Z, Galitzky J, Maoret JJ, Hanacek J, Pers TH, Bouloumie A, Stich V, Langin D. (2009). Macrophages and adipocytes in human obesity: Adipose tissue gene expression and insulin sensitivity during calorie restriction and weight stabilization. *Diabetes.* **58**:1558–67.
14. Kosteli A, Sugaru E, Haemmerle G, Martin JF, Lei J, Zechner R, Ferrante AW, Jr. (2010). Weight loss and lipolysis promote a dynamic immune response in murine adipose tissue. *The J Clin Investi.* **120**:3466–79.
15. Medrikova D, Jilkova ZM, Bardova K, Janovska P, Rossmeisl M, Kopecky J. (2012). Sex differences during the course of diet-induced obesity in mice: Adipose tissue expandability and glycemic control. *Inte J Obesity.* **36**:262–72.
16. Hossain MS, Chowdhury AA, Rahman MS, Nishimura K, Jisaka M, Nagaya T, Shono F, Yokota K. (2012). Stable expression of lipocalin-type prostaglandin D synthase in cultured preadipocytes impairs adipogenesis program independently of endogenous prostanoids. *Expe Cell Res.* **318**:408–15.
17. Lu S, Nishimura K, Hossain MA, Jisaka M, Nagaya T, Yokota K. (2004). Regulation and role of arachidonate cascade during changes in life cycle of adipocytes. *Appl Biochemi Biotechnol.* **118**:133–53.
18. Mendizabal Y, Llorens S, Nava E. (2013). Vasoactive effects of prostaglandins from the perivascular fat of mesenteric resistance arteries in WKY and SHROB rats. *Life Sci.* **93**:1023–32.
19. Borglum JD, Pedersen SB, Ailhaud G, Negrel R, Richelsen B. (1999). Differential expression of prostaglandin receptor mRNAs during adipose cell differentiation. *Prostaglandins Other Lipid Mediators.* **57**:305–17.
20. Horrillo R, Gonzalez-Periz A, Martinez-Clemente M, Lopez-Parra M, Ferre N, Titos E, Moran-Salvador E, Deulofeu R, Arroyo V, Claria J. (2010). 5-lipoxygenase activating protein signals adipose tissue inflammation and lipid dysfunction in experimental obesity. *J Immunol.* **184**:3978–87.

21. Sniderman AD, Lawler PR, Williams K, Thanassoulis G, de Graaf J, Furberg CD. (2012). The causal exposure model of vascular disease. *Clin Sci.* **122**:369–73.
22. Sniderman A, Kwiterovich PO. (2013). Update on the detection and treatment of atherogenic low-density lipoproteins. *Curr Opin Endocrinol, Diabetes, Obesity.* **20**:140–7.
23. Brunzell JD, Davidson M, Furberg CD, Goldberg RB, Howard BV, Stein JH, Witztum JL. (2008). Lipoprotein management in patients with cardiometabolic risk: Consensus conference report from the American Diabetes Association and the American College of Cardiology Foundation. *J Ame College Cardiol.* **51**:1512–24.
24. Toth PP, Grabner M, Punekar RS, Quimbo RA, Cziraky MJ, Jacobson TA. (2014). Cardiovascular risk in patients achieving low-density lipoprotein cholesterol and particle targets. *Atherosclerosis.* **235**:585–91.
25. Tousoulis D, Psarros C, Demosthenous M, Patel R, Antoniades C, Stefanadis C. (2014). Innate and adaptive inflammation as a therapeutic target in vascular disease: The emerging role of statins. *J Ame College Cardiol.* **63**: 2491–502.
26. Quehenberger O, Armando AM, Brown AH, Milne SB, Myers DS, Merrill AH, Bandyopadhyay S, Jones KN, Kelly S, Shaner RL, Sullards CM, Wang E, Murphy RC, Barkley RM, Leiker TJ, Raetz CR, Guan Z, Laird GM, Six DA, Russell DW, McDonald JG, Subramaniam S, Fahy E, Dennis EA. (2010). Lipidomics reveals a remarkable diversity of lipids in human plasma. *J Lipid Res.* **51**:3299–305.
27. Wang L, Sapuri-Butti AR, Aung HH, Parikh AN, Rutledge JC. (2008). Triglyceride-rich lipoprotein lipolysis increases aggregation of endothelial cell membrane microdomains and produces reactive oxygen species. *Ame J Physiol Heart Circul Physiol.* **295**:H237–44.
28. Wang L, Gill R, Pedersen TL, Higgins LJ, Newman JW, Rutledge JC. (2009). Triglyceride-rich lipoprotein lipolysis releases neutral and oxidized FFAs that induce endothelial cell inflammation. *J Lipid Res.* **50**:204–13.
29. Rosenson RS, Davidson MH, Hirsh BJ, Kathiresan S, Gaudet D. (2014). Genetics and causality of triglyceride-rich lipoproteins in atherosclerotic cardiovascular disease. *J Ame College Cardiol.* **64**:2525–40.
30. Aung HH, Lame MW, Gohil K, An CI, Wilson DW, Rutledge JC. (2013). Induction of ATF3 gene network by triglyceride-rich lipoprotein lipolysis products increases vascular apoptosis and inflammation. *Arteriosclerosis, Thrombosis, Vascu Biol.* **33**:2088–96.
31. Wang YI, Schulze J, Raymond N, Tomita T, Tam K, Simon SI, Passerini AG. (2011). Endothelial inflammation correlates with subject triglycerides and waist size after a high-fat meal. *America Journal of Physiology Heart and Circualtor Physiology.* 300:H784–91.

32. Sun C, Alkhoury K, Wang YI, Foster GA, Radecke CE, Tam K, Edwards CM, Facciotti MT, Armstrong EJ, Knowlton AA, Newman JW, Passerini AG, Simon SI. (2012). IRF-1 and miRNA126 modulate VCAM-1 expression in response to a high-fat meal. *Circul Res.* **111**:1054–64.
33. Gower RM, Wu H, Foster GA, Devaraj S, Jialal I, Ballantyne CM, Knowlton AA, Simon SI. (2011). CD11c/CD18 expression is upregulated on blood monocytes during hypertriglyceridemia and enhances adhesion to vascular cell adhesion molecule-1. *Arteriosclerosis, Thrombosis, Vasc Biol.* **31**:160–6.
34. Smith WL, DeWitt DL, Garavito RM. (2000). Cyclooxygenases: Structural, cellular, and molecular biology. *Ann Rev Biochemi.* **69**:145–82.
35. Ricciotti E, FitzGerald GA. (2011). Prostaglandins and inflammation. *Arteriosclerosis, Thrombosis, Vasc Biol.* **31**:986–1000.
36. Smyth EM, Grosser T, Wang M, Yu Y, FitzGerald GA. (2009). Prostanoids in health and disease. *J Lipid Res.* **50** Suppl:S423–8.
37. Liu M, Saeki K, Matsunobu T, Okuno T, Koga T, Sugimoto Y, Yokoyama C, Nakamizo S, Kabashima K, Narumiya S, Shimizu T, Yokomizo T. (2014). 12-Hydroxyheptadecatrienoic acid promotes epidermal wound healing by accelerating keratinocyte migration via the BLT2 receptor. *The J Exp Med.* **211**:1063–78.
38. Narumiya S, FitzGerald GA. (2001). Genetic and pharmacological analysis of prostanoid receptor function. *The J Clin Invest.* **108**:25–30.
39. Breyer RM, Bagdassarian CK, Myers SA, Breyer MD. (2001). Prostanoid receptors: subtypes and signaling. *Ann Rev Pharmacol Toxicol.* **41**:661–90.
40. Yuan C, Sidhu RS, Kuklev DV, Kado Y, Wada M, Song I, Smith WL. (2009). Cyclooxygenase allosterism, fatty acid-mediated cross-talk between monomers of cyclooxygenase homodimers. *The J Biol Chem.* **284**:10046–55.
41. Langenbach R, Morham SG, Tiano HF, Loftin CD, Ghanayem BI, Chulada PC, Mahler JF, Lee CA, Goulding EH, Kluckman KD, Kim HS, Smithies O. (1995). Prostaglandin synthase 1 gene disruption in mice reduces arachidonic acid-induced inflammation and indomethacin-induced gastric ulceration. *Cell.* **83**:483–92.
42. Langenbach R, Loftin C, Lee C, Tiano H. (1999). Cyclooxygenase knockout mice: models for elucidating isoform-specific functions. *Biochem Pharmacol.* **58**:1237–46.
43. Chen M, Boilard E, Nigrovic PA, Clark P, Xu D, Fitzgerald GA, Audoly LP, Lee DM. (2008). Predominance of cyclooxygenase 1 over cyclooxygenase 2 in the generation of proinflammatory prostaglandins in autoantibody-driven K/BxN serum-transfer arthritis. *Arthritis Rheumatism.* **58**:1354–65.
44. Wallace JL, McKnight W, Reuter BK, Vergnolle N. (2000). NSAID-induced gastric damage in rats: Requirement for inhibition of both cyclooxygenase 1 and 2. *Gastroenterology.* **119**:706–14.

45. Gilroy DW, Colville-Nash PR, Willis D, Chivers J, Paul-Clark MJ, Willoughby DA. (1999). Inducible cyclooxygenase may have anti-inflammatory properties. *Nat Medi.* **5**:698–701.
46. Patrignani P, Tacconelli S, Bruno A, Sostres C, Lanas A. (2011). Managing the adverse effects of nonsteroidal anti-inflammatory drugs. *Exp Rev Clin Pharmacol.* **4**:605–21.
47. Brune K, Furst DE. (2007). Combining enzyme specificity and tissue selectivity of cyclooxygenase inhibitors: Towards better tolerability? *Rheumatology.* **46**:911–9.
48. Grosser T, Fries S, FitzGerald GA. (2006). Biological basis for the cardiovascular consequences of COX-2 inhibition: Therapeutic challenges and opportunities. *The J Clin Invest.* **116**:4–15.
49. Brune K, Patrignani P. (2015). New insights into the use of currently available non-steroidal anti-inflammatory drugs. *J Pain Res.* **8**:105–18.
50. Funk CD. (2001). Prostaglandins and leukotrienes: Advances in eicosanoid biology. *Science.* **294**:1871–5.
51. Wang M, Zukas AM, Hui Y, Ricciotti E, Pure E, FitzGerald GA. (2006). Deletion of microsomal prostaglandin E synthase-1 augments prostacyclin and retards atherogenesis. *Proc Nat Acade Scie USA.* **103**:14507–12.
52. Kamei D, Yamakawa K, Takegoshi Y, Mikami-Nakanishi M, Nakatani Y, Oh-Ishi S, Yasui H, Azuma Y, Hirasawa N, Ohuchi K, Kawaguchi H, Ishikawa Y, Ishii T, Uematsu S, Akira S, Murakami M, Kudo I. (2004). Reduced pain hypersensitivity and inflammation in mice lacking microsomal prostaglandin e synthase-1. *The J Biol Chem.* **279**:33684–95.
53. Yao C, Sakata D, Esaki Y, Li Y, Matsuoka T, Kuroiwa K, Sugimoto Y, Narumiya S. (2009). Prostaglandin E2-EP4 signaling promotes immune inflammation through Th1 cell differentiation and Th17 cell expansion. *Nat Med.* **15**:633–40.
54. Kabashima K, Sakata D, Nagamachi M, Miyachi Y, Inaba K, Narumiya S. (2003). Prostaglandin E2-EP4 signaling initiates skin immune responses by promoting migration and maturation of Langerhans cells. *Nat Med.* **9**:744–9.
55. Kawabe J, Ushikubi F, Hasebe N. (2010). Prostacyclin in vascular diseases. Recent insights and future perspectives. *Circul J: Official J Jap Circul Soc.* **74**:836–43.
56. Higgs GA, Moncada S, Salmon JA, Seager K. (1983). The source of thromboxane and prostaglandins in experimental inflammation. *Brit J Pharmacol.* **79**:863–8.
57. Berkenkopf JW, Weichman BM. (1988). Production of prostacyclin in mice following intraperitoneal injection of acetic acid, phenylbenzoquinone and zymosan: Its role in the writhing response. *Prostaglandins.* **36**:693–709.

58. Pulichino AM, Rowland S, Wu T, Clark P, Xu D, Mathieu MC, Riendeau D, Audoly LP. (2006). Prostacyclin antagonism reduces pain and inflammation in rodent models of hyperalgesia and chronic arthritis. *The J Pharmacol Expe Therapeutics*. **319**:1043–50.
59. Bley KR, Bhattacharya A, Daniels DV, Gever J, Jahangir A, O'Yang C, Smith S, Srinivasan D, Ford AP, Jett MF. (2006). RO1138452 and RO3244794: Characterization of structurally distinct, potent and selective IP (prostacyclin) receptor antagonists. *Brit J Pharmacol*. **147**:335–45.
60. Urade Y, Ujihara M, Horiguchi Y, Ikai K, Hayaishi O. (1989). The major source of endogenous prostaglandin D2 production is likely antigen-presenting cells. Localization of glutathione-requiring prostaglandin D synthetase in histiocytes, dendritic, and Kupffer cells in various rat tissues. *J Immunol*. **143**:2982–9.
61. Tanaka K, Ogawa K, Sugamura K, Nakamura M, Takano S, Nagata K. (2000). Cutting edge: Differential production of prostaglandin D2 by human helper T cell subsets. *J Immunol*. **164**:2277–80.
62. Lewis RA, Soter NA, Diamond PT, Austen KF, Oates JA, Roberts LJ, (1982). 2nd. Prostaglandin D2 generation after activation of rat and human mast cells with anti-IgE. *J Immunol*. **129**:1627–31.
63. Spik I, Brenuchon C, Angeli V, Staumont D, Fleury S, Capron M, Trottein F, Dombrowicz D. (2005). Activation of the prostaglandin D2 receptor DP2/CRTH2 increases allergic inflammation in mouse. *J Immunol*. **174**:3703–8.
64. Hammad H, de Heer HJ, Soullie T, Hoogsteden HC, Trottein F, Lambrecht BN. (2003). Prostaglandin D2 inhibits airway dendritic cell migration and function in steady state conditions by selective activation of the D prostanoid receptor 1. *J Immunol*. **171**:3936–40.
65. Saleem S, Ahmad AS, Maruyama T, Narumiya S, Dore S. (2009). PGF(2alpha) FP receptor contributes to brain damage following transient focal brain ischemia. *Neurotox Res*. **15**:62–70.
66. Kunori S, Matsumura S, Mabuchi T, Tatsumi S, Sugimoto Y, Minami T, Ito S. (2009). Involvement of prostaglandin F 2 alpha receptor in ATP-induced mechanical allodynia. *Neuroscience*. **163**:362–71.
67. Nakahata N. (2008). Thromboxane A2: physiology/pathophysiology, cellular signal transduction and pharmacol. *Pharmacol Therapeutics*. **118**:18–35.
68. Montuschi P, Barnes PJ, Roberts LJ, 2nd. (2004). Isoprostanes: markers and mediators of oxidative stress. *FASEB J: Off Publ Fed Am Soc Exp Biol*. **18**:1791–800.
69. Audoly LP, Rocca B, Fabre JE, Koller BH, Thomas D, Loeb AL, Coffman TM, FitzGerald GA. (2000). Cardiovascular responses to the isoprostanes iPF(2alpha)-III and iPE(2)-III are mediated via the thromboxane A(2). receptor *in vivo*. *Circulation*. **101**:2833–40.

70. Francois H, Makhanova N, Ruiz P, Ellison J, Mao L, Rockman HA, Coffman TM. (2008). A role for the thromboxane receptor in L-NAME hypertension. *Am J Physiol Renal Physiol.* **295**:F1096–102.
71. Francois H, Athirakul K, Mao L, Rockman H, Coffman TM. (2004). Role for thromboxane receptors in angiotensin-II-induced hypertension. *Hypertension.* **43**:364–9.
72. Kobayashi T, Tahara Y, Matsumoto M, Iguchi M, Sano H, Murayama T, Arai H, Oida H, Yurugi-Kobayashi T, Yamashita JK, Katagiri H, Majima M, Yokode M, Kita T, Narumiya S. (2004). Roles of thromboxane A(2). and prostacyclin in the development of atherosclerosis in apoE-deficient mice. *The J Clini Invest.* **114**:784–94.
73. Kuhn H, O'Donnell VB. (2006). Inflammation and immune regulation by 12/15-lipoxygenases. *Prog Lipid Res.* **45**:334–56.
74. Anning PB, Coles B, Bermudez-Fajardo A, Martin PE, Levison BS, Hazen SL, Funk CD, Kuhn H, O'Donnell VB. (2005). Elevated endothelial nitric oxide bioactivity and resistance to angiotensin-dependent hypertension in 12/15-lipoxygenase knockout mice. *The Am J Pathol.* **166**:653–62.
75. Bleich D, Chen S, Zipser B, Sun D, Funk CD, Nadler JL. (1999). Resistance to type 1 diabetes induction in 12-lipoxygenase knockout mice. *The J Clinical Investi.* **103**:1431-6.
76. Huo Y, Zhao L, Hyman MC, Shashkin P, Harry BL, Burcin T, Forlow SB, Stark MA, Smith DF, Clarke S, Srinivasan S, Hedrick CC, Pratico D, Witztum JL, Nadler JL, Funk CD, Ley K. (2004). Critical role of macrophage 12/15-lipoxygenase for atherosclerosis in apolipoprotein E-deficient mice. *Circulation.* **110**:2024–31.
77. Hajek AR, Lindley AR, Favoreto S, Jr., Carter R, Schleimer RP, Kuperman DA. (2008). 12/15-Lipoxygenase deficiency protects mice from allergic airways inflammation and increases secretory IgA levels. *The J Allergy Clin Immunol.* **122**:633–9 e3.
78. Heydeck D, Thomas L, Schnurr K, Trebus F, Thierfelder WE, Ihle JN, Kuhn H. (1998). Interleukin-4 and -13 induce upregulation of the murine macrophage 12/15-lipoxygenase activity: Evidence for the involvement of transcription factor STAT6. *Blood.* **92**:2503–10.
79. Lundstrom SL, Yang J, Kallberg HJ, Thunberg S, Gafvelin G, Haeggstrom JZ, Gronneberg R, Grunewald J, van Hage M, Hammock BD, Eklund A, Wheelock AM, Wheelock CE. (2012). Allergic asthmatics show divergent lipid mediator profiles from healthy controls both at baseline and following birch pollen provocation. *PloS One.* **7**:e33780.
80. Miller YI, Chang MK, Funk CD, Feramisco JR, Witztum JL. (2001). 12/15-lipoxygenase translocation enhances site-specific actin polymerization in macrophages phagocytosing apoptotic cells. *The J Biol Chem.* **276**:19431–9.

81. Morgan AH, Hammond VJ, Sakoh-Nakatogawa M, Ohsumi Y, Thomas CP, Blanchet F, Piguet V, Kiselyov K, O'Donnell VB. (2015). A novel role for 12/15-lipoxygenase in regulating autophagy. *Redox Biol.* **4**:40–7.
82. Radmark O, Samuelsson B. (2010). Regulation of the activity of 5-lipoxygenase, a key enzyme in leukotriene biosynthesis. *Biochemi Biophysi Res Commun.* **396**:105–10.
83. Machida I, Matsuse H, Kondo Y, Kawano T, Saeki S, Tomari S, Obase Y, Fukushima C, Kohno S. (2004). Cysteinyl leukotrienes regulate dendritic cell functions in a murine model of asthma. *J Immunol.* **172**:1833–8.
84. Poeckel D, Funk CD. (2010). The 5-lipoxygenase/leukotriene pathway in preclinical models of cardiovascular disease. *Cardiovasc Res.* **86**:243–53.
85. Corser-Jensen CE, Goodell DJ, Freund RK, Serbedzija P, Murphy RC, Farias SE, Dell'Acqua ML, Frey LC, Serkova N, Heidenreich KA. (2014). Blocking leukotriene synthesis attenuates the pathophysiology of traumatic brain injury and associated cognitive deficits. *Exp Neurol.* **256**:7–16.
86. Farias S, Frey LC, Murphy RC, Heidenreich KA. (2009). Injury-related production of cysteinyl leukotrienes contributes to brain damage following experimental traumatic brain injury. *J Neurotrauma.* **26**:1977–86.
87. Joshi YB, Pratico D. (2014). The 5-lipoxygenase pathway: oxidative and inflammatory contributions to the Alzheimer's disease phenotype. *Front Cellular Neurosci.* **8**:436.
88. Zhang HP, Jia CE, Lv Y, Gibson PG, Wang G. (2014). Montelukast for prevention and treatment of asthma exacerbations in adults: Systematic review and meta-analysis. *Allergy Asthma Proc: The off J Regional State Allergy Soc.* **35**:278–87.
89. Liu M, Yokomizo T. (2015). The role of leukotrienes in allergic diseases. *Allergol Inte Official J Jap Soc Allergol.* **64**:17–26.
90. Pace-Asciak CR. (2015). Pathophysiology of the hepoxilins. *Biochimica et Biophysica acta.* **1851**:383–396.
91. Bunting S, Gryglewski R, Moncada S, Vane JR. (1976). Arterial walls generate from prostaglandin endoperoxides a substance (prostaglandin X) which relaxes strips of mesenteric and coeliac ateries and inhibits platelet aggregation. *Prostaglandins.* **12**:897–913.
92. Karim S, Habib A, Levy-Toledano S, Maclouf J. (1996). Cyclooxygenase-1 and -2 of endothelial cells utilize exogenous or endogenous arachidonic acid for transcellular production of thromboxane. *The J Biol Chem.* **271**:12042–8.
93. Capra V, Rovati GE, Mangano P, Buccellati C, Murphy RC, Sala A. (2015). Transcellular biosynthesis of eicosanoid lipid mediators. *Biochimica et Biophysica Acta.* **1851**:377–382.
94. Fabre JE, Goulet JL, Riche E, Nguyen M, Coggins K, Offenbacher S, Koller BH. (2002). Transcellular biosynthesis contributes to the production of

leukotrienes during inflammatory responses *in vivo. The J Clin invest.* **109**:1373–80.

95. Zarini S, Gijón MA, Ransome AE, Murphy RC, Sala A. Transcellular biosynthesis of leukotrienes *in vivo* during mouse peritoneal inflammation. *Proc Natl Acad Sci USA.* **106:** 8296–8301.
96. Forsman H, Onnheim K, Andreasson E, Dahlgren C. (2011). What formyl peptide receptors, if any, are triggered by compound 43 and lipoxin A4? *Scandi J Immunol.* **74**:227–34.
97. Hanson J, Ferreiros N, Pirotte B, Geisslinger G, Offermanns S. (2013). Heterologously expressed formyl peptide receptor 2 (FPR2/ALX) does not respond to lipoxin A(4). *Biochemi Pharmacol.* **85**:1795–802.
98. Serhan CN. (2010). Novel lipid mediators and resolution mechanisms in acute inflammation: to resolve or not? *The Am J Pathol.* **177**:1576–91.
99. Serhan CN, Chiang N, Van Dyke TE. (2008). Resolving inflammation: Dual anti-inflammatory and pro-resolution lipid mediators. *Nat Rev Immunol.* **8**:349–61.
100. Buckley CD, Gilroy DW, Serhan CN. (2014). Proresolving lipid mediators and mechanisms in the resolution of acute inflammation. *Immunity.* **40**:315–27.
101. Colas RA, Shinohara M, Dalli J, Chiang N, Serhan CN. (2014). Identification and signature profiles for pro-resolving and inflammatory lipid mediators in human tissue. *Am J Physiol Cell Physiol.* **307**:C39–54.
102. Catella F, Healy D, Lawson JA, FitzGerald GA. (1986). 11-Dehydrothromboxane B2: A quantitative index of thromboxane A2 formation in the human circulation. *Proc Nat Acad Scie USA.* **83**:5861–5.
103. Ferreiros N, Homann J, Labocha S, Grossmann N, Hahn JS, Brune B, Geisslinger G. (2014). Lipoxin A(4): Problems with its determination using reversed phase chromatography-tandem mass spectrometry and confirmation with chiral chromatography. *Talanta.* **127**:82–7.
104. Rouzer CA, Marnett LJ. (2011). Endocannabinoid oxygenation by cyclooxygenases, lipoxygenases, and cytochromes P450: Cross-talk between the eicosanoid and endocannabinoid signaling pathways. *Chem Rev.* **111**:5899–921.
105. Kozak KR, Prusakiewicz JJ, Rowlinson SW, Marnett LJ. (2002). Enantiospecific, selective cyclooxygenase-2 inhibitors. *Bioorganic Med Chem Lett.* **12**:1315–8.
106. Kozak KR, Rowlinson SW, Marnett LJ. (2000). Oxygenation of the endocannabinoid, 2-arachidonylglycerol, to glyceryl prostaglandins by cyclooxygenase-2. *The J Biol Chem.* **275**:33744–9.
107. Edgemond WS, Hillard CJ, Falck JR, Kearn CS, Campbell WB. (1998). Human platelets and polymorphonuclear leukocytes synthesize oxygenated derivatives of arachidonylethanolamide (anandamide): Their affinities for

cannabinoid receptors and pathways of inactivation. *Molecular Pharmacol.* **54**:180–8.

108. van der Stelt M, van Kuik JA, Bari M, van Zadelhoff G, Leeflang BR, Veldink GA, Finazzi-Agro A, Vliegenthart JF, Maccarrone M. (2002). Oxygenated metabolites of anandamide and 2-arachidonoylglycerol: conformational analysis and interaction with cannabinoid receptors, membrane transporter, and fatty acid amide hydrolase. *J Med Chemi.* **45**:3709–20.
109. Basu S. (2010). Fatty acid oxidation and isoprostanes: Oxidative strain and oxidative stress. *Prostaglandins, Leukotrienes, Essential Fatty Acids.* **82**:219–25.
110. Clark SR, Thomas CP, Hammond VJ, Aldrovandi M, Wilkinson GW, Hart KW, Murphy RC, Collins PW, O'Donnell VB. (2013). Characterization of platelet aminophospholipid externalization reveals fatty acids as molecular determinants that regulate coagulation. *Proc Nat Acad Sci USA.* **110**:5875–80.
111. Thomas CP, Clark SR, Hammond VJ, Aldrovandi M, Collins PW, O'Donnell VB. (2014). Identification and quantification of aminophospholipid molecular species on the surface of apoptotic and activated cells. *Nat Protoc.* **9**:51–63.
112. Bochkov VN, Oskolkova OV, Birukov KG, Levonen AL, Binder CJ, Stockl J. (2010). Generation and biological activities of oxidized phospholipids. *Antioxidants Redox Signali.* **12**:1009–59.
113. Berliner JA, Territo MC, Sevanian A, Ramin S, Kim JA, Bamshad B, Esterson M, Fogelman AM. (1990). Minimally modified low density lipoprotein stimulates monocyte endothelial interactions. *The J Clin Invest.* **85**:1260–6.
114. Watson AD, Leitinger N, Navab M, Faull KF, Horkko S, Witztum JL, Palinski W, Schwenke D, Salomon RG, Sha W, Subbanagounder G, Fogelman AM, Berliner JA. (1997). Structural identification by mass spectrometry of oxidized phospholipids in minimally oxidized low density lipoprotein that induce monocyte/endothelial interactions and evidence for their presence *in vivo*. *The J Biol Chem.* **272**:13597–607.
115. Clark SR, Guy CJ, Scurr MJ, Taylor PR, Kift-Morgan AP, Hammond VJ, Thomas CP, Coles B, Roberts GW, Eberl M, Jones SA, Topley N, Kotecha S, O'Donnell VB. (2011). Esterified eicosanoids are acutely generated by 5-lipoxygenase in primary human neutrophils and in human and murine infection. *Blood.* **117**:2033–43.
116. Hammond VJ, Morgan AH, Lauder S, Thomas CP, Brown S, Freeman BA, Lloyd CM, Davies J, Bush A, Levonen AL, Kansanen E, Villacorta L, Chen YE, Porter N, Garcia-Diaz YM, Schopfer FJ, O'Donnell VB. (2012). Novel keto-phospholipids are generated by monocytes and macrophages, detected in cystic fibrosis, and activate peroxisome proliferator-activated receptor-gamma. *The J Biol Chem.* **287**:41651–66.

117. Maskrey BH, Bermudez-Fajardo A, Morgan AH, Stewart-Jones E, Dioszeghy V, Taylor GW, Baker PR, Coles B, Coffey MJ, Kuhn H, O'Donnell VB. (2007). Activated platelets and monocytes generate four hydroxyphosphatidylethanolamines via lipoxygenase. *The J Biol Chem.* **282**:20151–63.
118. Morgan AH, Dioszeghy V, Maskrey BH, Thomas CP, Clark SR, Mathie SA, Lloyd CM, Kuhn H, Topley N, Coles BC, Taylor PR, Jones SA, O'Donnell VB. (2009). Phosphatidylethanolamine-esterified eicosanoids in the mouse: tissue localization and inflammation-dependent formation in Th-2 disease. *The J Biol Chem.* **284**:21185–91.
119. Morgan LT, Thomas CP, Kuhn H, O'Donnell VB. (2010). Thrombin-activated human platelets acutely generate oxidized docosahexaenoic-acid-containing phospholipids via 12-lipoxygenase. *Biochem J.* **431**:141–8.
120. Thomas CP, Morgan LT, Maskrey BH, Murphy RC, Kuhn H, Hazen SL, Goodall AH, Hamali HA, Collins PW, O'Donnell VB. (2010). Phospholipid-esterified eicosanoids are generated in agonist-activated human platelets and enhance tissue factor-dependent thrombin generation. *The J Biol Chem.* **285**:6891–903.
121. Aldrovandi M, Hammond VJ, Podmore H, Hornshaw M, Clark SR, Marnett LJ, Slatter DA, Murphy RC, Collins PW, O'Donnell VB. (2013). Human platelets generate phospholipid-esterified prostaglandins via cyclooxygenase-1 that are inhibited by low dose aspirin supplementation. *J Lipid Res.* **54**:3085–97.
122. Choi JW, Herr DR, Noguchi K, Yung YC, Lee CW, Mutoh T, Lin ME, Teo ST, Park KE, Mosley AN, Chun J. (2010). LPA receptors: subtypes and biological actions. *Ann Rev Pharmacol Toxicol.* **50**:157–86.
123. Yung YC, Stoddard NC, Chun J. (2014). LPA receptor signaling: pharmacology, physiology, and pathophysiology. *J Lipid Res.* **55**:1192–1214.
124. Eichholtz T, Jalink K, Fahrenfort I, Moolenaar WH. (1993). The bioactive phospholipid lysophosphatidic acid is released from activated platelets. *Biochem J.* **291** (Pt 3):677–80.
125. Tanaka M, Okudaira S, Kishi Y, Ohkawa R, Iseki S, Ota M, Noji S, Yatomi Y, Aoki J, Arai H. (2006). Autotaxin stabilizes blood vessels and is required for embryonic vasculature by producing lysophosphatidic acid. *The J Biol Chem.* **281**:25822–30.
126. Spiegel S, Milstien S. (2011). The outs and the ins of sphingosine-1-phosphate in immunity. *Nat Rev Immunol.* **11**:403–15.
127. Lee MJ, Van Brocklyn JR, Thangada S, Liu CH, Hand AR, Menzeleev R, Spiegel S, Hla T. (1998). Sphingosine-1-phosphate as a ligand for the G protein-coupled receptor EDG-1. *Science.* **279**:1552–5.
128. Liu Y, Wada R, Yamashita T, Mi Y, Deng CX, Hobson JP, Rosenfeldt HM, Nava VE, Chae SS, Lee MJ, Liu CH, Hla T, Spiegel S, Proia RL. (2000). Edg-1,

the G protein-coupled receptor for sphingosine-1-phosphate, is essential for vascular maturation. *The J Clin Invest.* **106**:951–61.

129. Kihara Y, Mizuno H, Chun J. (2015). Lysophospholipid receptors in drug discovery. *Exp Cell Res.* **333**(2): 171–7.
130. Herzog BH, Fu J, Wilson SJ, Hess PR, Sen A, McDaniel JM, Pan Y, Sheng M, Yago T, Silasi-Mansat R, McGee S, May F, Nieswandt B, Morris AJ, Lupu F, Coughlin SR, McEver RP, Chen H, Kahn ML, Xia L. (2013). Podoplanin maintains high endothelial venule integrity by interacting with platelet CLEC-2. *Nature.* **502**:105–9.
131. Henry B, Ziobro R, Becker KA, Kolesnick R, Gulbins E. (2013). Acid sphingomyelinase. *Handbook Exp Pharmacol.* 77–88.
132. Bruni A, Bigon E, Battistella A, Boarato E, Mietto L, Toffano G. (1984). Lysophosphatidylserine as histamine releaser in mice and rats. *Agents Actions.* **14**:619–25.
133. Iwashita M, Makide K, Nonomura T, Misumi Y, Otani Y, Ishida M, Taguchi R, Tsujimoto M, Aoki J, Arai H, Ohwada T. (2009). Synthesis and evaluation of lysophosphatidylserine analogues as inducers of mast cell degranulation. Potent activities of lysophosphatidylthreonine and its 2-deoxy derivative. *J Med Chem.* **52**:5837–63.
134. Bellini F, Bruni A. (1993). Role of a serum phospholipase A1 in the phosphatidylserine-induced T cell inhibition. *FEBS Lett.* **316**:1–4.
135. van der Kleij D, Latz E, Brouwers JF, Kruize YC, Schmitz M, Kurt-Jones EA, Espevik T, de Jong EC, Kapsenberg ML, Golenbock DT, Tielens AG, Yazdanbakhsh M. (2002). A novel host-parasite lipid cross-talk. Schistosomal lyso-phosphatidylserine activates toll-like receptor 2 and affects immune polarization. *The J Biol Chem.* **277**:48122–9.
136. Sugo T, Tachimoto H, Chikatsu T, Murakami Y, Kikukawa Y, Sato S, Kikuchi K, Nagi T, Harada M, Ogi K, Ebisawa M, Mori M. (2006). Identification of a lysophosphatidylserine receptor on mast cells. *Biochem Biophys Res Commun.* **341**:1078–87.
137. Henstridge CM, Balenga NA, Ford LA, Ross RA, Waldhoer M, Irving AJ. (2009). The GPR55 ligand L-alpha-lysophosphatidylinositol promotes RhoA-dependent Ca2+ signaling and NFAT activation. *FASEB J: Offi Publ Fed Am Soc Exp Biol.* **23**:183–93.
138. Makide K, Uwamizu A, Shinjo Y, Ishiguro J, Okutani M, Inoue A, Aoki J. (2014). Novel lysophosphoplipid receptors: their structure and function. *J Lipid Res.* **55**:1986–95.
139. Hawkins PT, Stephens LR. (2015). PI3K signalling in inflammation. *Biochimica et Biophysica acta.* **1851**:882–897.
140. Moroi AJ, Watson SP. (2015). Impact of the PI3-kinase/Akt pathway on ITAM and hemITAM receptors: Haemostasis, platelet activation and antithrombotic therapy. *Biochem Pharmacol.* **94**:186–94.

141. Hsu AC, Starkey MR, Hanish I, Parsons K, Haw TJ, Howland LJ, Barr I, Mahony JB, Foster PS, Knight DA, Wark PA, Hansbro PM. (2015). Targeting PI3K-p110alpha Suppresses influenza viral infection in chronic obstructive pulmonary disease. *Am J Respir Crit Care Med.* **191**:1012–23.
142. Wymann M. (2012). PI3Ks-drug targets in inflammation and cancer. *Subcellular Biochem.* **58**:111–81.
143. Riehle RD, Cornea S, Degterev A. (2013). Role of phosphatidylinositol 3,4,5-trisphosphate in cell signaling. *Adv Expe Med Biol.* **991**:105–39.
144. O'Donnell VB, Murphy RC, Watson SP. (2014). Platelet lipidomics: modern day perspective on lipid discovery and characterization in platelets. *Circul Res.* **114**:1185–203.
145. Maceyka M, Spiegel S. (2014). Sphingolipid metabolites in inflammatory disease. *Nature.* **510**:58–67.
146. Hannun YA, Obeid LM. (2008). Principles of bioactive lipid signalling: Lessons from sphingolipids. *Nat Rev Molecular Cell Biol.* **9**:139–50.
147. Cyster JG, Schwab SR. (2012). Sphingosine-1-phosphate and lymphocyte egress from lymphoid organs. *Ann Rev Immunol.* **30**:69–94.
148. Rivera J, Proia RL, Olivera A. (2008). The alliance of sphingosine-1-phosphate and its receptors in immunity. *Nat Rev Immunol.* **8**:753–63.
149. Lamour NF, Wijesinghe DS, Mietla JA, Ward KE, Stahelin RV, Chalfant CE. (2011). Ceramide kinase regulates the production of tumor necrosis factor alpha (TNFalpha) via inhibition of TNFalpha-converting enzyme. *The J Biolo Chem.* **286**:42808–17.
150. Bishop-Bailey D. (2015). Nuclear receptors in vascular biology. *Curr Atherosclerosis Reports.* **17**:507.
151. Kerley CP, Elnazir B, Faul J, Cormican L. (2015). Vitamin D as an adjunctive therapy in asthma. Part 2: A review of human studies. *Pulmonary pharmacol Therapeutics.* **32**: 75–92.
152. van Neerven S, Kampmann E, Mey J. (2008). RAR/RXR and PPAR/RXR signaling in neurological and psychiatric diseases. *Prog Neurobiol.* **85**:433–51.
153. Berger J, Moller DE. (2002). The mechanisms of action of PPARs. *Ann Rev Med.* **53**:409–35.
154. Lefterova MI, Haakonsson AK, Lazar MA, Mandrup S. (2014). PPARgamma and the global map of adipogenesis and beyond. *Trends Endocrinol Metabolism: TEM.* **25**:293–302.
155. Tontonoz P, Spiegelman BM. (2008). Fat and beyond: the diverse biology of PPARgamma. *Ann Rev Biochem.* **77**:289–312.
156. Lefterova MI, Zhang Y, Steger DJ, Schupp M, Schug J, Cristancho A, Feng D, Zhuo D, Stoeckert CJ, Jr., Liu XS, Lazar MA. (2008). PPARgamma and C/EBP factors orchestrate adipocyte biology via adjacent binding on a genome-wide scale. *Genes Develop.* **22**:2941–52.

157. Nielsen R, Pedersen TA, Hagenbeek D, Moulos P, Siersbaek R, Megens E, Denissov S, Borgesen M, Francoijs KJ, Mandrup S, Stunnenberg HG. (2008). Genome-wide profiling of PPARgamma:RXR and RNA polymerase II occupancy reveals temporal activation of distinct metabolic pathways and changes in RXR dimer composition during adipogenesis. *Genes Develop.* **22**:2953–67.
158. Schopfer FJ, Cole MP, Groeger AL, Chen CS, Khoo NK, Woodcock SR, Golin-Bisello F, Motanya UN, Li Y, Zhang J, Garcia-Barrio MT, Rudolph TK, Rudolph V, Bonacci G, Baker PR, Xu HE, Batthyany CI, Chen YE, Hallis TM, Freeman BA. (2010). Covalent peroxisome proliferator-activated receptor gamma adduction by nitro-fatty acids: Selective ligand activity and anti-diabetic signaling actions. *The J Biol Chem.* **285**:12321–33.
159. Schupp M, Lazar MA. (2010). Endogenous ligands for nuclear receptors: digging deeper. *The J Biol Chem.* **285**:40409–15.
160. Chakravarthy MV, Lodhi IJ, Yin L, Malapaka RR, Xu HE, Turk J, Semenkovich CF. (2009). Identification of a physiologically relevant endogenous ligand for PPARalpha in liver. *Cell.* **138**:476–88.
161. Jump DB, Botolin D, Wang Y, Xu J, Christian B, Demeure O. (2005). Fatty acid regulation of hepatic gene transcription. *The J Nutr.* **135**:2503–6.
162. Martin PG, Guillou H, Lasserre F, Dejean S, Lan A, Pascussi JM, Sancristobal M, Legrand P, Besse P, Pineau T. (2007). Novel aspects of PPARalpha-mediated regulation of lipid and xenobiotic metabolism revealed through a nutrigenomic study. *Hepatology.* **45**:767–77.
163. Delerive P, De Bosscher K, Besnard S, Vanden Berghe W, Peters JM, Gonzalez FJ, Fruchart JC, Tedgui A, Haegeman G, Staels B. (1999). Peroxisome proliferator-activated receptor alpha negatively regulates the vascular inflammatory gene response by negative cross-talk with transcription factors NF-kappaB and AP-1. *The J Biol Chem.* **274**:32048–54.
164. Delerive P, Martin-Nizard F, Chinetti G, Trottein F, Fruchart JC, Najib J, Duriez P, Staels B. (1999). Peroxisome proliferator-activated receptor activators inhibit thrombin-induced endothelin-1 production in human vascular endothelial cells by inhibiting the activator protein-1 signaling pathway. *Circulation Research.* **85**:394–402.
165. Hiukka A, Maranghi M, Matikainen N, Taskinen MR. (2010). PPARalpha: an emerging therapeutic target in diabetic microvascular damage. *Nat Rev Endocrinol.* **6**:454–63.
166. Contreras AV, Torres N, Tovar AR. (2013). PPAR-alpha as a key nutritional and environmental sensor for metabolic adaptation. *Adv Nutr.* **4**:439–52.
167. Ali FY, Davidson SJ, Moraes LA, Traves SL, Paul-Clark M, Bishop-Bailey D, Warner TD, Mitchell JA. (2006). Role of nuclear receptor signaling in platelets: Antithrombotic effects of PPARbeta. *FASEB J: Off Publ Federation Am Soc Exp Biol.* **20**:326–8.

168. Li Y, Connolly M, Nagaraj C, Tang B, Balint Z, Popper H, Smolle-Juettner FM, Lindenmann J, Kwapiszewska G, Aaronson PI, Wohlkoenig C, Leithner K, Olschewski H, Olschewski A. (2012). Peroxisome proliferator-activated receptor-beta/delta, the acute signaling factor in prostacyclin-induced pulmonary vasodilation. *Am J Resp Cell Molecular Biol.* **46**:372–9.
169. Olson EJ, Pearce GL, Jones NP, Sprecher DL. (2012). Lipid effects of peroxisome proliferator-activated receptor-delta agonist GW501516 in subjects with low high-density lipoprotein cholesterol: characteristics of metabolic syndrome. *Arteriosclerosis, Thrombosis, Vasc Biol.* **32**:2289–94.
170. Ooi EM, Watts GF, Sprecher DL, Chan DC, Barrett PH. (2011). Mechanism of action of a peroxisome proliferator-activated receptor (PPAR)-delta agonist on lipoprotein metabolism in dyslipidemic subjects with central obesity. *The J Clin Endocrinol Metabolism.* **96**:E1568–76.
171. Mackenzie LS, Lione L. (2013). Harnessing the benefits of PPARbeta/delta agonists. *Life Sci.* **93**:963–7.
172. Collins JL, Fivush AM, Watson MA, Galardi CM, Lewis MC, Moore LB, Parks DJ, Wilson JG, Tippin TK, Binz JG, Plunket KD, Morgan DG, Beaudet EJ, Whitney KD, Kliewer SA, Willson TM. (2002). Identification of a nonsteroidal liver X receptor agonist through parallel array synthesis of tertiary amines. *J Med Chem.* **45**:1963–6.
173. Spann NJ, Garmire LX, McDonald JG, Myers DS, Milne SB, Shibata N, Reichart D, Fox JN, Shaked I, Heudobler D, Raetz CR, Wang EW, Kelly SL, Sullards MC, Murphy RC, Merrill AH, Jr., Brown HA, Dennis EA, Li AC, Ley K, Tsimikas S, Fahy E, Subramaniam S, Quehenberger O, Russell DW, Glass CK. (2012). Regulated accumulation of desmosterol integrates macrophage lipid metabolism and inflammatory responses. *Cell.* **151**:138–52.
174. Hu X, Li S, Wu J, Xia C, Lala DS. (2003). Liver X receptors interact with corepressors to regulate gene expression. *Molecular Endocrinol.* **17**:1019–26.
175. Huuskonen J, Fielding PE, Fielding CJ. (2004). Role of p160 coactivator complex in the activation of liver X receptor. *Arteriosclerosis, Thrombosis Vascu Biol.* **24**:703–8.
176. Svensson S, Ostberg T, Jacobsson M, Norstrom C, Stefansson K, Hallen D, Johansson IC, Zachrisson K, Ogg D, Jendeberg L. (2003). Crystal structure of the heterodimeric complex of LXRalpha and RXRbeta ligand-binding domains in a fully agonistic conformation. *The EMBO J.* **22**:4625–33.
177. Peet DJ, Janowski BA, Mangelsdorf DJ. (1998). The LXRs: A new class of oxysterol receptors. *Curr Opin Genet Develop.* **8**:571–5.
178. Hong C, Tontonoz P. (2014). Liver X receptors in lipid metabolism: opportunities for drug discovery. *Nat Rev Drug Discovery.* **13**:433–44.

179. Joseph SB, Castrillo A, Laffitte BA, Mangelsdorf DJ, Tontonoz P. (2003). Reciprocal regulation of inflammation and lipid metabolism by liver X receptors. *Nat Medi.* **9**:213–9.
180. Balazy M. (2004). Eicosanomics: Targeted lipidomics of eicosanoids in biological systems. *Prostaglandins Other Lipid Mediators.* **73**:173–80.
181. Han X, Yang K, Gross RW. (2012). Multi-dimensional mass spectrometry-based shotgun lipidomics and novel strategies for lipidomic analyses. *Mass Spectro Rev.* **31**:134–78.
182. Bligh EG, Dyer WJ. (1959). A rapid method of total lipid extraction and purification. *Canad J Biochemis Physiol.* **37**:911–7.
183. Dworski R, Roberts LJ, 2nd, Murray JJ, Morrow JD, Hartert TV, Sheller JR. (2001). Assessment of oxidant stress in allergic asthma by measurement of the major urinary metabolite of F2-isoprostane, 15-F2t-IsoP (8-iso-PGF2alpha). *Clin Exp Allergy:J Brit Soc Allergy Clin Immunol.* **31**:387–90.
184. Jabr S, Gartner S, Milne GL, Roca-Ferrer J, Casas J, Moreno A, Gelpi E, Picado C. (2013). Quantification of major urinary metabolites of PGE2 and PGD2 in cystic fibrosis: Correlation with disease severity. *Prostaglandins, Leukotrienes, Essential Fatty Acids.* **89**:121–6.
185. Murray JJ, Nowak J, Oates JA, FitzGerald GA. (1990). Platelet-vessel wall interactions in individuals who smoke cigarettes. *Adv Exp Medi Biol.* **273**:189–98.
186. Neath SX, Jefferies JL, Berger JS, Wu AH, McConnell JP, Boone JL, McCullough PA, Jesse RL, Maisel AS. (2014). The current and future landscape of urinary thromboxane testing to evaluate atherothrombotic risk. *Rev Cardiovas Medi.* **15**:119–30.

Chapter 4
Reactive Oxygen Species

Ulla G. Knaus*

1. Introduction

Polymorphonuclear leukocytes (PMNs) and the inflammatory response to infection or injury have been connected for decades. While recognized for their efficient clearance of pathogens and particulate matter, the increased recruitment, prolonged activation, and delayed apoptosis of PMNs has been always closely linked to impaired resolution of inflammatory processes leading to chronic inflammation. The main chemical mediators contributing to both beneficial and detrimental consequences of PMN involvement are reactive oxygen species (ROS). The importance of ROS in the context of microbial killing is emphasized by the recurrent bacterial and fungal infections in patients with chronic granulomatous disease (CGD), a genetically heterogeneous disease that is characterized by abolished or severely reduced ROS production in innate immune cells.[1–3] Exaggerated inflammation on the other hand has been connected to oxidative stress, an imbalance between ROS generating and ROS degrading systems[4] and the preferred approach for alleviating oxidative damage involved antioxidant therapy. This notion is

*Conway Institute, School of Medicine, University College Dublin, Dublin, Ireland.

now debated, not just because currently available antioxidants did not deliver as promised.[5–7] In the last decade the importance of ROS in normal physiology and the contribution of the microenvironment including macrophages, specific T lymphocyte populations, and the stroma in promoting and resolving inflammation became evident.[6,8–11] Almost all of the cell types in this niche are capable of producing ROS via various enzymes. The ROS levels generated by these cells are much lower than the oxidative burst by PMNs. In immune cells as well as other cell types, the primary reactive species, superoxide and hydrogen peroxide, are now considered signaling molecules that regulate redox relays, protein kinase pathways, transcription factor and GTPase activity, lipid-mediated signaling, and the overall redox balance during changes in oxygen supply (hypoxia, hyperoxia).[12] Disrupted signaling circuits may account for the hyperinflammation observed in CGD patients lacking superoxide production,[13,14] although other functional changes in ROS-deficient immune cells may contribute to the phenotype. To date, detecting oxidative damage in inflammation is still retrospective, impeding a clear distinction between ROS as cause or consequence of disease. Importantly, not all ROS are equal in their chemical reactivity, stability (half-life), localization, and ability in inducing long-range effects. Progress in determining the species and quantity of ROS produced together with identifying their source and localization will facilitate a disease-centered risk–benefit analysis and will provide a rationale when and which targeted interventions are appropriate.

2. Reactive oxygen species

Atmospheric oxygen, the third most abundant chemical element in the universe, is of vital importance for all aerobic organisms. Oxygen is a diradical containing two unpaired electrons with parallel spin states. This chemical structure imposes a kinetic barrier towards reduction due to the need for spin inversion when dioxygen accepts electrons during an oxidation reaction. Acceptance of four electrons reduces oxygen to water, but partial reduction states occur, resulting in one-electron (radical) and two-electron (nonradi-

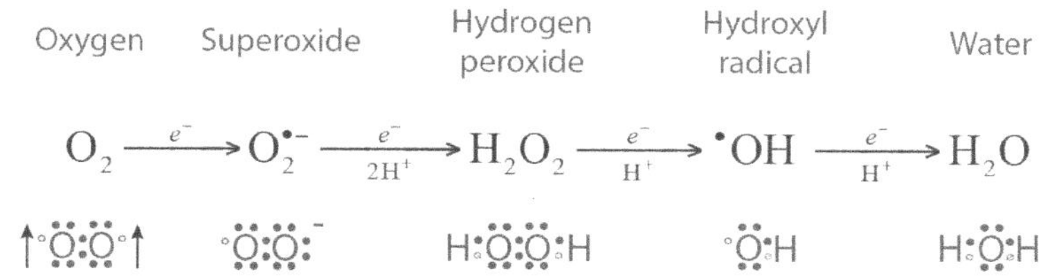

Fig. 1. Sequential reduction of oxygen.

cal) oxygen metabolites (Fig. 1). Physiologically relevant ROS are the initial products superoxide ($O_2^{\bullet-}$) and hydrogen peroxide (H_2O_2), and their secondary reactive products are hydroxyl radical ($^{\bullet}OH$) and hypochlorous acid (HOCl). When nitric oxide radicals ($^{\bullet}NO$) are present, highly reactive adducts including peroxynitrite ($ONOO^-$) and nitrogen dioxide ($^{\bullet}NO_2$) can be generated. Although the term ROS is widely used, which might be appropriate in the context of living systems as long as the reactive entity being produced cannot be unequivocally identified, this idiom fails to discriminate between highly divergent oxygen-derived species. Only physiologically relevant species in the inflammatory disease context will be discussed here.

2.1. *Superoxide*

The initial product formed by molecular oxygen accepting a single electron is superoxide ($O_2^{\bullet-}$). It has a short half-life (10^{-6}s)[15] and acts as reductant with metal complexes (e.g., cytochrome c), but $O_2^{\bullet-}$ can also oxidize and inactivate iron–sulfur [4Fe–4S] clusters of aconitase or dehydratases, thereby promoting the formation of secondary oxygen species when free iron is released. The reactivity of $O_2^{\bullet-}$ with other radicals in the direct vicinity is rapid, for example by forming $ONOO^-$ and $^{\bullet}NO_2$ when encountering $^{\bullet}NO$. These reactive nitrogen species (RNS) are highly reactive, oxidizing proteins that contain transition metal centers such as peroxidases and modifying tyrosine residues (3-nitrotyrosine).[16,17] In a hydrophilic environment, two $O_2^{\bullet-}$ molecules will interact in a coupled oxidation–reduction reaction called dismutation, which can occur spontaneously or is catalyzed by superoxide dismutases (SOD; see antioxidant systems). The dismutation product is a non-radical termed hydrogen peroxide (H_2O_2). The location of $O_2^{\bullet -}$ generation is central to its reactivity, as a hydrophobic microenvironment increases the chemical reactivity and may even permit penetration of the protonated, uncharged hydroperoxyl ($HO_2^{\bullet}$) molecule through cell membranes, potentially by passing through channels.[18]

2.2. *Hydrogen peroxide*

H_2O_2 has a lower reduction potential but longer half-life (10^{-5}s) than other ROS.[15] H_2O_2 is predominantly formed by dismutation of $O_2^{\bullet -}$, but direct divalent reduction of oxygen without a measurable intermediate has been reported.[19] H_2O_2 is kinetically slow in most oxidation reaction except for its reaction rate with heme proteins and iron–sulfur clusters.[20] The low reactivity and non-radical nature permits H_2O_2 to traverse eukaryotic and prokaryotic membranes and biological fluids, either by diffusion or via membrane-incorporated water channels (aquaporins).[21] By transmitting extracellular signals, H_2O_2 acts as a second messenger in redox-mediated pathways. The degradation of H_2O_2 to oxygen and water is accomplished by the enzyme catalase (CAT), but other means for H_2O_2 removal exist (e.g., glutathione peroxidase). On the other hand, when transition metal ions such as Fe(II) are present, a Fenton reaction will take place, resulting in decomposition of H_2O_2 to hydroxyl radical ($^{\bullet}OH$) and hydroxide ion (HO^-). Additionally, peroxidases catalyze the reaction of H_2O_2 with halides, leading to the formation of highly reactive hypohalous acids (selected reactions are listed below).

$$2O_2^{\bullet -} + 2H^+ \xrightarrow{\text{SOD}} O_2 + H_2O$$

$$O_2^{\bullet -} + [4Fe - 4S]^{2+} + 2H^+ \rightarrow [4Fe - 4S]^{3+} + H_2O_2$$

$$O_2^{\bullet -} + NO^{\bullet} \rightarrow ONOO^- \rightarrow {}^{\bullet}NO_2 + {}^{\bullet}OH$$

$$2H_2O_2 \xrightarrow{CAT} 2H_2O + O_2$$
$$H_2O_2 + Fe^{2+} \rightarrow Fe^{3+} + {}^{\bullet}OH + HO^-$$
$$H_2O_2 + Fe^{3+} \rightarrow Fe^{2+} + {}^{\bullet}OOH + H^+$$
$$H_2O_2 + O_2^{\bullet-} \rightarrow {}^{\bullet}OH + HO^- + O_2$$
$$H_2O_2 + Cl^- \xrightarrow{MPO} HOCl + HO^- \xrightarrow{RNH_2} RNHCl$$
$$H_2O_2 + CpI(MPO) \rightarrow CpII(MPO) + O_2^{\bullet-} + H^+$$
$$H_2O_2 + NO_2^- \xrightarrow{MPO} {}^{\bullet}NO_2$$

2.3. *Hydroxyl radical*

Hydroxyl radicals (${}^{\bullet}OH$) have a very short half-life (10^{-9}s)[22] and are the most reactive biologically-derived chemicals. Their generation is not only accomplished by a Fenton reaction, but also by the interaction of $O_2^{\bullet-}$ with HOCl, the predominant hypohalous acid generated in the PMN phagosome during phagocytosis. Due to the high reactivity of this radical, only targets in the immediate vicinity will be oxidized. The ${}^{\bullet}OH$ species is likely responsible for DNA damage including single- and double-strand breaks, DNA–DNA intrastrand adducts, and DNA–protein crosslinks. The nucleobase guanine is most susceptible to oxidation, resulting in the products 8-hydroxyguanine (8-OHG) and 8-hydroxydeoxyguanosine (8-OHdG). These species are highly mutagenic and can lead to GC-AT transversions. Hydroxyl radicals are also involved in lipid peroxidation, leading to the main products malondialdehyde (MDA) and 4-hydroxy-2-nonenal (4-HNE).[23]

2.4. *Hypochlorous acid*

A microenvironment containing H_2O_2, a peroxidase, and a halide (Cl^-, I^-, Br^-) or pseudohalide (SCN^-) in sufficient concentration will promote the generation of hypohalous acids. Well-characterized mammalian peroxidases are myeloperoxidase (MPO, in PMNs)[24,25] and eosinophil peroxidase (EPO, in eosinophils). MPO is exclusively expressed in the myeloid lineage, with neutrophils containing the majority of the enzyme. During phagocytosis MPO is released from azurophilic (primary) granules into the phagosome. MPO participates in prooxidant and antioxidant activities, catalyzing the generation of HOCl and radicals, but also utilizing NADPH oxidase-derived $O_2^{\bullet -}$ and H_2O_2 to regenerate redox intermediates and to produce oxygen. HOCl is considered the main bactericidal component in the phagosome, and a constant supply of superoxide (~17 μM), H_2O_2 (~2–3 μM) and chloride (~20–70 mM) is required to drive its production (concentrations indicate the steady state).[20,26,27] In the respiratory tract lactoperoxidase (LPO) may utilize H_2O_2 released from lung epithelial cells to catalyze hypothiocyanite ($OSCN^-$) formation and subsequent sulfhydryl oxidation.[28]

2.5. *Oxidative protein modification*

The redox proteome links reversible and irreversible covalent modifications induced by ROS or by the overall redox state of cells, tissues, or organisms to the structure and function of proteins. Understanding this redox footprint in terms of protein function (enzyme activity, complex formation, localization) and the implications of oxidative modifications for development or progression of disease is still in progress. While a global readout such as bacterial or host protein oxidation in the phagosome is more amendable to analysis, *in vivo* analysis of tissue injury due to oxidative stress is retrospective without addressing cause and effect. Understanding the source, species, concentration, and localization of ROS at different stages of disease will generate the knowledge required for therapeutic intervention. Some of the most common oxidative modifications of proteins detected in eukaryotes and prokaryotes are listed here.

For H_2O_2, a two-electron oxidant and a common signaling mediator, low-pKa (4–5) thiols (RSH) are the preferred oxidation target at physiological pH as the reactive cysteine thiol exists then as thiolate anion (S^-). Oxidation of reactive thiols generates a range of cysteine oxidation products. The chemical nature of the modification is dependent on proximity of the target to the ROS source (H_2O_2 concentration) and the duration of H_2O_2 production, starting with conversion to sulfenic acid (RSOH) and disulfides, followed by irreversible oxidation to sulfinic acid (RSO_2H) and sulfonic acid (RSO_3H).[29] Reduction of sulfenic acid by reducing agents including glutathione (GSH), glutaredoxins (GRX), and thioredoxin (TRX) permits recycling and provides regulated inhibition/activation cycles for protein tyrosine phosphatases and peroxiredoxins. HOCl can also oxidize cysteine to higher oxidation states such as sulfenic acids and disulfides, but additionally catalyzes formation of sulfenyl chlorides, sulfinamides, and sulfonamides as well as oxidation of the amino acid methionine to methionine sulfoxide.[20,30] HOCl-mediated oxidation of amine groups leads to formation of chloramines, which react with thiol groups and give rise to 3-chlorotyrosine and 3,5-dichlorotyrosine via transchlorination. Oxidation of substrates in the presence of a peroxidase will remove a single electron, thereby generating a free radical that can further react with ROS (e.g., $O_2^{\bullet-}$, H_2O_2), creating organic hydroperoxides and lipid peroxidation. Tyrosine residues in proteins are not only prone to nitration, but will also be modified by oxidation to tyrosine hydroperoxide, 3,4-dihydroxyphenylalanine (DOPA), and dityrosine.[31] Oxidation of tryptophan residues by HOCl or $^{\bullet}OH$ leads to formation of *N*-formylkynurenine, 3-hydroxy-kynurenine, kynurenine, and hydroxytryptophan.[32] Even histidines can be modified by hydroxyl radicals, for example to 2-oxo-histidine or 4-hydroxy glutamate.[33]

3. Oxidant–antioxidant balance

Redox homeostasis describes a physiological state in which generation of ROS and their conversion or removal by antioxidant systems or radical scavengers are in equilibrium. Excess of ROS production by altered mitochondrial function, upregulation of ROS sources, or failure of antioxidant systems is considered the hallmark of oxidative stress and subsequent pathophysiological consequences including prolonged chronic inflammation, tissue injury, and fibrosis. Contrary to this long-held notion, ROS deficiency arising by deleting a ROS source (e.g., NADPH oxidase in mice) or by mutational inactivation (e.g., CGD or other disease-associated patient variants) compromises not only pathogen control but also triggers non-resolving inflammation and serves as a risk factor for injury and delayed wound healing.[13,34,35] Therefore, maintaining ROS signaling is important for the management of inflammation and for many related disorders including metabolic, neurodegenerative, and cardiovascular disease.

Antioxidants are not solely removing ROS and preventing ROS signaling, but often convert one oxygen-derived species into another species or form redox or protein interaction relays, thereby impacting biological systems in myriad ways. Enzymes with "antioxidant" activity are themselves regulated by redox and posttranslational mechanisms and can interact with each other or other signaling molecules. Therefore, their reactivity, distribution, and recycling will depend on the cellular and environmental context. The most important enzymatic antioxidant systems in mammalian cells will be discussed here.

Although $O_2^{\bullet-}$, the initial oxygen reduction product, can dismutate spontaneously to O_2 and H_2O_2 (~10^5 $M^{-1}s^{-1}$), this process requires that two $O_2^{\bullet-}$ molecules react with each other. The enzyme catalyzing this reaction far more efficiently was discovered in 1969 and termed superoxide dismutase (SOD).[36,37] Dismutation in the presence of SOD is rapid (~$3–7 \times 10^9$ $M^{-1}s^{-1}$), with diffusion of $O_2^{\bullet-}$ to the active site of SOD being the rate-limiting step.[38,39] Three SODs are present in mammalian cells, namely SOD1 (dimeric CuZnSOD in cytoplasm, peroxisomes, and mitochondrial intermembrane space), SOD2 (tetrameric MnSOD in the mitochondrial matrix), and SOD3 (EC-SOD, extracellular CuZnSOD as glycosylated tetramer). While SOD1 variants are causative for familial forms of the neurodegenerative disease amyotrophic lateral sclerosis (ALS), it is still a matter of debate if the change in redox status or the propensity of these variants for aggregation and structural instability impact the severity of the disease.[40] Overexpression of SOD2 in tumors has been associated with increased H_2O_2 levels, enhanced proliferation and neuroendocrine differentiation, and reduced TRAIL-induced apoptosis.[41,42]

The decomposition of H_2O_2 to H_2O and O_2 is catalyzed by the enzyme catalase (CAT), a tetramer with four porphyrin heme groups. The reaction is optimal at pH 7 and takes place in peroxisomes and mitochondria of mammalian cells.[43] H_2O_2 is also converted to H_2O by the structurally diverse family of glutathione peroxidases (GPx1-8).[44] GPx catalyzes the oxidation of reduced monomeric glutathione (GSH) via H_2O_2, leading to glutathione disulfide (GSSH) and H_2O. GSSH is then rapidly reduced to GSH by the NADPH-dependent glutathione reductase. The ratio of GSH to GSSH at a certain time point is often used as an indicator of oxidative stress. Mammalian cells contain in the steady state a high concentration of GSH (up to 10 m*M*), which will be either redox recycled or synthesized.[45] The de novo synthesis of not only GSH, but many genes involved in the antioxidant defense and redox signaling is under control of the master regulator nuclear factor erythroid 2 (NFE2)-related factor 2 (NRF2), a member of the basic region leucine zipper transcription factors. Regulatory mechanisms including oxidative inhibition of NRF2 ubiquitination by modifying specific cysteine thiols on NRF2 and its partner protein KEAP1 (Kelch-like erythroid cell-derived protein with CNC homology-associated protein 1) permit NRF2 translocation to the nucleus and binding to a DNA sequence called antioxidant response element (ARE). ARE-containing genes control redox homeostasis (e.g., GPx2, TRX, PRX1, PRX6, HO-1) and drug metabolism.[46–48]

Peroxiredoxins (PRX1-6) remove H_2O_2, lipid peroxides and peroxynitrite by reversible oxidation of an active site cysteine in PRX (pKa thiol 5–6; rate constant for H_2O_2 reactivity 10^5–10^8 $M^{-1}s^{-1}$) to sulfenic acid followed by formation of a disulfide bridge.[49] Subsequent reduction of PRXs is accomplished by interaction with reduced thioredoxin (TRX). Multiple levels of regulation exist for PRXs. For example, PRX1 activity is negatively controlled by tyrosine phosphorylation, while PRX2 can be inactivated by hyperoxidation.[50] PRX2 can participate directly in cytokine-induced STAT3 signaling by transducing an upstream H_2O_2 signal via a redox relay from oxidized PRX2 to STAT3. Oxidized STAT3 oligomers showed altered transcriptional activity.[51] The endoplasmatic reticulum (ER)-resident PRX4 participates in protein folding by protein-disulfide isomerase (PDI) and ER oxidoreductin 1 (ERO1),[52] while a mitochondrial PRX3-TRX system likely removes H_2O_2 originating from the mitochondrial respiratory chain.[53] Sulfiredoxin (SRX), an oxidoreductase reacting on sulfur groups, reduces hyperoxidized PRX from sulfinic (inactive) to sulfenic (active) acid in an ATP-dependent manner.[54]

Another antioxidant mechanism involves the thioredoxin system, which in mammals consists of three thioredoxin (TRX) isoforms, three flavin-containing thioredoxin reductase (TRXR) isoforms, and an electron donor (NADPH).[55] TRX, a disulfide reductase, reduces oxidized proteins via its active site cysteine motif Cys–Gly–Pro–Cys. Oxidized TRX is then converted back to its reduced form via TRXR by electron transfer originating from NADPH to TRXR-FAD. Besides TRX, TRXR can directly reduce lipid hydroperoxides, PDIs, and molecules with antioxidant capacity such as ubiquinone. Oxidant–antioxidant relays extend even to RNS, with multilayered crosstalk between •NO and TRX.[56] TRX1 is localized in the cytoplasm, plasma membrane, and nucleus and can act as H_2O_2 sensor controlling ROS-induced signaling to the MAP kinases c-Jun N-terminal kinase (JNK) and p38. The reduced form of TRX1 binds to the N-terminal region of apoptosis signal-regulating kinase 1 (ASK1, *MAP3K5*), a mitogen-activated protein kinase (MAPK) kinase kinase that activates downstream MAPKs, thereby inhibiting ASK1 activity in the ASK1 signalosome. In conditions of oxidant generation due to NADPH oxidase activation, ER stress, or pathogen sensing, TRX1 will be oxidized, leading to dissociation from ASK1. Structural changes then permit oligomerization and autophosphorylation of ASK1, leading to full kinase activity.[57] Increased ROS levels also induce the release of the thioredoxin interacting protein, TXNIP, from reduced TRX1. TXNIP shuttles then into the mitochondria and binds to oxidized TRX2, inducing the release of ASK1, leading to mitochondrial dysfunction and apoptosis.[58]

4. ROS sources

Generation of oxygen-derived species, mainly $O_2^{\bullet-}$, is often the by-product of ionizing radiation or of enzymatic and chemical reactions with oxygen and/or water. Redox cycling agents such as paraquat, menadione, certain drugs, and xenobiotics can react with flavoenzymes such as cytochrome P450 reductase or complex I of the mitochondrial electron transport chain (ETC), generating radicals that then will react spontaneously with oxygen to generate $O_2^{\bullet-}$. The high reactivity of some of these compounds together with the abundance of potential flavin-containing proteins makes it difficult to pinpoint when and where ROS are being generated. Examples for enzymes that produce ROS as by-product (i.e., secondary enzymatic product) of their primary metabolic function are the mitochondrial respiratory chain, xanthine oxidase, monoamine oxidase, lysyl oxidase, lipoxygenase, and cyclooxygenase. We will discuss here briefly some of these sources, although the overall focus will be on the family of NADPH oxidases, specialized enzymes whose only known function is the tightly regulated generation of ROS.

4.1. *H_2O_2 as secondary enzymatic product*

The primary function of xanthine oxidase (*XDH*) is catalyzing the conversion of hypoxanthine to xanthine and further to uric acid, but under certain inflammatory conditions the enzyme's dehydrogenase activity can act as a ROS generator. In tissues at low oxygen concentrations or in hypoxic conditions, xanthine oxidase seems to produce H_2O_2 and not superoxide.[59] Monoamine oxidases (*MAO*) are flavin-containing amine oxidoreductases that catalyze the oxidative deamination of monoamines. As MAOA/B are located in the outer membrane of mitochondria (Fig. 2), and as H_2O_2 will be constantly generated during their catalytic cycle, their enzymatic activity will likely alter mitochondrial signaling, for example in alternatively activated macrophages.[60] The copper-containing lysyl oxidase (*LOX*, *LOXL1/2*) family is involved in matrix crosslinking and transcription by oxidizing peptidyl lysine residues. LOX gener-

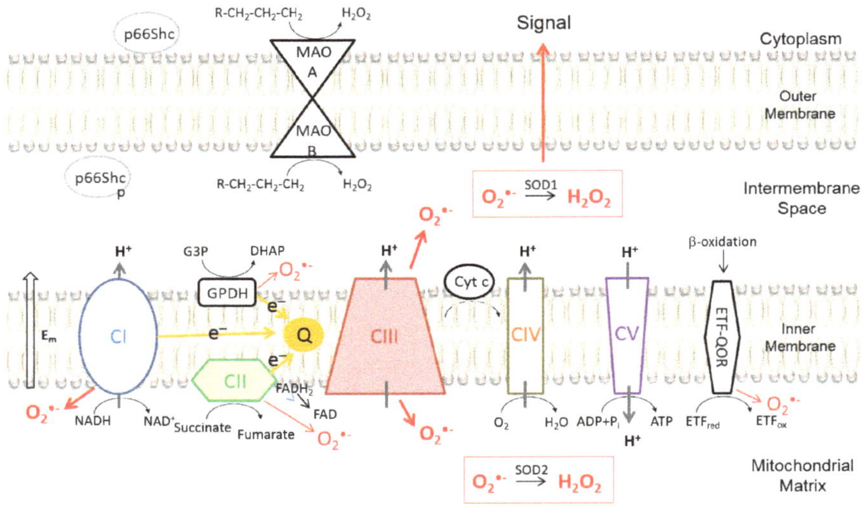

Fig. 2. Overview of mtROS production by ETC complexes and other sources. Complexes I (CI), II (CII), and III (CIII) can generate $O_2^{\bullet -}$, which will be converted to H_2O_2 by superoxide dismutases (SODs) (Q, coenzyme Q). $O_2^{\bullet -}$ is also produced by α-glycerophosphate dehydrogenase (GPDH) converting glycerol-3-phosphate (G3P) to dihydroxyacetone phosphate (DHAP) and by electron transferring flavoprotein (ETF)-ubiquinone oxidoreductase (QOR), while H_2O_2 is generated by monoaminooxidase (MAO) A/B. p66Shc may act as H_2O_2 source in the inner membrane space or as antioxidant in the cytoplasm.

ates H_2O_2 as by-product and some members are considered tumor suppressors.[61]

4.2. *Prokaryotic H_2O_2*

Although the focus here is on mammalian ROS sources, in certain environments such as mucosal surfaces of the gastrointestinal tract, vaginal tract, nasal passages, pulmonary tract, or on skin surfaces, a close relationship between the mammalian host and the microbiota is required for homeostasis, prevention of disease, and resolution of insults. In this mutually beneficial relationship between eukaryotic host and colonizing prokaryotes, H_2O_2 generated by probiotic bacteria, in particular *Lactobacillus*, or by pathogens such as *Streptococcus* will serve as signaling molecule, mimicking H_2O_2 release from the mucosa upon bacterial sensing. How the rate and duration of H_2O_2 production compares between prokaryotic and eukaryotic sources *in vivo* is unknown. The enzymes responsible for commensal H_2O_2 production remain undefined, with the exception an FMN oxidoreductase in *L. johnsonii*.[62]

4.3. $O_2^{\bullet-}$ as secondary enzymatic product — Mitochondrial electron transport chain

Mitochondria are essential organelles that consume molecular oxygen in order to generate energy (ATP) by oxidative phosphorylation (OXPHOS). This process is accomplished by the electron transport chain (ETC) that consists of complex I–V (CI–V) and electron carriers generated by the Krebs cycle (NADH, $FADH_2$), which provide the electrons that drive proton gradients at the inner membrane towards CV (ATP synthase). Mitochondria also act as sensors for oxygen availability, calcium influx, carbohydrate and fatty acid metabolism, and generate superoxide. Although complexes I and III are the main producers of superoxide, other mitochondrial proteins such as MAOB, glycerol-3-phosphate dehydrogenase (GPDH), and the electron transferring flavoprotein ubiquinone oxidoreductase (ETF-QOR) can generate mitochondrial ROS (mtROS) (Fig. 2).[63,64] The role of p66Shc (*SHC*) seems to be controversial. Phosphorylated p66Shc can translocate to the mitochondria and oxidize cytochrome c in certain cell types, thereby increasing mtROS,[65] while in other circumstances a feedback loop exists, where NRF2-upregulated p66Shc in its cytosolic, phosphorylated form will stimulate NRF2-dependent transcription of antioxidant defense genes.[66]

Superoxide generation by the ETC depends on the local O_2 concentration, the protonmotive force (Δp), the $NADH/NAD^+$ ratio, and the $CoQH_2/CoQ$ ratio.[63] In normal circumstances when the ETC works efficiently and ATP production is high, the "leak" of electrons that can react with O_2 will be very low (1–2%). In these conditions superoxide dismutation by SODs and removal of

H_2O_2 by mitochondrial antioxidant systems such as PRX/TRX and GSH/GSSG-GPx will be sufficient to keep the mtROS concentration at 10–200 p*M*.[63] More electrons will escape from the ETC, in particular from iron-sulfur centers and FMN at CI, or from unstable ubisemiquinone in the coenzyme Q (CoQ) cycle of CIII, when (i) the ATP production is low, causing high Δp and a pool of reduced CoQ, or when (ii) the $NADH/NAD^+$ ratio is high in the mitochondrial matrix. Triggers for ETC malfunction can be changes in the rate of O_2 consumption or availability, or alterations in the membrane potential ($\Delta\Psi_m$). The ETC is considered a large supercomplex, where association between CI, CIII, and CIV in stoichiometric ratio takes place, which likely facilitates CoQ channeling in the electron transfer between CI and CIII.[67] CI consists of 45 proteins and is the entry point for electrons from NADH to a FMN cofactor, which transfers them via several iron-sulfur centers to the CoQ reduction site. CIII interacts transiently with CoQ, moving electrons from the CoQ pool to cytochrome c. In a reconstituted assay system, supercomplex organization limited superoxide generation by CI.[68] CI is the major superoxide source, either when the $NADH/NAD^+$ ratio increases or when reverse electron transport (RET) occurs. Elevated $\Delta\Psi_m$, high Δp, and a reduced CoQ pool favor RET, bringing electrons back from $CoQH_2$ into CI. Reverse operation from CII to CI may contribute to ischemia–reperfusion injury.[69] Electron escape from CIII and subsequent $O_2^{\bullet-}$ expulsion to the matrix or intermembrane space has been linked to a decrease in O_2 supply (under 5%, termed hypoxia). Albeit counterintuitive, mtROS generation increased in hypoxic conditions[70] and inhibited prolyl hydroxylase (PHD) activity, leading to stabilization of the transcription factor HIF-1α.[71] A specific phenomenon that might represent a housekeeping task, a signaling function, or damage control during mtROS accumulation is mtROS-induced mtROS release (RIRR) by ATP synthase. ATP synthase drives not only ATP synthesis during OXPHOS, the enzyme can also turn into an ATPase during ischemia,[72] and dimerize in order to form the mitochondrial pore.[73] The signal(s) leading to RIRR are still unknown and their origins are unidentified.[74]

The ETC supercomplex has likely association partners that provide regulatory input in mtROS generation, but these proteins have not yet been identified or their mode of action is unknown. For example, the glucose-regulated NOD-like receptor (NLR) protein NLRX1 (NOD5) interacts with the CIII subunit UQCRC2 in the mitochondrial matrix. NLRX1 may take part in adjusting mitochondrial activity in resting conditions to the overall cellular metabolism, and was reported to participate in basal mtROS generation by a yet undetermined mechanism.[75] The importance of mtROS in altering transcription and cellular signaling responses is now accepted, and the notion of uncontrolled "leakage" of electrons to O_2 needs to be revisited. Still many questions remain including how much mtROS will be produced *in vivo* (and in which cell types), which ETC complex or other mitochondrial proteins are responsible for mtROS production, and how various sources of ROS may regulate each other. Identification of regulatory proteins in the ETC supercomplex that can limit electron escape, but will not alter $\Delta\Psi_m$ or ATP generation, may provide a means for interfering with mtROS generation via small molecules that will modify the activity of these proteins. This approach will permit determining if mtROS generation can be directly controlled by specific on–off switches that respond to particular extracellular stimuli.

4.4. $O_2^{\bullet-}$ and H_2O_2 as primary enzymatic product — NADPH oxidases

The importance of ROS in redox regulation of numerous signaling pathways and of almost every cellular function should be reflected by the presence of a specialized enzyme that controls in a spatiotemporal manner the generation of ROS. To fulfill this role, this enzyme will require a complex regulatory network that is responsive to metabolic needs and extracellular stimuli and is expressed in all cell types. Integration of multiple responses to achieve ROS-dependent tasks that are essential for cells and tissues will necessitate several levels of regulation and/or, more efficiently, a number of such enzymes harboring different regulatory mechanisms that can be integrated into an interconnected ROS signaling network. The family of nicotinamide adenine dinucleotide phosphate (NADPH) oxidases (NOX/DUOX), conserved from fungi and plants to mammals, fulfills these criteria.[76] While the members of this family may not always show high sequence homology, the overall structural features of the enzyme's catalytic core that permits the transfer of electrons from cytoplasmic NADPH to FAD and across the membrane via two low potential hemes to molecular oxygen are conserved. The reduction of O_2 generates $O_2^{\bullet-}$ or in some cases H_2O_2 (by a yet undetermined mechanism) in the extracellular space, endosomal lumen, or phagosome, depending on the type of membrane that incorporates the oxidase.

4.4.1. *NOX/DUOX structural organization*

The basic NOX structure consists of six transmembrane (TM) α-helices connected by outside (A, C, E) and inside (B, D) loops and an extended cytosolic carboxyl (C) terminus that contains two non-covalently bound flavin adenine dinucleotide (FAD) and four NADPH binding sites (Fig. 3).[76] In mammalian NOX2 (*CYBB*, $gp91^{phox}$) the FAD-binding domain was mapped approximately to amino acid residues 335–345 (isoalloxazine moiety) and 350–360 (ribityl chain), and the NADPH-binding domain to residues 406–416 (pyrophosphate), 442–447 (ribose), 504–508 (adenine), and 535–539 (nicotinamide).[76,77] Two non-identical hemes with midpoint redox potentials of –225 mV and –265 mV are coordinated non-covalently via two histidine pairs located in transmembrane (TM) helix three and five.[78,79] The axial histidine ligands for mammalian NOX2 have been conclusively identified at the inner face of the membrane (His101 to His209 for –225 mV heme) and near the outer face of the membrane (His115 and His222 for –265 mV heme).[79,80] Sequence and domain comparisons show conservation of this bis-histidinyl arrangement and the spacing between histidines in both membrane domains (13 residues in TM3, 12 residues

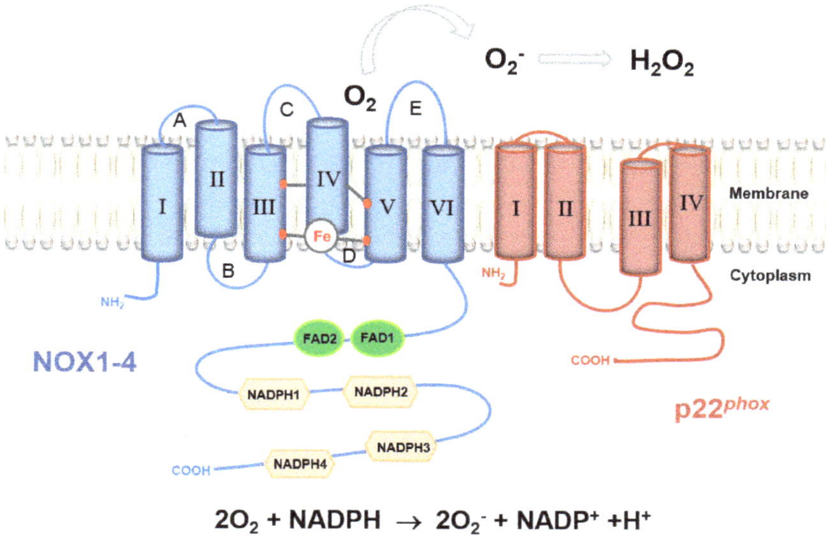

Fig. 3. Schematic model of the NOX-p22^{phox} dimer. Two flavin adenine dinucleotide (FAD) and four nicotinamide adenine dinucleotide phosphate (NADPH) domains are located in the NOX C-terminus.

in TM5).[76] Heme incorporation during biosynthesis of NOX2 is a prerequisite for formation of a heterodimer with the transmembrane protein p22^{phox} (*CYBA*), which is likely due to conformational changes taking place in NOX2 upon heme ligation.[81] While the NOX2 heme placement model is supported by observations in model cell lines and in patients expressing *CYBB* variants (see CGD) that stemmed from a single amino acid change at the aforementioned histidine residues and eliminates both NOX2 and p22^{phox} expression in polymorphonuclear leukocytes (PMNs),[80,82,83] the stepwise heme incorporation and its role in complex formation and protein stability of other NADPH oxidases has not yet been explored.

The family of mammalian NADPH oxidases is comprised of seven members termed NOX1-5 and DUOX1-2 enzymes.[84–89] While the structural organization of NOX1-4 follows closely the NOX domain paradigm, NOX5 and DUOX1/2 contain several

Ca^{2+}-binding EF-hand motifs in their extended N termini. The overall structure and activation mechanism of NOX5 harboring four EF-hand motifs is conserved in plant NADPH oxidases of the Rboh family,[90] while the amino terminus of DUOX includes a paired EF-hand followed by an additional helical membrane-spanning segment that connects to a sizeable (~600 amino acids) ectodomain with peroxidase homology. The peroxidase-like domains in human DUOX and *Drosophila melanogaster* Duox lack amino acids required for heme incorporation and peroxidase activity, while *Caenorhabditis elegans* Duox can serve as H_2O_2 source and functional peroxidase.[91,92]

All NOX/DUOX enzymes except for NOX5 require a partner protein for formation of a membrane-incorporated heterodimer, which is essential for complex stability, correct cellular localization, and catalytic activity of the oxidase. The transmembrane proteins $p22^{phox}$, DUOXA1, and DUOXA2 serve as dimerization partners for NOX1-4, DUOX1, and DUOX2, respectively.[93–98] The structure of $p22^{phox}$ has not been solved, and while predictions differ between 2–4 TM helices,[99–101] mutational analysis favors the 4 TM helix model with N and C termini localized in the cytosol.[101,102] Detailed analysis of a single $p22^{phox}$ point mutation in the penultimate TM helix and its influence on NOX1,2,4-$p22^{phox}$ assembly, localization, and ROS generation revealed that complex formation of NOX family members with $p22^{phox}$ differs.[101]

DUOXA proteins are 5 TM helix-spanning proteins featuring an extracellular N-terminus, several glycosylation sites in the first extracellular loop, and a cytosolic C-terminus. The *DUOXA* and *DUOX* genes are located contiguously on chromosome 15 with *DUOX1* and *DUOX2* being oriented in a head-to-head configuration with *DUOXA1* and *DUOXA2*, respectively. Therefore, each pair (*DUOX1–DUOXA1*, *DUOX2–DUOXA2*) shares a core promoter region, which is reflected in their coordinated expression.[94,103] NOX5, which is absent in rodents, may either not require complex formation, may be stabilized by intramolecular interaction between the N- and C-termini of the protein, or may homodimerize.[104,105]

4.4.2. *NOX2 assembly and activation*

The membrane-bound core of NADPH oxidases requires either assembly with several cytosolic components for activity (NOX1-3), or is mainly regulated by calcium mobilization and phosphorylation (NOX5, DUOX1/2), or is considered constitutively active and transcriptionally regulated (NOX4). The cytosolic proteins essential for NOX2-mediated $O_2^{\bullet-}$ generation have been identified and confirmed by analyzing inherited gene defects in CGD patients, by gene deletion studies in mice, and by reconstitution of oxidase function in model cell lines. The phagocyte oxidase expressed in human PMNs consists of the NOX2-p22^{phox} complex, the cytosolic proteins p47^{phox} (*NCF1*), p67^{phox} (*NCF2*), p40^{phox} (*NCF4*), and the GTP-binding protein RAC2.[106–110] In other cell types, the highly homologous GTPase RAC1 will be utilized.[111] In an amphiphile-activated cell-free oxidase system, $O_2^{\bullet-}$ production, measured as cytochrome c reduction, was achieved by reconstitution of the minimal enzyme complex, adding purified p47^{phox}, p67^{phox}, and RAC1/2 to neutrophil membranes or to a relipidated and reflavinated NOX2-p22^{phox} complex.[112] This experimental setup has greatly contributed to our understanding of NOX2 assembly and activation.

The regulatory components p47^{phox}, p67^{phox}, and p40^{phox} of the human NOX2 NADPH oxidase were identified as proteins absent or mutationally inactivated in the neutrophil cytosol of patients with autosomal recessive forms of CGD.[2,113–115] All three proteins are characterized by several motifs and domains that permit intra- and intermolecular protein–protein and protein–lipid interactions. In p47^{phox} an N-terminal *phox* homology (PX) domain is followed by tandem Src homology (SH3) domains, an autoinhibitory region (AIR) and a proline-rich region (PRR). Two SH3 domains are also present in p67^{phox}, but they are separated by a Phox and Bem1 (PB1) domain. The N-terminal part of p67^{phox} contains four tetratricopeptide repeats (TPR) and an activation domain (AD). In p40^{phox}, a single SH3 domain separates the N-terminal PX domain from a C-terminal PB1 domain.[116] Protein interactions commonly occur between SH3 domains and PRR motifs, between supercoiled TPR regions and diverse protein sequences, between PB1 domains of distinct proteins to facilitate oligomerization, and between cytoplasmic lipid-binding modules (PX) and phosphoinositides in membrane compartments,[117–120] while the other motifs present are restricted to oxidase-associated proteins.

In resting neutrophils, the cytosolic proteins form a pre-assembled complex that obscures interaction sites and underpins the inactive state of the NOX2 oxidase. To accomplish this, the tandem SH3 domains of $p47^{phox}$ are masked by intramolecular interaction with the AIR domain together with conformational changes that render the PX domain inaccessible. The $p47^{phox}$ PRR region is bound to the second SH3 domain of $p67^{phox}$. $P67^{phox}$ attaches to $p40^{phox}$ via PB1 domains present in both proteins, while intramolecular interaction between the PB1 and the PX domain in $p40^{phox}$ suppresses binding of $p40^{phox}$ to membranes containing phosphatidylinositol 3-phosphate.[121] The NOX2-based phagocyte oxidase can be activated either by soluble agonists such as pathogen-associated molecular patterns (PAMPs) or by phagocytosis of bacteria, fungi, or opsonized particles. In the blood stream or during migration into tissues, PMNs can be exposed to priming agents and/or activating stimuli (Fig. 4). Priming agents such as LTB4, PAF, LPS, TNF-α, GM-CSF, integrin

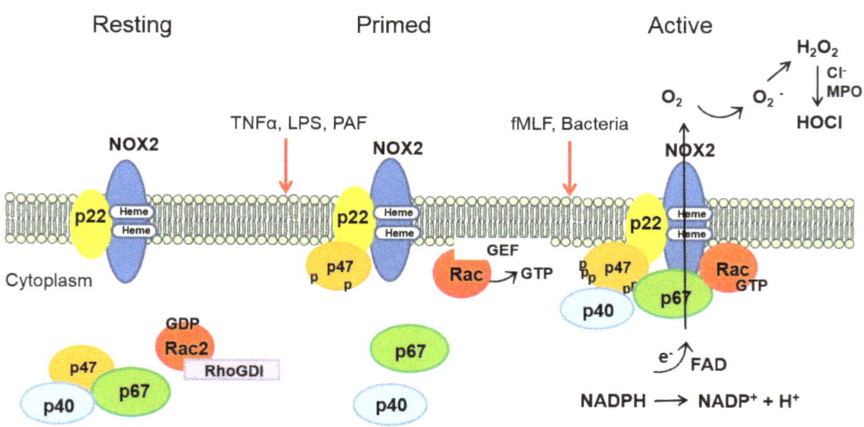

Fig. 4. Sequential assembly of the NOX2 NADPH oxidase. Stages shown are dormant in resting polymorphonuclear leukocytes (PMNs), the primed state, and full PMN activation. Definitions are myeloperoxidase (MPO), for NOX complex please see text and glossary.

β_2 agonists, and matrix components will lead to a pre-activated (primed) state of the oxidase.[122] For TNF-α-mediated priming, the sequence of events includes phosphorylation of $p47^{phox}$ Ser345 by p38/ERK1/2, leading to a conformational change that permits binding of a peptidyl prolyl *cis–trans* isomerase.[123] TNF-α, similar to other priming agents, will not trigger NOX2 activation or sizeable $O_2^{\bullet-}$ production, but potentiates oxidase activity markedly when an activating stimulus (e.g., bacterial peptide fMLF, complement fragment C5a) is encountered. This second agent will induce several additional signals including activation of protein kinase C, thereby promoting $p47^{phox}$ phosphorylation on neighboring (Ser315, Ser320, Ser328) and other (Ser359, Ser370) sites, and subsequent opening and exposure of the tandem SH3 domains.[124] Both SH3 domains are required for binding to a PRR domain located in the C-terminus of $p22^{phox}$ (amino acids 151–160). This stepwise opening of the masked $p47^{phox}$ conformation permits regulated disassembly of the cytosolic complex, followed by translocation and docking at the membrane-bound complex. During the full activation of the oxidase, multiple additional phosphorylations and novel protein–protein/lipid interactions occur, which are required for NOX2 assembly and activation including (i) phosphorylation of $p47^{phox}$ serine residues, enhanced accessibility of the $p47^{phox}$ PX domain, and binding to phosphatidylinositol 3,4-biphosphate, and acidic phospholipids in membranes, (ii) $p67^{phox}$ translocation and $p67^{phox}$ $SH3_2$ binding to the $p47^{phox}$ PRR, (iii) activation of RAC and (iv) binding of the $p67^{phox}$ TPR to GTP-RAC. The GTP-binding protein RAC1/2 is activated by soluble agents or phagosome closure and will translocate to the membrane independently. RAC activation proceeds by translocation of the inactive cytosolic GDP-RAC/RHOGDI complex to the membrane, dissociation of RAC from RHOGDI, GDP to GTP exchange by an exchange factor (GEF), and coordinated association of processed (geranylgeranylated) RAC with the membrane, $p67^{phox}$ and NOX2.[125] While $p47^{phox}$ can be viewed as an adapter protein assembling the oxidase, RAC-GTP binding to $p67^{phox}$ is essential for NOX2 catalytic activity[126] and may permit interaction of the $p67^{phox}$ AD domain with the NOX2-$p22^{phox}$ complex to initiate electron transfer. The protein $p40^{phox}$ is not required for NOX2 oxidase activity upon soluble stimuli, but augments the phagocytic respiratory burst markedly by translocation and binding to phagosomal, phosphatidylinositol 3-phosphate-containing membranes via its high-affinity PX domain.[127,128]

4.4.3. *Regulation of other NOX/DUOX family members*

The mechanisms regulating activation of other NADPH oxidase family members either resemble the multimeric NOX2 complex (e.g., NOX1/3) or show very distinct characteristics. The NOX1-p22^{phox} heterodimer assembles with active RAC-GTP and the cytosolic components NOXO1 and NOXA1, paralogs of p47^{phox} and p67^{phox}, respectively, on membrane compartments when an activating stimulus occurs.[98] Albeit the domain architecture and presumably the adapter function of NOXO1 is comparable to p47^{phox}, the absence of the masking AIR domain permits binding of NOXO1 to p22^{phox} in unstimulated cells, leading to a basal level of $O_2^{\bullet-}$ generation that can be enhanced by appropriate stimuli. The transcriptional upregulation of NOXO1 expression by cytokines and PAMPs may serve as an additional means of controlling basal and stimulated NOX1 activity.[129,130] The NOXA1 domain structure is similar to p67^{phox}, but this protein lacks the SH3 domain located in the middle of p67^{phox}. The regulation of NOX3 is comparable to NOX1 in reconstituted cell lines with NOXO1 and NOXA1 being the preferred partner proteins, although p47^{phox} and p67^{phox} proteins can substitute.[131,132] Inactivating mutations in NOXO1 (or NOX3) lead to severe balance defects in mice due to impaired otoconia formation, supporting NOXO1 as essential protein for NOX3 activation.[133]

The regulation of the catalytic activity of the other NADPH oxidase family members differs substantially from NOX1-3. NOX4 seems to be mainly transcriptionally regulated, forming a constitutively active NOX4-p22^{phox} heterodimer. Transcriptional NOX4 upregulation has been observed via the hypoxia–HIF-1α axis, TGF-β-mediated signaling, or endoplasmatic reticulum stress to name a few examples.[134–136] Activation of NOX5 is regulated by stimuli enhancing Ca^{2+} mobilization or Ca^{2+} influx from the extracellular milieu. Binding of Ca^{2+} to the two tandem EF-hand motifs may cause a conformational change, which results in intramolecular interaction between the N and C termini of NOX5, leading to electron flow. As the *in vitro* EC_{50} for Ca^{2+} is too high for *in vivo* activation of the enzyme, mechanisms for calcium sensitization will be necessary. This can be accomplished by modifying the NOX5 C-terminus, either by phosphorylation of serine and threonine residues or by binding of calmodulin, an EF-hand containing protein, or other proteins including chaperones.[137,138] Likewise, Ca^{2+}-activated DUOX/DUOXA complexes seem to require additional regulatory mechanisms. A negative signal is provided by NOXA1 binding to a proline-rich domain located in the C-terminus of DUOX1. This interaction suppressed basal H_2O_2 generation and was released by Ca^{2+} flux.[139] Activating signals may require G protein-coupled receptor signaling to phospholipase C (PLC)-β and PKC as reported in *Drosophila*.[140] Further, both inhibitory and activating DUOX1 phosphorylation sites have been reported.[141] Of particular interest is the yet unresolved observation that DUOX1/2 and NOX4 enzymes release as final product H_2O_2 instead of $O_2^{\bullet-}$.[95–97] The E-loop of NOX4 and the interaction between the N-terminus of DUOXA and the A-loop of DUOX were implicated in intramolecular conversion of $O_2^{\bullet-}$,[142–144] but these mutational studies will require mechanistic details when structural information regarding heterodimer formation will be available.

4.4.4. *ROS deficiency due to NADPH oxidase variants including CGD*

NADPH oxidases are widely expressed in many tissues, but most of them show tissue-specific expression patterns. Unique expression correlates with irreplaceable function in ROS-related disorders that can be directly linked to inactivating mutations in patient cohorts or in mice (naturally occurring, chemically induced, or genetically modified). For example, many variants with loss of function or reduced function of the NOX2 complex have been identified, leading to

X-linked or autosomal recessive CGD, an inherited disorder characterized by recurrent pulmonary infections, hyperinflammation, and gastrointestinal complications.[1,145,146] CGD patients seem to be particularly susceptible to infections with catalase-positive bacteria (e.g., *S. aureus*, Burkholderia, and Nocardia species) and fungi (e.g., Aspergillus and Candida species). Patients harboring NOX2 complex variants with reduced $O_2^{\bullet-}$ generation that remains above the threshold of causing characteristic CGD are susceptible to developing pediatric inflammatory bowel disease (IBD).[13,147] Missense mutations in *NOX1* or *DUOX2* constitute a similar risk factor for very early-onset IBD.[148] Reduced H_2O_2 production by *DUOX2* and *DUOXA2* variants is associated with permanent or transient congenital hypothyroidism due to a defect in iodine organification.[149] CGD and hypothyroidism are also observed in knockout or mutant mice, indicating that these mouse models can mimic human disease.[13]

5. ROS in immunity and inflammation

5.1. *Mitochondrial ROS in immunity and inflammation*

The interest in mtROS triggering redox signaling and driving proinflammatory cytokine production has increased in the last couple of years. In infections, viruses often target the mitochondria by altering Ca^{2+} homeostasis, $\Delta\Psi_m$ (mitochondrial membrane potential), antiviral defense pathways, and apoptosis.[150] Changes in mtROS levels are frequently observed as a secondary effect, but one can envision direct interaction of viral components with ETC regulators or proteins connected to the ETC. For example, the CIII-associated NLRX1 protein was reported as a direct binding partner of the Influenza A virus polymerase basic protein 1-frame 2 (PB1-F2) protein, thereby stabilizing $\Delta\Psi_m$ and attenuating macrophage apoptosis.[151] One can imagine that such protective effects can be subverted, leading to increased electron escape, mtROS generation, and cell death. On the other hand, mtROS can provide protection in bacterial host defense as recently shown for ECSIT, a protein associated with CI assembly at the inner mitochondrial membrane.[152] Upon Toll-like receptor (TLR1,2,4) activation, ECSIT translocated to the outer mitochondrial membrane, followed by binding to TRAF6 and polyubiquitination. Gene deletion experiments in macrophages indicated that ECSIT is involved in TLR-induced mtROS generation and was required for bacterial killing of intracellular *Salmonella* Typhimurium.[153] Antimicrobial signaling also involves sensor proteins located in the outer mitochondrial membrane, and even if these proteins do not directly participate in mtROS generation, their signaling responses will be negatively or positively regulated by changes in $\Delta\Psi_m$, Ca^{2+} mobilization, and mtROS release.[154] One of these proteins is the RIG-like helicase receptor (RLR) protein MAVS, which participates in the response to RNA viruses by stimulating NF-κB-mediated transcription and the type I interferon response.[155] MAVS can induce recruitment and oligomerization of NLRP3 at the outer mitochondrial membrane leading to caspase-1 activation.[156,157] Thus, mtROS release could directly affect assembly and activation of the NLRP3 inflammasome. While mtROS have been connected to transcriptional upregulation of NLRP3,[158,159] they lead also to oxidation of mtDNA, which when released can serve as stimulus for NLRP3 inflammasome activation.[160,161] In accordance, the antioxidant MitoQ, a mitochondria-targeted derivative of ubiquinone, decreased the production of the proinflammatory cytokines IL-1β and IL-18 by suppressing NLRP3 inflammasome activation.[162] Inflammasome-independent upregulation of proinflammatory IL-6 and TNF-α by LPS-stimulated mtROS production has been reported for TNF receptor-associated periodic syndrome (TRAPS), an autosomal dominant autoinflammatory disease.[163]

Infections, nutrient deprivation, or hypoxia are stressors that mediate autophagy, induce ROS generation, and trigger redox imbalance. While an apparent connection exists between ROS and autophagic processes, neither the source of ROS nor the oxygen species generated are conclusively identified. Metabolic stressors leading to canonical autophagy alter the efficiency of the mitochondrial respiratory chain and decrease the availability of NADPH, a required cofactor for antioxidant relays in the mitochondria. Increased mtROS might be responsible for oxidation of the autophagy protein ATG4, inactivating its delipidating activity on LC3, thereby permitting elongation of the autophagosome.[164] Albeit many reports connect mtROS to autophagy, mechanistic details are still scarce.[165,166]

5.2. *NOX2-derived ROS in immunity and inflammation*

While NADPH oxidases expressed at mucosal surfaces of barrier epithelia such as DUOX1, DUOX2, or NOX1, and even NOX4 and NOX5 participate in inflammatory disease, tissue injury, and fibrosis, mechanistic details and their contribution to the inflammatory process are not yet fully established, and hence their input will not be discussed herein. The role of NOX2-derived ROS in inflammatory disease centers on innate immune cell functions in acute and chronic inflammation. Neutrophil recruitment and activation is a key event in providing host defense, infection control, and restoring tissue homeostasis, but when the switch from the proinflammatory to the resolving program does not occur properly, tissue damage, chronic inflammation, and autoimmunity will arise. Early on, the primary function of the NOX2-dependent phagocyte oxidative burst was recognized as a crucial protective mechanism for pathogen control as superoxide-deficient CGD patients present with recurrent fungal and bacterial infections. Phagocytes recruited to sites of infection engulf microbes by a regulated, actin-dependent process termed phagocytosis. During this process, priming-induced fusion of NOX2-$p22^{phox}$ containing specific and secretory granules with the plasma membrane occurs. Invagination of these membranes and closure of the compartment forms a single-layer membrane around the microbe. The membrane-bound NOX2-$p22^{phox}$ heterodimer is incorporated into the phagosomal membrane by facing its assembly site towards the cytosol, so that the reduction of molecular oxygen and $O_2^{\bullet-}$ generation will occur inside the phagosome. Activation of RAC2, complete assembly of the oxidase, and electron flow will commence upon phagosome closure.[167] Contents of granules including MPO catalyzing HOCl production or antimicrobial peptides are released into the phagosome and contribute to microbial killing.[24,168] Oxidative mechanisms such as methionine oxidation and protein chlorination as well as protease-dependent mechanisms cooperate in damaging microbial proteins and DNA.[169,170] Although HOCl production is essential for microbial killing in neutrophils, the importance of NOX2, but not of MPO, for an overall effective host defense is apparent. Mutational inactivation of NOX2 (X-CGD) or in genes required for NOX2 complex formation (AR-CGD) cause CGD with severe consequences for patients, while MPO deficiency will usually not give rise to clinical manifestations. This difference seems not to be connected to the antimicrobial activity of neutrophil extracellular traps (NETs) as NET formation is dependent on MPO (and in many cases on NOX2),[171,172] but is likely due to NOX2-dependent ROS-mediated processes in macrophages and dendritic cells. A role for NOX2 was reported in LC3-associated phagocytosis (LAP), a process that requires assembly of certain autophagy proteins at the phagosome membrane.[173,174] NADPH oxidase colocalized also with LC3 to fused, multicellular vacuoles in colonic goblet cells. The secretory function (i.e., mucus secretion) of goblet cells was dependent on NOX-derived ROS.[175] Both of these processes utilize NOX and certain autophagy mediators without displaying the hallmarks of canonical autophagy. Macrophage NOX2 activity is not only essential for microbial killing upon phagocytosis, but also for chemotaxis,[176] macrophage lineage skewing, and many intracellular signaling processes such as Toll-like receptor- and G-protein-coupled receptor-driven pathways.[177] In dendritic cells, NOX2 activity seems to be primarily required for maintaining a neutral pH in the phagosome, thereby permitting efficient antigen digestion and peptide cross-presentation, thus linking innate to adaptive immunity.[178]

Albeit exaggerated ROS production by NOX2 has long been considered proinflammatory and NOX2 activity was linked to inflammatory disease including acute lung injury or chronic arthritis,[4] animal studies and observations in CGD patients point increasingly to a protective, anti-inflammatory role of this oxidase that is essential for resolution of inflammation. CGD patients present commonly with granulomas, colitis, and lupus-like syndromes and their immune cells produce significantly increased levels of chemokines and proinflammatory cytokines (IL-8, IL-6, TNF-α).[13,179,180] In mice, Nox2 limits systemic inflammation induced by PAMPs (LPS, zymosan) or by danger-associated molecular patterns (DAMPs) such as uric acid crystals or endogenous substances released by damaged cells.[181–187] The protective effect of Nox2-derived ROS was connected to decreased neutrophil recruitment to sites of damage and activation of Nrf2-mediated transcription.[182,184] A recent report identified overproduction of IL-1α and subsequently G-CSF as drivers of increased neutrophil and macrophage influx in sterile peritoneal inflammation in Nox2 (*Cybb*$^{-/-}$)-deficient mice.[181] The molecular mechanism of how NOX2-derived $O_2^{\bullet-}$ alters specific transcriptional pathways, dampens inflammation, and contributes to resolution of inflammatory processes is not yet defined. One can easily envision an interplay between several different immune cell populations, or between phagocytic cells and other cell types. For example, in the intestinal mucosa ROS production by activated neutrophils will activate hypoxia-inducible factor 1 (HIF-1) in the epithelial cell layer lining the gut by consuming the limited supply of oxygen at the mucosal surface. HIF-1 will then induce a protective response that contributes to tissue repair.[35]

6. Outlook

New insights gained over the past decade have led to a reevaluation of oxidative stress as an essential orchestrator of inflammatory disease. Large-scale sequencing efforts on patient populations to elucidate the genetic basis for disease together with human primary cell analysis, advanced animal models (e.g., defined missense mutations reflecting CGD genotypes by CRISPR/Cas9 approach), and novel tools for ROS detection have improved our understanding of beneficial and detrimental effects of ROS. Important tasks are still lying ahead such as (i) developing precise methods for localized detection of a defined reactive species and synchronously its ROS source *in vivo*, (ii) identifying specific inhibitors in order to target a particular ROS source, and (iii) determining how critical ROS are for disease and at which time point ROS generation will initiate, ameliorate, or amplify inflammation. Advanced animal models that permit manipulating a particular ROS source in a spatiotemporal manner and cell/organoid-based studies performed at relevant oxygen concentrations will help making progress on this front. ROS generated by various sources feed into redox relays and signaling circuits, and thus quantitative systems biology models might be indispensable to understand how various ROS-generating systems interact with each other and influence each other. Recent studies show communication between mtROS, NOX/DUOX enzymes, and other ROS sources,[188–191] although mechanistic details are still limited. Integration of ROS signals and ROS converting/degrading enzymes in a spatiotemporal manner will inform us where and when to intervene in inflammatory disorders, which may likely include both enhancing and inhibiting a specific ROS-generating system.

Acknowledgments

Our work has been supported for many years by the National Institutes of Health (USA) and recently by Science Foundation Ireland (Ireland). Assistance by Dr L. Alvarez for preparation of chemical equations is gratefully acknowledged.

Glossary of acronyms and abbreviations

ARE	Antioxidant response element
ASK1	N-terminal region of apoptosis signal-regulating kinase 1; *MAP3K5*
CAT	Catalase
CGD	Chronic granulomatous disease
DAMP	Danger-associated molecular pattern
DUOX	Dual oxidase
DUOXA	Dual oxidase maturation factor
ETC	Electron transport chain
ETF-QOR	Electron transferring flavoprotein ubiquinone oxidoreductase
EPO	Eosinophil peroxidase

FAD	Flavin adenine dinucleotide
GPx	Glutathione peroxidase
GPDH	Glycerol-3-phosphate dehydrogenase
GSH	Glutathione
GSSH	Glutathione disulfide
H_2O_2	Hydrogen peroxide
HIF-1	Hypoxia-inducible factor-1
HOCl	Hypochlorous acid
IBD	Inflammatory bowel disease
LAP	LC3-associated phagocytosis
LOX	Lysyl oxidase
LPO	Lactoperoxidase
MAO	Monoamine oxidase
mtROS	Mitochondrial reactive oxygen species
MPO	Myeloperoxidase
NADPH	Nicotinamide adenine dinucleotide phosphate
NET	Neutrophil extracellular trap
NLRP3	NLR family, Pyrin Domain Containing 3
NO	Nitric oxide
NOX	NADPH oxidase
NOX1	*NOX1*
NOX2	*CYBB*, glycoprotein (gp)91^{phox}
NOX3	*NOX3*
NOX4	*NOX4*
NOX5	*NOX5*
NOXA1	NADPH oxidase activator 1
NOXO1	NADPH oxidase organizer 1
NRF	Nuclear factor erythroid 2 (NFE2)-related factor
$O_2^{\bullet-}$	Superoxide radical
$^{\bullet}OH$	Hydroxyl radical
$ONOO^-$	Peroxynitrite
OXPHOS	Oxidative phosphorylation
$p22^{phox}$	*CYBA*
$p47^{phox}$	Neutrophil cytosolic factor 1 (*NCF1*)
$p67^{phox}$	Neutrophil cytosolic factor 2 (*NCF2*)
$p40^{phox}$	Neutrophil cytosolic factor 4 (*NCF4*)

PAMP	Pathogen-associated molecular pattern
PB1	Phox and Bem1 domain
PDI	Protein-disulfide isomerase
PMN	Polymorphonuclear
PRR	Proline-rich domain
PRX	Peroxiredoxin
PX	Phox homology domain
RAC	RAS-related C3 botulinum toxin substrate (RHO GTPase family)
RET	Reverse electron transport
RHOGDI	RHO GDP dissociation inhibitor
RNS	Reactive nitrogen species
ROS	Reactive oxygen species
SH3	Src homology domain
SOD	Superoxide dismutase
TPR	Tetratricopeptide repeats
TRX	Thioredoxin
XO	Xanthine oxidase; *XDH*

References

1. Holland SM. (2013). Chronic granulomatous disease. *Hematology/oncology clinics of North America*. **27**(1):89–99, viii.
2. Nunoi H, Rotrosen D, Gallin JI, Malech HL. (1988). Two forms of autosomal chronic granulomatous disease lack distinct neutrophil cytosol factors. *Science*. **242**(4883):1298–1301.
3. Segal AW. (1987). Absence of both cytochrome b-245 subunits from neutrophils in X-linked chronic granulomatous disease. *Nature*. **326**(6108): 88–91.
4. Mittal M, Siddiqui MR, Tran K, Reddy SP, Malik AB. (2014). Reactive oxygen species in inflammation and tissue injury. *Antioxid Redox Signal*. **20**(7):1126–1167.
5. Giorgio M. (2015). Oxidative stress and the unfulfilled promises of antioxidant agents. *Ecancermedicalscience* **9**: 556.
6. Kawagishi H, Finkel T. (2014). Unraveling the truth about antioxidants: ROS and disease: finding the right balance. *Nat Med*. **20**(7):711–713.
7. Schmidt HH, Stocker R, Vollbracht C, Paulsen G, Riley D, Daiber A *et al.* (2015). Antioxidants in Translational Medicine. *Antioxid Redox Signal*. **23**(14):1130–1143.

8. Murphy MP, Holmgren A, Larsson NG, Halliwell B, Chang CJ, Kalyanaraman B *et al.* (2011). Unraveling the biological roles of reactive oxygen species. *Cell Metabol.* **13**(4):361–366.
9. Ortega-Gomez A, Perretti M, Soehnlein O. (2013). Resolution of inflammation: an integrated view. *EMBO Mol Med.* **5**(5):661–674.
10. Serhan CN, Brain SD, Buckley CD, Gilroy DW, Haslett C, O'Neill LA *et al.* (2007). Resolution of inflammation: state of the art, definitions and terms. *FASEB J.* **21**(2):325–332.
11. Zuo L, Zhou T, Pannell BK, Ziegler AC, Best TM. (2015). Biological and physiological role of reactive oxygen species — the good, the bad and the ugly. *Acta Physiol.* **214**(3):329–348.
12. Holmstrom KM, Finkel T. (2014). Cellular mechanisms and physiological consequences of redox-dependent signalling. *Nat Rev Mol Cell Biol.* **15**(6):411–421.
13. O'Neill S, Brault J, Stasia MJ, Knaus UG. (2015). Genetic disorders coupled to ROS deficiency. *Redox Biol* **6**: 135–156.
14. Rieber N, Hector A, Kuijpers T, Roos D, Hartl D. (2012). Current concepts of hyperinflammation in chronic granulomatous disease. *Clin Develop Immunol* **2012**: 252460.
15. Giorgio M, Trinei M, Migliaccio E, Pelicci PG. (2007). Hydrogen peroxide: a metabolic by-product or a common mediator of ageing signals? *Nat Rev Mol Cell Biol.* **8**(9):722–728.
16. Bashan N, Kovsan J, Kachko I, Ovadia H, Rudich A. (2009). Positive and negative regulation of insulin signaling by reactive oxygen and nitrogen species. *Physiol Rev.* **89**(1):27–71.
17. Weidinger A, Kozlov AV. (2015). Biological Activities of Reactive Oxygen and Nitrogen Species: Oxidative Stress versus Signal Transduction. *Biomolecules.* **5**(2):472–484.
18. Salvador A, Sousa J, Pinto RE. (2001). Hydroperoxyl, superoxide and pH gradients in the mitochondrial matrix: A theoretical assessment. *Free Radic Biol Med.* **31**(10):1208–1215.
19. McCormick ML, Buettner GR, Britigan BE. (1998). Endogenous superoxide dismutase levels regulate iron-dependent hydroxyl radical formation in Escherichia coli exposed to hydrogen peroxide. *J Bacteriol.* **180**(3):622–625.
20. Winterbourn CC. (2013). The biological chemistry of hydrogen peroxide. *Methods Enzymol* **528**: 3–25.
21. Bienert GP, Chaumont F. (2014). Aquaporin-facilitated transmembrane diffusion of hydrogen peroxide. *Biochim Biophys Acta.* **1840**(5):1596–1604.
22. Pryor WA. (1986). Oxy-radicals and related species: their formation, lifetimes, and reactions. *Ann Rev Physiol* **48**: 657–667.

23. Ayala A, Munoz MF, Arguelles S. (2014). Lipid peroxidation: production, metabolism, and signaling mechanisms of malondialdehyde and 4-hydroxy-2-nonenal. *Oxid Med Cell Longev* **2014**: 360–438.
24. Nauseef WM. (2014). Myeloperoxidase in human neutrophil host defence. *Cell Microbiol.* **16**(8):1146–1155.
25. Klebanoff SJ, Kettle AJ, Rosen H, Winterbourn CC, Nauseef WM. (2013). Myeloperoxidase: a front-line defender against phagocytosed microorganisms. *J Leukoc Biol.* **93**(2):185–198.
26. Kettle AJ, Anderson RF, Hampton MB, Winterbourn CC. (2007). Reactions of superoxide with myeloperoxidase. *Biochemistry.* **46**(16):4888–4897.
27. Paumann-Page M, Furtmuller PG, Hofbauer S, Paton LN, Obinger C, Kettle AJ. (2013). Inactivation of human myeloperoxidase by hydrogen peroxide. *Arch Biochem Biophys.* **539**(1):51–62.
28. Bafort F, Parisi O, Perraudin JP, Jijakli MH. (2014). Mode of action of lactoperoxidase as related to its antimicrobial activity: A review. *Enzyme Res* **2014**:517–564.
29. Paulsen CE, Carroll KS. (2013). Cysteine-mediated redox signaling: chemistry, biology, and tools for discovery. *Chem Rev.* **113**(7):4633–4679.
30. Lo Conte M, Carroll KS. (2013). The redox biochemistry of protein sulfenylation and sulfinylation. *J Biol Chem.* **288**(37):26480–26488.
31. Houee-Levin C, Bobrowski K, Horakova L, Karademir B, Schoneich C, Davies MJ *et al.* (2015). Exploring oxidative modifications of tyrosine: An update on mechanisms of formation, advances in analysis and biological consequences. *Free Radic Res.* **49**(4):347–373.
32. Perdivara I, Deterding LJ, Przybylski M, Tomer KB. (2010). Mass spectrometric identification of oxidative modifications of tryptophan residues in proteins: chemical artifact or post-translational modification? *J Am Soc Mass Spect.* **21**(7):1114–1117.
33. Schoneich C. (2000). Mechanisms of metal-catalyzed oxidation of histidine to 2-oxo-histidine in peptides and proteins. *J Pharmaceut Biomed Anal.* **21**(6):1093–1097.
34. Alam A, Leoni G, Wentworth CC, Kwal JM, Wu H, Ardita CS *et al.* (2014). Redox signaling regulates commensal-mediated mucosal homeostasis and restitution and requires formyl peptide receptor 1. *Mucosal Immunol.* 7(3):645–655.
35. Campbell EL, Bruyninckx WJ, Kelly CJ, Glover LE, McNamee EN, Bowers BE *et al.* (2014). Transmigrating neutrophils shape the mucosal microenvironment through localized oxygen depletion to influence resolution of inflammation. *Immunity.* **40**(1):66–77.
36. McCord JM, Fridovich I. (1969a). Superoxide dismutase. An enzymic function for erythrocuprein (hemocuprein). *J Biol Chem.* **244**(22):6049–6055.

37. McCord JM, Fridovich I. (1969b). The utility of superoxide dismutase in studying free radical reactions. I. Radicals generated by the interaction of sulfite, dimethyl sulfoxide, and oxygen. *J Biol Chem.* **244**(22):6056–6063.
38. Miller AF. (2012). Superoxide dismutases: ancient enzymes and new insights. *FEBS Lett.* **586**(5):585–595.
39. Sheng Y, Abreu IA, Cabelli DE, Maroney MJ, Miller AF, Teixeira M *et al.* (2014). Superoxide dismutases and superoxide reductases. *Chem Rev.* **114**(7):3854–3918.
40. Pratt AJ, Shin DS, Merz GE, Rambo RP, Lancaster WA, Dyer KN *et al.* (2014). Aggregation propensities of superoxide dismutase G93 hotspot mutants mirror ALS clinical phenotypes. *Proc Natl Acad Sci USA.* **111**(43):E4568–4576.
41. Mohr A, Buneker C, Gough RP, Zwacka RM. (2008). MnSOD protects colorectal cancer cells from TRAIL-induced apoptosis by inhibition of Smac/DIABLO release. *Oncogene.* **27**(6):763–774.
42. Quiros-Gonzalez I, Sainz RM, Hevia D, Mayo JC. (2011). MnSOD drives neuroendocrine differentiation, androgen independence, and cell survival in prostate cancer cells. *Free Radic Biol Med.* **50**(4):525–536.
43. Zhou Z, Kang YJ. (2000). Cellular and subcellular localization of catalase in the heart of transgenic mice. *J Histochem Cytochem.* **48**(5):585–594.
44. Brigelius-Flohe R, Maiorino M. (2013). Glutathione peroxidases. *Biochim Biophys Acta.* **1830**(5):3289–3303.
45. Lushchak VI. (2012). Glutathione homeostasis and functions: potential targets for medical interventions. *J Amino Acid* **2012**:736–837.
46. Iwaoka M, Katakura A, Mishima J, Ishihara Y, Kunwar A, Priyadarsini KI. (2015). Mimicking the lipid peroxidation inhibitory activity of phospholipid hydroperoxide glutathione peroxidase (GPx4) by using fatty acid conjugates of a water-soluble selenolane. *Molecules.* **20**(7):12364–12375.
47. Ma Q. (2013). Role of nrf2 in oxidative stress and toxicity. *Ann Rev Pharmacol Toxicol* **53**: 401–426.
48. Tebay LE, Robertson H, Durant ST, Vitale SR, Penning TM, Dinkova-Kostova AT *et al.* (2015). Mechanisms of activation of the transcription factor Nrf2 by redox stressors, nutrient cues, and energy status and the pathways through which it attenuates degenerative disease. *Free Radic Biol Med.* **88**(Pt B): 108–146.
49. Nagy P, Karton A, Betz A, Peskin AV, Pace P, O'Reilly RJ *et al.* (2011). Model for the exceptional reactivity of peroxiredoxins 2 and 3 with hydrogen peroxide: a kinetic and computational study. *J Biol Chem.* **286**(20):18048–18055.
50. Rhee SG, Woo HA, Kil IS, Bae SH. (2012). Peroxiredoxin functions as a peroxidase and a regulator and sensor of local peroxides. *J Biol Chem.* **287**(7):4403–4410.

51. Sobotta MC, Liou W, Stocker S, Talwar D, Oehler M, Ruppert T *et al.* (2015). Peroxiredoxin-2 and STAT3 form a redox relay for H2O2 signaling. *Nat Chem Biol.* **11**(1):64–70.
52. Kakihana T, Araki K, Vavassori S, Iemura S, Cortini M, Fagioli C *et al.* (2013). Dynamic regulation of Ero1alpha and peroxiredoxin 4 localization in the secretory pathway. *J Biol Chem.* **288**(41):29586–29594.
53. Lowes DA, Galley HF. (2011). Mitochondrial protection by the thioredoxin-2 and glutathione systems in an in vitro endothelial model of sepsis. *Biochem J.* **436**(1):123–132.
54. Jeong W, Bae SH, Toledano MB, Rhee SG. (2012). Role of sulfiredoxin as a regulator of peroxiredoxin function and regulation of its expression. *Free Radic Biol Med.* **53**(3):447–456.
55. Collet JF, Messens J. (2010). Structure, function, and mechanism of thioredoxin proteins. *Antioxid Redox Signal.* **13**(8):1205–1216.
56. Benhar M. (2015). Nitric oxide and the thioredoxin system: A complex interplay in redox regulation. *Biochim Biophys Acta.* **1850**(12):2476–2484.
57. Soga M, Matsuzawa A, Ichijo H. (2012). Oxidative Stress-Induced Diseases via the ASK1 Signaling Pathway. *Int J Cell Biol* **2012**:439–587.
58. Yoshihara E, Masaki S, Matsuo Y, Chen Z, Tian H, Yodoi J. (2014). Thioredoxin/Txnip: redoxisome, as a redox switch for the pathogenesis of diseases. *Front Immunol* **4**: 514.
59. Kelley EE, Khoo NK, Hundley NJ, Malik UZ, Freeman BA, Tarpey MM. (2010). Hydrogen peroxide is the major oxidant product of xanthine oxidase. *Free Radic Biol Med.* **48**(4):493–498.
60. Cathcart MK, Bhattacharjee A. (2014). Monoamine oxidase A (MAO-A): A signature marker of alternatively activated monocytes/macrophages. *Inflamm Cell Signal.* **1**(4).
61. Iturbide A, Garcia de Herreros A, Peiro S. (2015). A new role for LOX and LOXL2 proteins in transcription regulation. *Febs J.* **282**(9):1768–1773.
62. Hertzberger R, Arents J, Dekker HL, Pridmore RD, Gysler C, Kleerebezem M *et al.* (2014). H(2)O(2) production in species of the Lactobacillus acidophilus group: a central role for a novel NADH-dependent flavin reductase. *Appl Environ Microbiol.* **80**(7):2229–2239.
63. Murphy MP. (2009). How mitochondria produce reactive oxygen species. *Biochem J.* **417**(1):1–13.
64. Waypa GB, Smith KA, Schumacker PT. (2016). O2 sensing, mitochondria and ROS signaling: The fog is lifting. *Mol Aspects Med* **47–48**:76–89.
65. Pinton P, Rimessi A, Marchi S, Orsini F, Migliaccio E, Giorgio M *et al.* (2007). Protein kinase C beta and prolyl isomerase 1 regulate mitochondrial effects of the life-span determinant p66Shc. *Science.* **315**(5812):659–663.

66. Miyazawa M, Tsuji Y. (2014). Evidence for a novel antioxidant function and isoform-specific regulation of the human p66Shc gene. *Mol Biol Cell.* **25**(13):2116–2127.
67. Lenaz G, Tioli G, Falasca AI, Genova ML. (2016). Complex I function in mitochondrial supercomplexes. *Biochim Biophys Acta.* Jan 25.
68. Maranzana E, Barbero G, Falasca AI, Lenaz G, Genova ML. (2013). Mitochondrial respiratory supercomplex association limits production of reactive oxygen species from complex I. *Antioxid Redox Signal.* **19**(13):1469–1480.
69. Chouchani ET, Pell VR, Gaude E, Aksentijevic D, Sundier SY, Robb EL *et al.* (2014). Ischaemic accumulation of succinate controls reperfusion injury through mitochondrial ROS. *Nature.* **515**(7527):431–435.
70. Waypa GB, Marks JD, Guzy RD, Mungai PT, Schriewer JM, Dokic D *et al.* (2013). Superoxide generated at mitochondrial complex III triggers acute responses to hypoxia in the pulmonary circulation. *Am J Respir Crit Care Med.* **187**(4):424–432.
71. Chandel NS, Maltepe E, Goldwasser E, Mathieu CE, Simon MC, Schumacker PT. (1998). Mitochondrial reactive oxygen species trigger hypoxia-induced transcription. *Proc Natl Acad Sci USA.* **95**(20):11715–11720.
72. St-Pierre J, Brand MD, Boutilier RG. (2000). Mitochondria as ATP consumers: cellular treason in anoxia. *Proc Natl Acad Sci USA.* **97**(15):8670–8674.
73. Giorgio V, von Stockum S, Antoniel M, Fabbro A, Fogolari F, Forte M *et al.* (2013). Dimers of mitochondrial ATP synthase form the permeability transition pore. *Proc Natl Acad Sci USA.* **110**(15):5887–5892.
74. Zorov DB, Juhaszova M, Sollott SJ. (2014). Mitochondrial reactive oxygen species (ROS) and ROS-induced ROS release. *Physiol Rev.* **94**(3):909–950.
75. Soares F, Tattoli I, Rahman MA, Robertson SJ, Belcheva A, Liu D *et al.* (2014). The mitochondrial protein NLRX1 controls the balance between extrinsic and intrinsic apoptosis. *J Biol Chem.* **289**(28):19317–19330.
76. Kawahara T, Quinn MT, Lambeth JD. (2007). Molecular evolution of the reactive oxygen-generating NADPH oxidase (Nox/Duox) family of enzymes. *BMC Evol Biol* **7**: 109.
77. Davis AR, Mascolo PL, Bunger PL, Sipes KM, Quinn MT. (1998). Cloning and sequencing of the bovine flavocytochrome b subunit proteins, gp91-phox and p22-phox: Comparison with other known flavocytochrome b sequences. *J Leukoc Biol.* **64**(1):114–123.
78. Cross AR, Rae J, Curnutte JT. (1995). Cytochrome b-245 of the neutrophil superoxide-generating system contains two nonidentical hemes. Potentiometric studies of a mutant form of gp91phox. *J Biol Chem.* **270**(29):17075–17077.

79. Yu L, Quinn MT, Cross AR, Dinauer MC. (1998). Gp91(phox) is the heme binding subunit of the superoxide-generating NADPH oxidase. *Proc Natl Acad Sci USA*. **95**(14):7993–7998.
80. Biberstine-Kinkade KJ, DeLeo FR, Epstein RI, LeRoy BA, Nauseef WM, Dinauer MC. (2001). Heme-ligating histidines in flavocytochrome b(558):identification of specific histidines in gp91(phox). *J Biol Chem*. **276**(33):31105–31112.
81. Yu L, Zhen L, Dinauer MC. (1997). Biosynthesis of the phagocyte NADPH oxidase cytochrome b558. Role of heme incorporation and heterodimer formation in maturation and stability of gp91phox and p22phox subunits. *J Biol Chem*. **272**(43):27288–27294.
82. Heyworth PG, Curnutte JT, Rae J, Noack D, Roos D, van Koppen E *et al.* (2001). Hematologically important mutations: X-linked chronic granulomatous disease (second update). *Blood Cells Mol Dis*. **27**(1):16–26.
83. Roos D, de Boer M, Kuribayashi F, Meischl C, Weening RS, Segal AW *et al.* (1996). Mutations in the X-linked and autosomal recessive forms of chronic granulomatous disease. *Blood*. **87**(5):1663–1681.
84. Banfi B, Molnar G, Maturana A, Steger K, Hegedus B, Demaurex N *et al.* (2001). A Ca(2+)-activated NADPH oxidase in testis, spleen, and lymph nodes. *J Biol Chem*. **276**(40):37594–37601.
85. Bedard K, Krause KH. (2007). The NOX family of ROS-generating NADPH oxidases: physiology and pathophysiology. *Physiol Rev*. **87**(1):245–313.
86. De Deken X, Wang D, Many MC, Costagliola S, Libert F, Vassart G *et al.* (2000). Cloning of two human thyroid cDNAs encoding new members of the NADPH oxidase family. *J Biol Chem*. **275**(30):23227–23233.
87. Dupuy C, Ohayon R, Valent A, Noel-Hudson MS, Deme D, Virion A. (1999). Purification of a novel flavoprotein involved in the thyroid NADPH oxidase. Cloning of the porcine and human cdnas. *J Biol Chem*. **274**(52):37265–37269.
88. Geiszt M, Kopp JB, Varnai P, Leto TL. (2000). Identification of renox, an NAD(P)H oxidase in kidney. *Proc Natl Acad Sci USA*. **97**(14):8010–8014.
89. Suh YA, Arnold RS, Lassegue B, Shi J, Xu X, Sorescu D *et al.* (1999). Cell transformation by the superoxide-generating oxidase Mox1. *Nature*. **401**(6748):79–82.
90. Torres MA, Dangl JL. (2005). Functions of the respiratory burst oxidase in biotic interactions, abiotic stress and development. *Curr Opin Plant Biol*. **8**(4):397–403.
91. Hurd TR, Liang FX, Lehmann R. (2015). Curly Encodes Dual Oxidase, Which Acts with Heme Peroxidase Curly Su to Shape the Adult Drosophila Wing. *PLoS Genet*. **11**(11):e1005625.

92. Meitzler JL, Ortiz de Montellano PR. (2009). Caenorhabditis elegans and human dual oxidase 1 (DUOX1) “peroxidase” domains: insights into heme binding and catalytic activity. *J Biol Chem.* **284**(28):18634–18643.
93. Dinauer MC, Pierce EA, Bruns GA, Curnutte JT, Orkin SH. (1990). Human neutrophil cytochrome b light chain (p22-phox). Gene structure, chromosomal location, and mutations in cytochrome-negative autosomal recessive chronic granulomatous disease. *J Clin Invest.* **86**(5):1729–1737.
94. Grasberger H, Refetoff S. (2006). Identification of the maturation factor for dual oxidase. Evolution of an eukaryotic operon equivalent. *J Biol Chem.* **281**(27):18269–18272.
95. Luxen S, Noack D, Frausto M, Davanture S, Torbett BE, Knaus UG. (2009). Heterodimerization controls localization of Duox-DuoxA NADPH oxidases in airway cells. *J Cell Sci.* **122**(Pt 8):1238–1247.
96. Martyn KD, Frederick LM, von Loehneysen K, Dinauer MC, Knaus UG. (2006). Functional analysis of Nox4 reveals unique characteristics compared to other NADPH oxidases. *Cell Signal.* **18**(1):69–82.
97. Morand S, Ueyama T, Tsujibe S, Saito N, Korzeniowska A, Leto TL. (2009). Duox maturation factors form cell surface complexes with Duox affecting the specificity of reactive oxygen species generation. *FASEB J.* **23**(4): 1205–1218.
98. Ueyama T, Geiszt M, Leto TL. (2006). Involvement of Rac1 in activation of multicomponent Nox1- and Nox3-based NADPH oxidases. *Mol Cell Biol.* **26**(6):2160–2174.
99. Meijles DN, Howlin BJ, Li JM. (2012). Consensus in silico computational modelling of the p22phox subunit of the NADPH oxidase. *Comput Biol Chem* **39**: 6–13.
100. Taylor RM, Burritt JB, Baniulis D, Foubert TR, Lord CI, Dinauer MC *et al.* (2004). Site-specific inhibitors of NADPH oxidase activity and structural probes of flavocytochrome b: characterization of six monoclonal antibodies to the p22phox subunit. *J Immunol.* **173**(12):7349–7357.
101. von Lohneysen K, Noack D, Jesaitis AJ, Dinauer MC, Knaus UG. (2008). Mutational analysis reveals distinct features of the Nox4-p22 phox complex. *J Biol Chem.* **283**(50):35273–35282.
102. Zhu Y, Marchal CC, Casbon AJ, Stull N, von Lohneysen K, Knaus UG *et al.* (2006). Deletion mutagenesis of p22phox subunit of flavocytochrome b558: identification of regions critical for gp91phox maturation and NADPH oxidase activity. *J Biol Chem.* **281**(41):30336–30346.
103. Hulur I, Hermanns P, Nestoris C, Heger S, Refetoff S, Pohlenz J *et al.* (2011). A single copy of the recently identified dual oxidase maturation factor (DUOXA) 1 gene produces only mild transient hypothyroidism in a patient with a novel biallelic DUOXA2 mutation and monoallelic DUOXA1 deletion. *J Clin Endocrinol Metab.* **96**(5):E841–845.

104. Banfi B, Tirone F, Durussel I, Knisz J, Moskwa P, Molnar GZ *et al.* (2004). Mechanism of Ca2+ activation of the NADPH oxidase 5 (NOX5). *J Biol Chem.* **279**(18):18583–18591.
105. Kawahara T, Jackson HM, Smith SM, Simpson PD, Lambeth JD. (2011). Nox5 forms a functional oligomer mediated by self-association of its dehydrogenase domain. *Biochemistry.* **50**(12):2013–2025.
106. Clark RA, Malech HL, Gallin JI, Nunoi H, Volpp BD, Pearson DW *et al.* (1989). Genetic variants of chronic granulomatous disease: prevalence of deficiencies of two cytosolic components of the NADPH oxidase system. *N Engl J Med.* **321**(10):647–652.
107. Dinauer MC, Orkin SH, Brown R, Jesaitis AJ, Parkos CA. (1987). The glycoprotein encoded by the X-linked chronic granulomatous disease locus is a component of the neutrophil cytochrome b complex. *Nature.* **327**(6124):717–720.
108. Knaus UG, Heyworth PG, Evans T, Curnutte JT, Bokoch GM. (1991). Regulation of phagocyte oxygen radical production by the GTP-binding protein Rac 2. *Science.* **254**(5037):1512–1515.
109. Segal AW, Jones OT. (1978). Novel cytochrome b system in phagocytic vacuoles of human granulocytes. *Nature.* **276**(5687):515–517.
110. Wientjes FB, Hsuan JJ, Totty NF, Segal AW. (1993). p40phox, a third cytosolic component of the activation complex of the NADPH oxidase to contain src homology 3 domains. *Biochem J.* **296**(**Pt** 3):557–561.
111. Abo A, Pick E, Hall A, Totty N, Teahan CG, Segal AW. (1991). Activation of the NADPH oxidase involves the small GTP-binding protein p21rac1. *Nature.* **353**(6345):668–670.
112. Pick E. (2014). Cell-free NADPH oxidase activation assays: "*in vitro* veritas". *Methods Mol Biol* **1124**: 339–403.
113. Matute JD, Arias AA, Wright NA, Wrobel I, Waterhouse CC, Li XJ *et al.* (2009). A new genetic subgroup of chronic granulomatous disease with autosomal recessive mutations in p40 phox and selective defects in neutrophil NADPH oxidase activity. *Blood.* **114**(15):3309–3315.
114. Tsunawaki S, Mizunari H, Nagata M, Tatsuzawa O, Kuratsuji T. (1994). A novel cytosolic component, p40phox, of respiratory burst oxidase associates with p67phox and is absent in patients with chronic granulomatous disease who lack p67phox. *Biochem Biophys Res Commun.* **199**(3):1378–1387.
115. Volpp BD, Nauseef WM, Clark RA. (1988). Two cytosolic neutrophil oxidase components absent in autosomal chronic granulomatous disease. *Science.* **242**(4883):1295–1297.
116. Kawahara T, Lambeth JD. (2007). Molecular evolution of Phox-related regulatory subunits for NADPH oxidase enzymes. *BMC Evol Biol.* **7**(1):178.

117. Cortajarena AL, Regan L. (2006). Ligand binding by TPR domains. *Protein Sci.* **15**(5):1193–1198.
118. Kaneko T, Li L, Li SS. (2008). The SH3 domain — a family of versatile peptide- and protein-recognition module. *Front Biosci* **13**: 4938–4952.
119. Mas C, Norwood SJ, Bugarcic A, Kinna G, Leneva N, Kovtun O *et al.* (2014). Structural basis for different phosphoinositide specificities of the PX domains of sorting nexins regulating G-protein signaling. *J Biol Chem.* **289**(41):28554–28568.
120. Moscat J, Diaz-Meco MT, Albert A, Campuzano S. (2006). Cell signaling and function organized by PB1 domain interactions. *Mol Cell.* **23**(5):631–640.
121. Sumimoto H. (2008). Structure, regulation and evolution of Nox-family NADPH oxidases that produce reactive oxygen species. *FEBS J.* **275**(13):3249–3277.
122. El-Benna J, Dang PM, Gougerot-Pocidalo MA. (2008). Priming of the neutrophil NADPH oxidase activation: role of p47phox phosphorylation and NOX2 mobilization to the plasma membrane. *Semin Immunopathol.* **30**(3):279–289.
123. Boussetta T, Gougerot-Pocidalo MA, Hayem G, Ciappelloni S, Raad H, Arabi Derkawi R *et al.* (2010). The prolyl isomerase Pin1 acts as a novel molecular switch for TNF-alpha-induced priming of the NADPH oxidase in human neutrophils. *Blood.* **116**(26):5795–5802.
124. El-Benna J, Dang PM, Gougerot-Pocidalo MA, Marie JC, Braut-Boucher F. (2009). p47phox, the phagocyte NADPH oxidase/NOX2 organizer: structure, phosphorylation and implication in diseases. *Exp Mol Med.* **41**(4):217–225.
125. Pick E. (2014). Role of the Rho GTPase Rac in the activation of the phagocyte NADPH oxidase: Outsourcing a key task. *Small GTPases* **5**: e27952.
126. Diekmann D, Abo A, Johnston C, Segal AW, Hall A. (1994). Interaction of Rac with p67phox and regulation of phagocytic NADPH oxidase activity. *Science.* **265**(5171):531–533.
127. Ellson CD, Gobert-Gosse S, Anderson KE, Davidson K, Erdjument-Bromage H, Tempst P *et al.* (2001). PtdIns(3)P regulates the neutrophil oxidase complex by binding to the PX domain of p40(phox). *Nat Cell Biol.* **3**(7):679–682.
128. Suh CI, Stull ND, Li XJ, Tian W, Price MO, Grinstein S *et al.* (2006). The phosphoinositide-binding protein p40phox activates the NADPH oxidase during FcgammaIIA receptor-induced phagocytosis. *J Exp Med.* **203**(8):1915–1925.
129. Kawahara T, Kohjima M, Kuwano Y, Mino H, Teshima-Kondo S, Takeya R *et al.* (2005). Helicobacter pylori lipopolysaccharide activates Rac1 and transcription of NADPH oxidase Nox1 and its organizer

NOXO1 in guinea pig gastric mucosal cells. *Am J Physiol Cell Physiol.* **288**(2):C450–457.
130. Kuwano Y, Tominaga K, Kawahara T, Sasaki H, Takeo K, Nishida K *et al.* (2008). Tumor necrosis factor alpha activates transcription of the NADPH oxidase organizer 1 (NOXO1) gene and upregulates superoxide production in colon epithelial cells. *Free Radic Biol Med.* **45**(12):1642–1652.
131. Cheng G, Ritsick D, Lambeth JD. (2004). Nox3 regulation by NOXO1, p47phox, and p67phox. *J Biol Chem.* **279**(33):34250–34255.
132. Nakano Y, Banfi B, Jesaitis AJ, Dinauer MC, Allen LA, Nauseef WM. (2007). Critical roles for p22phox in the structural maturation and subcellular targeting of Nox3. *Biochem J.* **403**(1):97–108.
133. Kiss PJ, Knisz J, Zhang Y, Baltrusaitis J, Sigmund CD, Thalmann R *et al.* (2006). Inactivation of NADPH oxidase organizer 1 results in severe imbalance. *Current Biol.* **16**(2):208–213.
134. Cucoranu I, Clempus R, Dikalova A, Phelan PJ, Ariyan S, Dikalov S *et al.* (2005). NAD(P)H oxidase 4 mediates transforming growth factor-beta1-induced differentiation of cardiac fibroblasts into myofibroblasts. *Circulation Res.* **97**(9):900–907.
135. Diebold I, Petry A, Hess J, Gorlach A. (2010). The NADPH oxidase subunit NOX4 is a new target gene of the hypoxia-inducible factor-1. *Mol Biol Cell.* **21**(12):2087–2096.
136. Wu RF, Ma Z, Liu Z, Terada LS. (2010). Nox4-derived H2O2 mediates endoplasmic reticulum signaling through local Ras activation. *Mol Cell Biol.* **30**(14):3553–3568.
137. Bedard K, Jaquet V, Krause KH. (2012). NOX5: from basic biology to signaling and disease. *Free Radic Biol Med.* **52**(4):725–734.
138. Chen F, Wang Y, Barman S, Fulton DJ. (2015). Enzymatic regulation and functional relevance of NOX5. *Curr Pharm Des.* **21**(41):5999–6008.
139. Pacquelet S, Lehmann M, Luxen S, Regazzoni K, Frausto M, Noack D *et al.* (2008). Inhibitory action of NoxA1 on dual oxidase activity in airway cells. *J Biol Chem.* **283**(36):24649–24658.
140. Lee KA, Kim B, Bhin J, Kim do H, You H, Kim EK *et al.* (2015). Bacterial uracil modulates Drosophila DUOX-dependent gut immunity via Hedgehog-induced signaling endosomes. *Cell Host Microbe.* **17**(2):191–204.
141. Rigutto S, Hoste C, Grasberger H, Milenkovic M, Communi D, Dumont JE *et al.* (2009). Activation of dual oxidases Duox1 and Duox2: differential regulation mediated by camp-dependent protein kinase and protein kinase C-dependent phosphorylation. *J Biol Chem.* **284**(11):6725–6734.
142. Hoste C, Dumont JE, Miot F, De Deken X. (2012). The type of DUOX-dependent ROS production is dictated by defined sequences in DUOXA. *Exp Cell Res.* **318**(18):2353–2364.

143. Takac I, Schroder K, Zhang L, Lardy B, Anilkumar N, Lambeth JD *et al.* (2011). The E-loop is involved in hydrogen peroxide formation by the NADPH oxidase Nox4. *J Biol Chem.* **286**(15):13304–13313.
144. Ueyama T, Sakuma M, Ninoyu Y, Hamada T, Dupuy C, Geiszt M *et al.* (2015). The extracellular A-loop of dual oxidases affects the specificity of reactive oxygen species release. *J Biol Chem.* **290**(10):6495–6506.
145. Kuhns DB, Alvord WG, Heller T, Feld JJ, Pike KM, Marciano BE *et al.* (2010). Residual NADPH oxidase and survival in chronic granulomatous disease. *N Engl J Med.* **363**(27):2600–2610.
146. van den Berg JM, van Koppen E, Ahlin A, Belohradsky BH, Bernatowska E, Corbeel L *et al.* (2009). Chronic granulomatous disease: the European experience. *PLoS ONE.* **4**(4):e5234.
147. Dhillon SS, Fattouh R, Elkadri A, Xu W, Murchie R, Walters T *et al.* (2014). Variants in nicotinamide adenine dinucleotide phosphate oxidase complex components determine susceptibility to very early onset inflammatory bowel disease. *Gastroenterology.* **147**(3):680–689 e682.
148. Hayes P, Dhillon S, O'Neill K, Thoeni C, Hui KY, Elkadri A *et al.* (2015). Defects in NADPH oxidase genes and in very early onset inflammatory bowel disease. *Cell Mol Gastroenterol Hepatol.* **1**(5):489–502.
149. Moreno JC, Bikker H, Kempers MJ, van Trotsenburg AS, Baas F, de Vijlder JJ *et al.* (2002). Inactivating mutations in the gene for thyroid oxidase 2 (THOX2) and congenital hypothyroidism. *N Engl J Med.* **347**(2):95–102.
150. Anand SK, Tikoo SK (2013). Viruses as modulators of mitochondrial functions. *Adv Virol* **2013**: 738–794.
151. Jaworska J, Coulombe F, Downey J, Tzelepis F, Shalaby K, Tattoli I *et al.* (2014). NLRX1 prevents mitochondrial induced apoptosis and enhances macrophage antiviral immunity by interacting with influenza virus PB1-F2 protein. *Proc Natl Acad Sci USA.* **111**(20):E2110–2119.
152. Vogel RO, Janssen RJ, van den Brand MA, Dieteren CE, Verkaart S, Koopman WJ *et al.* (2007). Cytosolic signaling protein Ecsit also localizes to mitochondria where it interacts with chaperone NDUFAF1 and functions in complex I assembly. *Genes Dev.* **21**(5):615–624.
153. West AP, Brodsky IE, Rahner C, Woo DK, Erdjument-Bromage H, Tempst P *et al.* (2011). TLR signalling augments macrophage bactericidal activity through mitochondrial ROS. *Nature.* **472**(7344):476–480.
154. Cloonan SM, Choi AM. (2013). Mitochondria: sensors and mediators of innate immune receptor signaling. *Curr Opin Microbiol.* **16**(3):327–338.
155. Koshiba T (2013). Mitochondrial-mediated antiviral immunity. *Biochim Biophys Acta.* **1833**(1):225–232.
156. Park S, Juliana C, Hong S, Datta P, Hwang I, Fernandes-Alnemri T *et al.* (2013). The mitochondrial antiviral protein MAVS associates with NLRP3 and regulates its inflammasome activity. *J Immunol.* **191**(8):4358–4366.

157. Subramanian N, Natarajan K, Clatworthy MR, Wang Z, Germain RN. (2013). The adaptor MAVS promotes NLRP3 mitochondrial localization and inflammasome activation. *Cell.* **153**(2):348–361.
158. Bauernfeind F, Bartok E, Rieger A, Franchi L, Nunez G, Hornung V. (2011). Cutting edge: reactive oxygen species inhibitors block priming, but not activation, of the NLRP3 inflammasome. *J Immunol.* **187**(2):613–617.
159. Zhou R, Yazdi AS, Menu P, Tschopp J. (2011). A role for mitochondria in NLRP3 inflammasome activation. *Nature.* **469**(7329):221–225.
160. Nakahira K, Haspel JA, Rathinam VA, Lee SJ, Dolinay T, Lam HC *et al.* (2011). Autophagy proteins regulate innate immune responses by inhibiting the release of mitochondrial DNA mediated by the NALP3 inflammasome. *Nat Immunol.* **12**(3):222–230.
161. Shimada K, Crother TR, Karlin J, Dagvadorj J, Chiba N, Chen S *et al.* (2012). Oxidized mitochondrial DNA activates the NLRP3 inflammasome during apoptosis. *Immunity.* **36**(3):401–414.
162. Dashdorj A, Jyothi KR, Lim S, Jo A, Nguyen MN, Ha J *et al.* (2013). Mitochondria-targeted antioxidant MitoQ ameliorates experimental mouse colitis by suppressing NLRP3 inflammasome-mediated inflammatory cytokines. *BMC Med* **11**: 178.
163. Bulua AC, Simon A, Maddipati R, Pelletier M, Park H, Kim KY *et al.* (2011). Mitochondrial reactive oxygen species promote production of proinflammatory cytokines and are elevated in TNFR1-associated periodic syndrome (TRAPS). *J Exp Med.* **208**(3):519–533.
164. Scherz-Shouval R, Shvets E, Elazar Z. (2007). Oxidation as a post-translational modification that regulates autophagy. *Autophagy.* **3**(4):371–373.
165. Filomeni G, De Zio D, Cecconi F. (2015). Oxidative stress and autophagy: the clash between damage and metabolic needs. *Cell Death Differ.* **22**(3):377–388.
166. Poillet-Perez L, Despouy G, Delage-Mourroux R, Boyer-Guittaut M. (2015). Interplay between ROS and autophagy in cancer cells, from tumor initiation to cancer therapy. *Redox Biol* **4**: 184–192.
167. Hoppe AD, Swanson JA. (2004). Cdc42, Rac1, and Rac2 display distinct patterns of activation during phagocytosis. *Mol Biol Cell.* **15**(8):3509–3519.
168. Winterbourn CC, Kettle AJ. (2013). Redox reactions and microbial killing in the neutrophil phagosome. *Antioxid Redox Signal.* **18**(6):642–660.
169. Green JN, Kettle AJ, Winterbourn CC. (2014). Protein chlorination in neutrophil phagosomes and correlation with bacterial killing. *Free Radic Biol Med* 77: 49–56.
170. Rosen H, Klebanoff SJ, Wang Y, Brot N, Heinecke JW, Fu X. (2009). Methionine oxidation contributes to bacterial killing by the myeloperoxidase system of neutrophils. *Proc Natl Acad Sci U S A.* **106**(44):18686–18691.

171. Bianchi M, Hakkim A, Brinkmann V, Siler U, Seger RA, Zychlinsky A *et al.* (2009). Restoration of NET formation by gene therapy in CGD controls aspergillosis. *Blood.* **114**(13):2619–2622.
172. Metzler KD, Fuchs TA, Nauseef WM, Reumaux D, Roesler J, Schulze I *et al.* (2011). Myeloperoxidase is required for neutrophil extracellular trap formation: implications for innate immunity. *Blood.* **117**(3):953–959.
173. Huang J, Canadien V, Lam GY, Steinberg BE, Dinauer MC, Magalhaes MA *et al.* (2009). Activation of antibacterial autophagy by NADPH oxidases. *Proc Natl Acad Sci USA.* **106**(15):6226–6231.
174. Martinez J, Malireddi RK, Lu Q, Cunha LD, Pelletier S, Gingras S *et al.* (2015). Molecular characterization of LC3-associated phagocytosis reveals distinct roles for Rubicon, NOX2 and autophagy proteins. *Nat Cell Biol.* **17**(7):893–906.
175. Patel KK, Miyoshi H, Beatty WL, Head RD, Malvin NP, Cadwell K *et al.* (2013). Autophagy proteins control goblet cell function by potentiating reactive oxygen species production. *EMBO J.* **32**(24):3130–3144.
176. Chaubey S, Jones GE, Shah AM, Cave AC, Wells CM. (2013). Nox2 is required for macrophage chemotaxis towards CSF-1. *PLoS ONE.* **8**(2):e54869.
177. Ogier-Denis E, Mkaddem SB, Vandewalle A. (2008). NOX enzymes and Toll-like receptor signaling. *Semin Immunopathol.* **30**(3):291–300.
178. Kotsias F, Hoffmann E, Amigorena S, Savina A. (2013). Reactive oxygen species production in the phagosome: impact on antigen presentation in dendritic cells. *Antioxid Redox Signal.* **18**(6):714–729.
179. Rosenzweig SD. (2008). Inflammatory manifestations in chronic granulomatous disease (CGD). *J Clin Immunol.* **28**(Suppl 1):S67–72.
180. Schappi MG, Jaquet V, Belli DC, Krause KH. (2008). Hyperinflammation in chronic granulomatous disease and anti-inflammatory role of the phagocyte NADPH oxidase. *Semin Immunopathol.* **30**(3):255–271.
181. Bagaitkar J, Pech NK, Ivanov S, Austin A, Zeng MY, Pallat S *et al.* (2015). NADPH oxidase controls neutrophilic response to sterile inflammation in mice by regulating the IL-1alpha/G-CSF axis. *Blood.* **126**(25):2724–2733.
182. Davidson BA, Vethanayagam RR, Grimm MJ, Mullan BA, Raghavendran K, Blackwell TS *et al.* (2013). NADPH oxidase and Nrf2 regulate gastric aspiration-induced inflammation and acute lung injury. *J Immunol.* **190**(4):1714–1724.
183. Han W, Li H, Cai J, Gleaves LA, Polosukhin VV, Segal BH *et al.* (2013). NADPH oxidase limits lipopolysaccharide-induced lung inflammation and injury in mice through reduction-oxidation regulation of NF-kappaB activity. *J Immunol.* **190**(9):4786–4794.

184. Kong X, Thimmulappa R, Kombairaju P, Biswal S. (2010). NADPH oxidase-dependent reactive oxygen species mediate amplified TLR4 signaling and sepsis-induced mortality in Nrf2-deficient mice. *J Immunol.* **185**(1):569–577.

185. Segal BH, Han W, Bushey JJ, Joo M, Bhatti Z, Feminella J *et al.* (2010). NADPH oxidase limits innate immune responses in the lungs in mice. *PLoS ONE.* **5**(3):e9631.

186. Whitmore LC, Goss KL, Newell EA, Hilkin BM, Hook JS, Moreland JG. (2014). NOX2 protects against progressive lung injury and multiple organ dysfunction syndrome. *Am J Physiol Lung Cell Mol Physiol.* **307**(1):L71–82.

187. Whitmore LC, Hilkin BM, Goss KL, Wahle EM, Colaizy TT, Boggiatto PM *et al.* (2013). NOX2 protects against prolonged inflammation, lung injury, and mortality following systemic insults. *J Innate Immun.* **5**(6):565–580.

188. Dikalov S. (2011). Cross talk between mitochondria and NADPH oxidases. *Free Radic Biol Med.* **51**(7):1289–1301.

189. Kroller-Schon S, Steven S, Kossmann S, Scholz A, Daub S, Oelze M *et al.* (2014). Molecular mechanisms of the crosstalk between mitochondria and NADPH oxidase through reactive oxygen species-studies in white blood cells and in animal models. *Antioxid Redox Signal.* **20**(2):247–266.

190. Nanduri J, Vaddi DR, Khan SA, Wang N, Makarenko V, Semenza GL *et al.* (2015). HIF-1alpha activation by intermittent hypoxia requires NADPH oxidase stimulation by xanthine oxidase. *PLoS ONE.* **10**(3):e0119762.

191. Rathore R, Zheng YM, Niu CF, Liu QH, Korde A, Ho YS *et al.* (2008). Hypoxia activates NADPH oxidase to increase [ROS]i and [Ca2+]i through the mitochondrial ROS-PKCepsilon signaling axis in pulmonary artery smooth muscle cells. *Free Radic Biol Med.* **45**(9):1223–1231.

Chapter 5
Leukocyte Adhesion

Klaus Ley*,† and Zhichao Fan*

Leukocyte adhesion is central to all forms of inflammation, because all leukocytes need to adhere to the vascular endothelium and transmigrate to get access to the site of inflammation.[1–4] The leukocyte adhesion cascade describes leukocyte recruitment through postcapillary venules. It consists of margination, rolling, arrest, spreading, intraluminal crawling, transendothelial migration, and migration into the tissue. This sequence of events is common for adhesion for many types of leukocytes in many organs and tissues. However, it is not universal: some leukocytes stop without rolling, and in some organs, capillaries rather than venules are the site of leukocyte adhesion. Leukocyte adhesion also occurs in lymphatics, to thrombi by adhesion to fibrin and platelets, to extracellular matrix proteins, and to epithelial cells. This chapter will cover most of the molecular mechanisms and biomechanical constraints of all these forms of leukocyte adhesion except those relevant to atherosclerosis. Chemokines are important regulators of leukocyte adhesion through integrins.

* La Jolla Institute for Allergy and Immunology.
† Department of Bioengineering, University of California San Diego.

1. Leukocyte adhesion molecules

1.1. *Integrins*

Integrins are activatable heterodimeric transmembrane molecules.[4–7] Most integrins have almost no affinity for their ligands unless activated by inside–out signaling. In leukocytes, the most important integrin activators are chemokines and other chemoattractants like C5a, formyl peptides, and leukotrienes. All these receptors are coupled by heterotrimeric G-proteins and are therefore called GPCRs.

All leukocytes (used here as a term encompassing all white blood cells) express one or more members of the β_2 (CD18) integrin family. In fact, β_2 integrins are also called leukocyte integrins, because they are leukocyte-specific and not expressed in other cells. The α subunits of all β_2 integrins contain an inserted I domain with homology to von Willebrand factor A domain. The I domain is the ligand binding site and, upon ligand binding, interacts with the β I-like domain through an "internal ligand" that is exposed when the integrin is activated and ligand is engaged. The β_2 subfamily has four members: lymphocyte function-associated antigen (LFA-1 or CD11a/CD18), macrophage-1 (Mac-1 or CD11b/CD18), $\alpha_X\beta_2$ integrin (CD11c/CD18), and $\alpha_D\beta_2$ integrin (CD11d/CD18). All leukocytes express LFA-1, although at different levels. Mac-1 is expressed on neutrophils, basophils, eosinophils, monocytes, and some activated T cell subsets. CD11c/CD18 is expressed on some monocytes, many macrophages, dendritic cells, as well as neutrophils, and some lymphocytes. CD11d/CD18 expression is found on neutrophils, some T cell subsets, monocytes, macrophages, and dendritic cells.

The ligand specificities of LFA-1 and CD11d/CD18 are relatively narrow; those of Mac-1 and CD11c/CD18 are broad (Table 1). LFA-1 binds InterCellular Adhesion Molecule 1 (ICAM-1, domain 1), 2, 3, 4, and 5. LFA-1 may also bind JAM-A.[8,9] Mac-1 also binds ICAM-1 (domain 3), 2, and 4 and a multitude of other ligands. Similar to Mac-1, CD11c/CD18 binds to multiple ligands beside ICAM-1, 2, 4 and Vascular cell adhesion protein 1 (VCAM-1), but

Table 1. β_2 integrins and part of their ligands.

	Alternative name	Main ligands
$\alpha_L\beta_2$	CD11a/CD18; LFA-1	ICAM-1[115–119]
		ICAM-2[29,120]
		ICAM-3[121]
		ICAM-4[122,123]
		ICAM-5[124,125]
		ESM-1[126]
		JAM-1[8]
		Telencephalin[127]
		Collagen[116]
$\alpha_M\beta_2$	CD11b/CD18; Mac-1	ICAM-1[128–130]
		ICAM-2[131]
		ICAM-4[122]
		Fibrinogen[132–134]
		Factor X[135]
		Collagen[116]
		iC3b[116,136]
		Heparin[137]
		GPIbα[138]
		JAM-3[63]
		Thy-1[139]
		Plasminogen[140]
		EPCR[141]
		Human leukocyte elastase[142]
		CNN1 (CYR61)[143,144]
		CNN2 (CTGF)[143]
		NIF[145]
		CD154 (CD40L)[146]
		Myeloperoxidase[147]
		LL-37 (cathelicidin)[148]
		Oligodeoxynucleotide[149]
		Denatured proteins[13]
$\alpha_X\beta_2$	CD11c/CD18; p150,95	ICAM-1[150,151]
		ICAM-2[152]
		ICAM-4[31]
		VCAM-1[152]
		Fibrinogen[151,153,154]

(*Continued*)

Table 1. (*Continued*)

	Alternative name	Main ligands
		Collagen[116]
		iC3b[116,151,155,156]
		Heparin[157]
		GPIbα[158]
		Thy-1[159]
		Plasminogen[160]
		Denatured proteins[13]
$\alpha_D\beta_2$	CD11d/CD18	ICAM-3[161]
		VCAM-1[162,163]
		Fibrinogen[164]
		Vitronectin[164]
		Cyr61[164]
		Plasminogen[164]

the affinities are poorly defined. CD11d binds ICAM-3, VCAM-1, and other ligands. CD11b/CD18 and CD11c/CD18 are also complement receptors (CR3 and CR4, respectively) and can bind denatured proteins, such as proteins coated on a foreign, non-biological surface as may occur in hemodialysis and implants.

As mentioned above, integrins require activation to become adhesive and bind ligand. This process is particularly well studied in β_2 integrins. For example, the dynamic range of the affinity of LFA-1 for ICAM-1 is estimated to change 10,000-fold from resting to fully activated.[10] β_2 integrin activation is initiated by signaling events triggered by chemokines binding their G-protein coupled receptors (GPCRs). Through signaling intermediates, kindlin-3 and talin-1 are brought to the plasma membrane, where they bind the cytoplasmic tail of the β_2 subunit. This induces two conformational changes: extension and high affinity (Figure 1). Extension and affinity change were originally thought to be interdependent, but recent work shows that the two processes can occur independent of each other.[11] The details of integrin activation are discussed in many excellent reviews.[4,5,7,12]

β_2 integrins are distributed all over the surface of leukocytes. However, extended and high-affinity (activated) β_2 integrins are concentrated in small clusters, most of which sit on the tips of microvilli. LFA-1 is expressed on the plasma membrane and has no intracellular stores, whereas Mac-1 is expressed on the plasma membrane and on the membrane of neutrophil tertiary and secretory granules (see Chapter 6 for more detail). LFA-1 is highest on lymphocytes and patrolling monocytes, but also expressed on all other leukocytes. LFA-1 is crucial for leukocyte arrest, the rapid adhesion from rolling that ensues when the leukocytes encounters an activating stimulus. Mac-1 expression is highest on neutrophils and increases further (~10-fold) after degranulation, when the intracellular pool of Mac-1 is mobilized. This and the vast range of ligands suggest that Mac-1 mainly functions in the extracellular space. In human, but not mouse, neutrophils Mac-1 is also involved in arrest. Like Mac-1, CD11c/CD18 can bind denatured proteins (hydrophobic amino acid sequences that are normally buried inside properly folded proteins).[13] Other than that, its function is unknown. The CD11c knockout mouse has some defects in lipid handling. The CD11d knockout mice showed defect in T cell function[14] and infectious and inflammatory responses, such as in malaria.[15]

Leukocytes express two α_4 integrins, $\alpha_4\beta_1$ (CD49d/CD29, Very Late Antigen-4, VLA-4) and $\alpha_4\beta_7$ (CD49d/β_7). The α_4 integrins can also be activated, but the dynamic range of affinity for ligand seems to be lower than β_2 integrins. $\alpha_4\beta_1$ is expressed on most leukocytes except naïve T and B cells and at low levels on neutrophils. $\alpha_4\beta_1$ integrin binds endothelial VCAM-1 and alternatively spliced fibronectin. This integrin is involved in chorioallantoic fusion; the knockout mouse is therefore embryonic lethal. Conditional knockout mice and blocking monoclonal antibodies have shown that $\alpha_4\beta_1$ integrin is important in monocyte, eosinophil, basophil, and activated lymphocyte trafficking. Although $\alpha_4\beta_1$ is low on neutrophils, its blockade causes defective neutrophil adhesion, transmigration, and diapedesis on vascular endothelial cells.[2]

$\alpha_4\beta_7$ is expressed by monocytes and antigen-experienced T and B cells. The main ligand for $\alpha_4\beta_7$ integrin is Mucosal Addressin Adhesion Molecule-1 (MAdCAM-1), which is exclusively expressed in the gastrointestinal tract. This organ specificity has spawned the

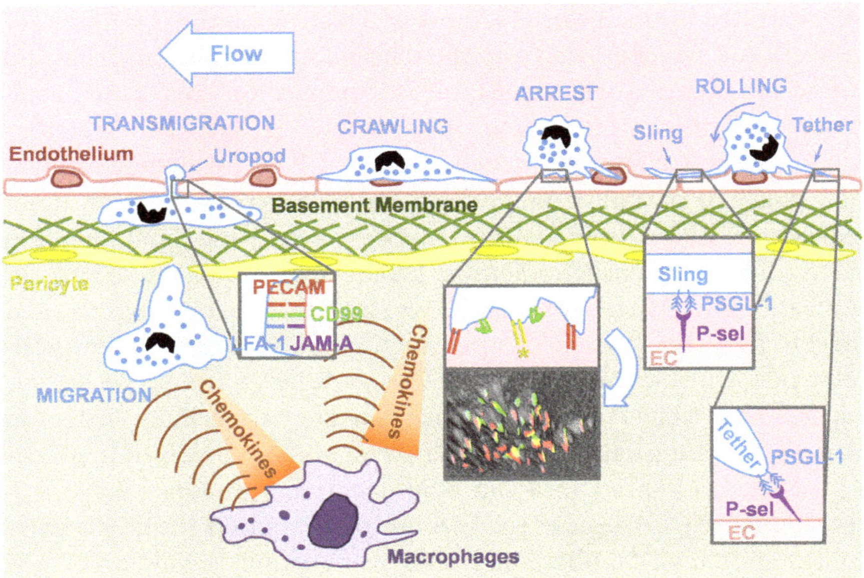

Fig. 1. Leukocyte recruitment. Most rolling leukocytes (blue, right) are neutrophils (indicated by pale granules and lobulated nucleus) and make long, thin tethers that stabilize selectin-mediated rolling by PSGL-1 binding endothelial P-selectin (insert). 10–15% of these tethers swing around and become slings, self-adhesive substrates (insert showing PSGL-1 bond to P-selectin) in front of the rolling cell. In response to chemokines immobilized on the endothelial surface, leukocytes arrest by activating β2 integrins (second cell from right). The top of the insert shows a schematic of integrin activation, where high affinity is green, extended is red, and extended high affinity is yellow. Only extended high-affinity integrin can bind ligands like ICAM-1 in trans (on the endothelial cell). The bottom of the insert shows live cell imaging data where the integrin conformations are detected by reporter antibodies and mapped on the bottom surface of the arresting neutrophil using total internal reflection microscopy (green, red, and yellow indicate the high-affinity, extended, and extended high-affinity β2 integrin, respectively). After arrest, neutrophils spread and start crawling on the endothelium until they find a suitable spot for transmigration. Transmigration preferentially occurs in a paracellular way, often in tricellular corners where three endothelial cells meet. The transmigrating cell forms a uropod enriched in PSGL-1, CD43, and tetraspanins. The uropod can nucleate adhesion of other leukocytes and may also detach. Transmigration spots are characterized by a weakened basement membrane (indicated by the less dense green hatches) and gaps between pericytes (yellow). The insert shows PECAM-1, CD99, and JAM-A, which

Fig. 1. (*Continued*) are key endothelial molecules for transmigration. After transmigration, the neutrophil changes shape again, develops a lamellipod in the front and a uropod in the rear and migrates in response to chemoattractant cytokines (chemokines), often produced by tissue resident macrophages (purple) and other tissue cells.

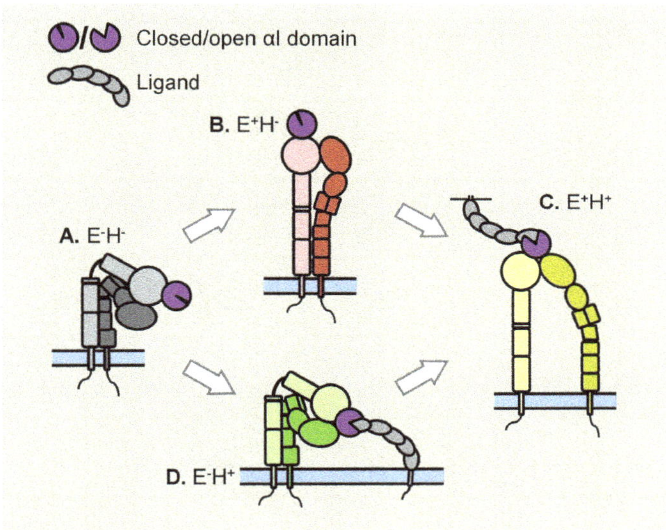

Fig. 2. Two pathways to integrin activation. Integrins (here: β2 integrins) exist in a low affinity bent conformation (not extended, E-; not high affinity, H-, αI domain (purple) closed, left, grey) on the plasma membrane of the leukocyte. Intracellular signaling pathways can result in extension (E+H-, middle top, red). In the classical switchblade mechanism, extension is followed by high affinity (E+H+, right, yellow) that can bind ligand in trans (on the endothelial cell). However, β2 integrins can also acquire high affinity first (E-H+, bottom, green), a conformation that results in ligand binding in cis (on the same leukocyte), followed by extension.

successful development of antibody-based drugs to combat intestinal inflammation.[16] Similar drugs targeting the α_4 integrin subunit are also effective against intestinal inflammation and multiple sclerosis, but these drugs can reactivate a latent virus in the brain that can cause lethal encephalitis. The β_7 integrin knockout mouse has severe defects in leukocyte recruitment to the intestines and Peyer's patches.

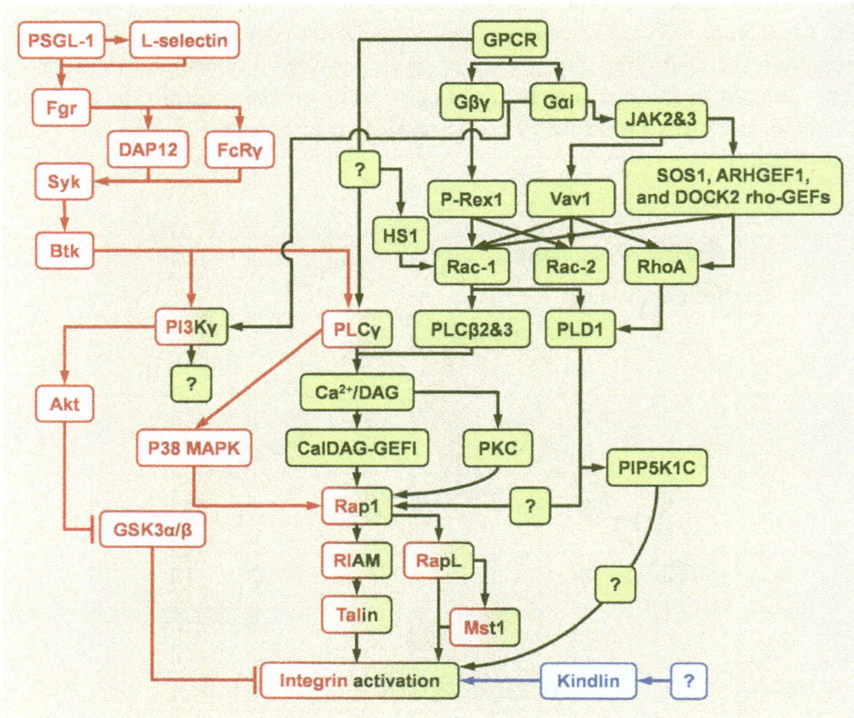

Fig. 3. Intracellular signaling affecting inside–out integrin activation. (a) (red): pathway starting with PSGL-1 and L-selectin on the leukocyte surface, triggered already during rolling, results in activation of the src kinase Fgr. Adapter molecules DAP12 and FcRγ provide ITAM domains to assemble and activate spleen tyrosine kinase (Syk), which activates Bruton's tyrosine kinase (Btk). Here, the pathway splits to PI3 kinase γ (PI3Kγ), which activates Akt that blocks GSK3α and β. These GSKs normally block integrin activation, so Akt relieves a key inactivator. The other pathway starts with phospholipase Cγ (PLCγ), which results in calcium flux and activates P38 MAP kinase (P38 MAPK) that activates the small GTPase Rap1. Rap1 recruits RIAM and talin, which directly binds the integrin β chain and triggers extension. (b) (green): chemokine-triggered integrin activation. The chemokine or other chemoattractant binds its cognate G-protein-coupled receptor (GPCR) expressed on the leukocyte surface. This leads to dissociation of Gαi from Gβγ. Gαi activates JAK2 and 3, which activates Vav1 and three guanosine nucleotide exchange factors for Rho: SOS1, ARHGEF1, and DOCK2. This results in activation of the small GTPase RhoA. Vav1 also participates in activating the small GTPases

Fig. 3. (*Continued*) Rac-1 and Rac-2. The Gβγ subunit activates P-Rex1, which also participates in activating Rac-1 and 2. Rac-1 and 2 activate PLCβ2 and 3, resulting in calcium flux (Ca^{2+}) and release of diacylglycerol (DAG). Both activate CalDAG-GEFI, the most important guanosine nucleotide exchange factor for Rap1. DAG also activates protein kinase C (PKC) that helps activate Rap1. Rac-1 and RhoA activate phospholipase D (PLD1), which in turn activates PIP5K1C. Rap1 also activates RapL, which activates Mst1 and may be involved in integrin activation. Molecules that are common to both the PSGL-1 and GPCR pathways are colored red and green. Unknown intermediate steps are indicated by question marks (?). Kindlin (in leukocytes: kindlin-3) is also required for integrin activation (blue), but nothing is known about how kindlin activation is triggered. Kindlin-3 binds integrin β chain at a site distinct from the talin binding site, but it is unclear how exactly kindlin affects integrin conformation.

$\alpha_E\beta_7$ is expressed on intraepithelial lymphocytes in the intestinal tract and on subsets of dendritic cells and T cells. It binds E-cadherin, a molecule expressed in epithelial cells. Hence, $\alpha_E\beta_7$ is thought to anchor leukocytes near or in epithelial cell monolayers. The α_E knockout mouse has no significant phenotype.

$\alpha_V\beta_3$ (CD51/CD61) is the only β_3 integrin expressed on leukocytes, also known as "Leukocyte Response Integrin". The other β_3 integrin is the platelet integrin $\alpha_{IIb}\beta_3$. $\alpha_V\beta_3$ is also expressed on endothelial cells. It binds fibronectin and other ligands. Its function on leukocytes is thought to enable activation of β_2 integrins, hence the name leukocyte response integrin.[17,18]

Activated lymphocytes express integrins that bind extracellular matrix molecules. Originally discovered as "very late antigens (VLA)" on T lymphocytes,[19] these integrins all have VLA names. Based on the expression pattern of their ligands, these integrins are thought to be important in lymphocyte migration in the interstitial space. With the exception of $\alpha_4\beta_1$ (see above), they are not involved in leukocyte adhesion to the endothelium. VLA-1 ($\alpha_1\beta_1$) and VLA-2 ($\alpha_2\beta_1$) are collagen receptors. Like β_2 integrins, they have I domains. The I domains contain the collagen binding sites. VLA-4 ($\alpha_4\beta_1$) and VLA-5 ($\alpha_5\beta_1$) are fibronectin receptors. They bind to different sites in the large fibronectin molecule: VLA-4 binds to the ILDV sequence and VLA-5 binds to the RGD sequence. VLA-6 ($\alpha_6\beta_1$) is a laminin receptor.

Neutrophils also express many of these VLAs, but they are stored in secretory granules and are expressed on the plasma membrane only after degranulation. Neutrophil $\alpha_6\beta_1$ integrin has been reported to be involved in transmigration through the vascular basement membrane.[20,21]

1.1.1. *Endothelial ligands for integrins*

InterCellular Adhesion Molecules (ICAMs) are the main ligands for β_2 integrins. ICAM-1 is expressed on all endothelial cells, where it is inducible (~3-fold) by inflammatory stimuli. ICAM-1 is also expressed on lymphocytes,[22] monocytes,[23] macrophages,[24] dendritic cells,[25] and neutrophils,[26] where it supports leukocyte–leukocyte aggregation. The LFA-1 interaction with ICAM-1 has a special role in stabilizing the immunological synapse[27] between a T cell and an antigen-presenting cell. On neutrophils, high-affinity (but not extended) LFA-1 has been shown to bind to ICAM-1 on the same cell, which constitutes a strong endogenous anti-adhesive mechanism. Several partial and complete ICAM-1 knockout mice have shown modest elevations in blood neutrophil numbers, suggesting that ICAM-1 is important but partially redundant with other adhesion molecules.[28]

ICAM-2 is expressed on endothelial cells and mouse,[29] but not human neutrophils. Its expression is not regulated by inflammatory stimuli. ICAM-3 is expressed on leukocytes, including human neutrophils, and involved in the endogenous anti-adhesive mechanism.[11] ICAM-4 was originally described as the Landsteiner–Wiener (LW) blood group antigen[30] and is expressed on red blood cells.[31] ICAM-4 is also a ligand for VLA-4[32] beside β_2 integrins. ICAM-5 is also known as telencephalin and expressed on neuronal cells.[33]

VCAM-1 is inducibly (~10-fold) expressed on endothelial cells, especially in arteries under pro-atherogenic conditions. VCAM-1 is also expressed on subsets of macrophages. Like $\alpha_4\beta_1$ integrin, the VCAM-1 knockout mouse is embryonic lethal because of failure of chorioallantoic fusion. Conditional knockout mice and antibody experiments have shown that VCAM-1 is of key importance for monocyte recruitment to atherosclerotic lesions.[34] It is also involved in lymphocyte homing to the central nervous system (CNS).

1.1.2. *ECM ligands for integrins*

The extracellular matrix is composed of collagens, fibronectin, fibrinogen, laminins, and elastin. Most collagens are bound by $\alpha_1\beta_1$ or $\alpha_2\beta_1$ and two of the four β_2 integrins (α_M and α_X, Table 1). Tissue fibronectin is adhesive for $\alpha_5\beta_1$. Fibrinogen bind three of the four β_2 integrins (α_M, α_X and α_D, Table 1). Most laminins bind $\alpha_6\beta_1$. Integrin-mediated adhesion is not required for leukocyte migration in tissues.[35] However, leukocytes and especially monocyte-derived macrophages can remodel interstitial extracellular matrix, for example, by contracting it, which is integrin-dependent.[36]

1.2. *Selectins*

Selectins are a small family of C-type lectins[37] that are involved in leukocyte rolling and signaling. Rolling is mediated by the rapid formation and breakage of transient bonds between the selectins and their glycoprotein ligands.[38]

L-selectin (CD62L) is expressed on all leukocytes. In monocytes, it is higher on classical (Ly-6C^{hi} in mice, CD14^{hi} in humans) than non-classical (Ly-6C^{lo} in mice, CD16+CD14^{lo} in humans) monocytes.[39–41] In lymphocytes, it is highest on naïve cells, and expression is lost after activation by both proteolytic shedding and transcriptional mechanisms. Proteolytic shedding by TNF-α-converting enzyme (TACE, also known as ADAM-17 or CD156b) is induced by inflammatory mediators. Soluble L-selectin is detectable in blood and has been proposed to be a biomarker, but is not currently used in clinical medicine. The function of soluble L-selectin, if any, is unknown.

Cell surface L-selectin is of key importance for naïve lymphocyte homing to lymph nodes and Peyer's patches. In L-selectin knockout mice, the recruitment defect is so severe that the lymph nodes are small and their structure is altered.[42] L-selectin binds to Peripheral node addressin (PNAd) on high endothelial venules. PNAd is a collection of glycoproteins characterized by a sulfated glucosamine.[43,44] Effectively, L-selectin ligand activity is regulated by the endothelial expression of glycosyl transferases and sulfotransferases. L-selectin also binds P-selectin glycoprotein ligand-1 (PSGL-1) on other leukocytes, which provides a mechanism for leukocyte–leukocyte interaction, also known as secondary tethering. On the neutrophil surface, L-selectin is in close proximity to PSGL-1, but does not appear to bind PSGL-1 in cis.[45] L-selectin is required for PSGL-1 signaling, a signaling pathway that ultimately leads to integrin extension.[46–48]

P-selectin (CD62P) is found in Weibel–Palade bodies of endothelial cells and α granules of platelets.[49] P-selectin is a homodimer. Secretagogues like histamine rapidly (~min) mobilize P-selectin by fusion of these granules with the plasma membrane. The phenotype of the P-selectin knockout mouse includes mild neutrophilia, suggesting that P-selectin is involved in baseline neutrophil trafficking. In many organs including the skin, skeletal muscle, and connective tissue, P-selectin is the main rolling molecule. The only known ligand for P-selectin is P-selectin glycoprotein ligand-1 (PSGL-1).[49]

E-selectin (CD62E) is not expressed on resting endothelial cells, but rapidly (1 h) induced by tumor necrosis factor (TNF) and other inflammatory stimuli by transcriptional mechanisms. E-selectin is mostly expressed on endothelial cells, but expression has been observed on some macrophages. E-selectin binds PSGL-1, but at a site different from the P-selectin binding site.[49,50] It also binds CD44 and ESL-1, a glycosylated FGF receptor.[49] The E-selectin knockout mouse has no spontaneous phenotype, but is protected from ischemic kidney injury.[51]

1.3. *Leukocyte ligands for selectins*

P-selectin glycoprotein ligand-1 (PSGL-1, CD162) was originally discovered as a ligand for P-selectin, but also binds L-selectin and

E-selectin. In addition, non-glycosylated PSGL-1 binds various chemokines.[52–54] The selectin binding affinity of PSGL-1 is regulated by glycosyl transferases and tyrosine sulfotransferases. Specifically, fucosyl transferase VII (FUT7) is critical for PSGL-1 binding to E-selectin, with a slight contribution of FUT4. Tyrosine sulfation improves the binding affinity of PSGL-1 for P-selectin and L-selectin. The phenotype of the PSGL-1 knockout mouse is similar to that of the P-selectin knockout mouse, suggesting that P-selectin binding is its most important function. PSGL-1 is expressed on all leukocytes, but is not functional on naïve T and B cells, because they lack expression of FUT7. FUT7 is rapidly induced in antigen-experienced T cells. FUT7 is constitutively expressed in myeloid cells, where PSGL-1 is constitutively active. In neutrophils, PSGL-1 binding is sufficient and probably required for β_2 integrin extension.[46–48] The signaling pathway from PSGL-1 engagement to β2 integrin extension has been studied in great detail.[45,47–49,55–61]

E-selectin also binds CD44 on leukocytes, but the glycosylation requirements have not been identified. A third ligand for E-selectin is ESL-1, a splice variant of an FGF receptor. Although one report suggested that PSGL-1, CD44, and ESL-1 account for all E-selectin binding to leukocytes, others have proposed that glycolipids can also bind E-selectin. Overall, E-selectin appears to be a promiscuous binder and mainly looks for glycoproteins decorated with sialyl-Lewis^x, a human blood group antigen that requires FUT7 expression. T-cell immunoglobulin and mucin domain 1 (TIM-1) is another reported ligand for P-selectin. It was reported to be involved in P-selectin-dependent T lymphocyte trafficking during inflammation and autoimmunity.[62]

1.4. *Immunoglobulin adhesion molecules*

JAM-A, B, C are short (2 Ig domains) transmembrane immunoglobulins mainly expressed on endothelial cells. They all support homotypic adhesion in trans, i.e., JAM-A binds JAM-A, JAM-B binds JAM-B, and JAM-C binds JAM-C. In addition, they can bind LFA-1 and Mac-1.[8,9,63–65]

Platelet-endothelial cell adhesion molecule-1 (PECAM-1, CD31) was the first endothelial adhesion molecule implicated in transendothelial migration. *In vitro* assays showed that human monocyte transmigration through endothelial monolayers was completely blocked by CD31 antibodies.[66] It came as a surprise when the CD31 knockout mouse had no leukocyte recruitment defect. Subsequently, it was shown that this is strongly dependent on the genetic background.[67] PECAM-1 binds PECAM-1 in trans. There is no evidence for other PECAM-1 ligands. The role of PECAM-1 in transendothelial migration has been studied in great detail and involves its recycling between intracellular stores and the plasma membrane.[165] The role of PECAM-1 on platelets is unknown. CD99 is a heavily O-glycosylated transmembrane protein that is also involved in transendothelial migration.[68]

2. Biomechanics of leukocytes adhesion under flow

In order to adhere to the endothelium, leukocytes must travel in the marginal zones of blood flow near the endothelial surface. Margination is a passive rheologic process governed by three mechanisms: red blood cell aggregation, leukocytes being pushed to the wall by overtaking erythrocytes, and a phenomenon that confines the streamlines of a small venule entering a large venule to a narrow zone near the endothelium.[38] Red cell aggregation only occurs in some species, and its importance in leukocyte recruitment is unknown. The other two margination mechanisms are operative in venules only. However, leukocyte rolling is inducible in large arteries. The mechanisms of margination in arteries, if any, are unknown.

Leukocyte adhesion has a strong preference for venules over arterioles. This is, in part, caused by preferential expression of P-selectin, E-selectin, and ICAM-1 in venules.[69] However, venules also have lower wall shear stress than arterioles, by a factor of 2–5. Wall shear stress is the force per unit area exerted by the flowing blood parallel to the endothelium in the direction of flow. It is measured in dyn/cm^2 or Pa, where 10 dyn/cm^2 = 1 Pa. The force on the leukocyte is approximately equal to the wall shear stress multiplied with the portion of its surface area that is exposed to the flow. So at 1 Pa (=1 N/m^2), a leukocyte with an area of 10 μm × 10 μm = 100 μm^2 experiences a force of 100 picoNewtons (1 pN is 10^{-12} N). The highest shear stress in mammals is observed in pre-capillary arterioles, where it can reach 10 Pa (100 dyn/cm^2). Although the blood flow velocity is highest in large arteries, shear stress is only intermediate, because their diameter is so large. Shear stress is directly proportional to flow velocity and blood viscosity and inversely proportional to vessel diameter. In large veins, wall shear stress can be very low (<0.1 Pa or <1 dyn/cm^2). Shear stress is also low in high endothelial venules of lymphatic organs.

Shear stress not only induces a forward force on the leukocyte, but also a torque. Torque is a force multiplied with a radius that tends to turn the object about its center. The torque is the main reason for leukocyte rolling. If there were only a forward force, leukocytes would slide, not roll. Rolling is a downstream rotational movement of leukocytes that is governed by a tenuous balance between the flow forces (wall shear stress times flow-exposed leukocyte surface area) and the molecular bonds. The binding of rolling leukocytes and endothelial cells is almost continuous, like a wheel rolling on a road. The slip, i.e., the difference in rotational and translational velocity, is very small, typically 2–5%.[70]

Neutrophils can form long, thin tethers in the rear. These structures distribute the load and facilitate rolling under shear.[71] Tethers can detach and form slings in front of the rolling neutrophil.[29,72] Slings can wrap around rolling cells and may contribute to more stable rolling under shear stress. The exact distribution of forces is still under active investigation, but rough estimates show that the typical number of 3–5 tethers per neutrophil can counterbalance the entire shear force and the entire torque.

Leukocyte arrest occurs when the adhesive forces are stronger than the propulsive shear forces and the torque. Typically, arrest happens when integrins are activated. However, arrest can also occur when wall shear stress drops, as may occur during inflammation, for example by thrombosis that impedes flow.

3. Adhesion cascade

The now classical adhesion cascade was first described in the 1990s, based on intravital microscopic observations. The elements of rolling, arrest, adhesion, spreading, and transendothelial migration were first defined for neutrophils, but have since been found to apply to other leukocytes as well. Differences in the specific adhesion molecules and chemoattractants that direct the trafficking of the various leukocyte subsets are detailed below.

Rolling is mediated by selectins, and its velocity can be modified (slowed) by transient β_2 or α_4 integrin binding. Slow rolling is induced by PSGL-1 engagement, which leads to β_2 integrin extension.[7,55] Although selectins are crucial for rolling, the viability of L-, P- and E-selectin triple knockout mice[73] demonstrate that rolling is not essential for survival.

Leukocyte arrest is usually triggered by integrin engagement. Integrin activation is most commonly triggered by chemokines and other chemoattractants. Many elements of the signaling pathway from the chemoattractant receptor (GPCR) to integrin activation are now known.[1,74,75]

After arrest, most leukocytes spread and migrate on the luminal surface of the endothelium. During spreading, integrins are engaged, and integrin outside–in signaling contributes to leukocyte activation. In HEV, spreading may not be necessary. Instead, naïve lymphocytes are engulfed by HEVs and transmigrate through the high endothelium in a transcellular fashion akin to transcytosis.

After spreading, neutrophils crawl[76,77] for short distances to find a suitable spot for transendothelial migration, which preferentially occurs at tricellular corners of endothelial cells or through the endothelial–endothelial contacts between two endothelial cells. The non-classical subset of monocytes (Ly6C^{lo}CX3CR1^{hi} in mice, CD14^{lo}CD16^{+} in humans) shows a characteristic patrolling behavior. They can migrate on the luminal surface of blood vessels for hundreds of microns, both in the direction of and against flow. There is evidence that classical monocytes are converted to non-classical monocytes through this migration on the endothelium by a Notch-dependent mechanism.[78]

Effector T lymphocytes also migrate along the endothelium, but with a bias in the upstream (against flow) direction. Most patrolling is LFA-1-dependent, but the details of the molecular mechanism and the biomechanics of patrolling are not known. Patrolling is thought to be an endothelial surveillance mechanism.[79]

When neutrophils find a suitable spot for transendothelial migration, they open the interendothelial junctions and traverse the endothelium to rest as flattened cells between the endothelium and the basement membrane. It takes about 10 min for a neutrophil to traverse the pericyte and basement membrane layers, which happens preferentially at "thin" spots with reduced laminin expression.[3] Neutrophils can also take a transendothelial pathway, but this is the exception rather than the rule.[80] By contrast, naïve lymphocytes routinely transcytose HEVs.[81] Little is known about the transendothelial migration of other leukocytes.

The adhesion cascade describes leukocyte adhesion in venules of many, but not all tissues. Skin venules certainly recruit leukocytes in this way. There is evidence that the leukocyte adhesion cascade is the mode of leukocyte recruitment in skeletal muscle, heart, connective tissue, the intestinal wall, joints, lymph nodes and Peyer's patches, bone marrow, and the meningeal microcirculation. However, the sequence of events, rolling, arrest, spreading, and transendothelial migration, is not strictly required. There are mouse models in which very little rolling is observed, yet leukocytes still get recruited and infiltrate tissues. To some extent, molecular defects in leukocyte adhesion are compensated by increased leukocyte numbers in the blood: if the adhesion cascade is disturbed, the bone marrow can adjust and put out more cells.[82] In fact, the neutrophilia observed in mice defective for individual leukocyte adhesion molecules provides an indirect measure of the importance of each of these molecules.[83] These compensatory mechanisms make the inflammatory system resilient.

3.1. *Deviations from the adhesion cascade*

Leukocyte adhesion does not proceed in the same way in all tissues. In the lung, no rolling is observed, and blocking or knocking out selectins has little or no effect on leukocyte recruitment to the lung.[2,84] In the liver, leukocyte recruitment in postcapillary venules follows the adhesion cascade, but many leukocytes enter the liver in sinusoids, where different adhesion mechanisms operate.[85–88] In the spleen, the circulatory system does not show the common arteriole-capillary-venule architecture. Very little is known about how leukocytes are recruited to the spleen. Knocking out or blocking selectins, integrins, or their ligands has little or no effect on the leukocyte content of the spleen. In the central nervous system, lymphocytes seem to stop abruptly, without prior rolling.[89,90]

4. Leukocyte subsets

Neutrophils are the front line cell for defense against bacterial, fungal, and viral intruders. Neutrophils roll on P-selectin (early) and E-selectin (within an hour after onset of inflammation). The main ligand for E- and P-selectin is PSGL-1. In PSGL-1 knockout mice, almost no P-selectin dependent rolling is observed, but the defect in E-selectin mediated rolling is minor. Triple blockade of PSGL-1, CD44, and ESL-1 abolishes almost all neutrophil rolling. Neutrophils express L-selectin and can enter inflamed lymph nodes by L-selectin–PNAd interactions. Most likely, L-selectin amplifies neutrophil recruitment by promoting interaction of neutrophils with already adherent neutrophils and with microparticles, both through L-selectin interactions with PSGL-1 in trans.[91] In neutrophils, L-selectin and PSGL-1 are both required for β_2 integrin extension.[45]

Neutrophils can arrest in response to the chemokines CXCL1, 2, 3, 5, 6, 7, and (in humans) 8, all of which bind CXCR1 and 2. They can also arrest in response to formyl peptides like N-formylmethionine-leucyl-phenylalanine (fMLP), which binds to formyl peptide receptor 1 (FPR1), complement C5a, which binds to CD88 (C5aR), and leukotriene B4, which binds to leukotriene B4 receptor 1 (BLTR1). Arrest is dependent on LFA-1 in mice. In human neutrophils, Mac-1 also contributes to arrest. The final steps of integrin activation leading to arrest involve talin-1 and kindlin-3 binding to the β_2 subunit.[92]

Neutrophils crawl in microvessels for limited distances (tens of microns) and then transmigrate. In mice, this crawling depends on Mac-1.[77] Neutrophil transendothelial migration is associated with their degranulation, which greatly increases the expression of Mac-1 and brings several β_1 integrins to the plasma membrane. Neutrophils use $\alpha_6\beta_1$ to traverse the basement membrane[20] and $\alpha_2\beta_1$ to migrate in the interstitial space.[93]

Naïve T and B cells have very restricted recruitment potential. They cannot bind to P- or E-selectin, because their PSGL-1 is not properly glycosylated. Their only rolling molecule is L-selectin, which mediates rolling on PNAd, expressed in lymph nodes. Their only adhesion molecule is LFA-1, which is activated when CCR7 encounters one of its ligands, CCL19 or CCL21. Thus, naïve lymphocytes can only traffic to secondary lymphatic organs.

T cells express either $\alpha\beta$ or $\gamma\delta$ T cell receptor (TCR). Those with $\alpha\beta$ receptors express either CD4 or CD8. CD4 T cells can differentiate to T-helper (Th) subsets known as Th1, Th2, Th17, TFH, and Treg, defined by characteristic transcription factors and cytokines. Th1, Th17, and Treg cells acquire functional PSGL-1 and can roll on both E- and P-selectin. Th2 cells have much less affinity for these selectins. Activated T cells lose L-selectin, but gain expression of many β_1 integrins (the VLAs), most prominently $\alpha_4\beta_1$. They also gain expression of CD44. Th1 cells typically arrest in response to the CXCR3 ligands CXCL9, 10, and 11. Some Th1 cells also express CCR5. Th2 cells express CLA, a ligand for E-selectin, and arrest in response to CCR4 ligands. Both Th17 and Treg cells express CCR6.

B cells can differentiate to plasma cells and produce antibodies of all isotypes. B cells express polymorphic B cell receptors (BCR), the CD45 isoform B220 and the immunoglobulin receptor CD19. When native B cells are exposed to antigens, they can be developed to at least five subsets:[94] the most abundant follicular B cells or B-2 cells ($CD5^-$, $CD19^{mid}$, $CD1d^{mid}$, $CD23^+$, $CD43^-$, IgM^{low}, IgD^{hi}), splenic marginal zone B cells ($CD5^-$, $CD19^{mid}$, $CD1d^{hi}$, $CD23^-$, $CD43^-$, IgM^{hi}, IgD^{low}), the two B-1 cell (the main producers of natural antibodies and participate in maintaining tissue homeostasis), subsets B-1a ($CD5^+$, $CD19^{hi}$, $CD1d^{mid}$, $CD23^-$, $CD43^+$, IgM^{hi},

IgD^{low}) and B-1b ($CD5^-$, $CD19^{hi}$, $CD1d^{mid}$, $CD23^-$, $CD43^+$, IgM^{hi}, IgD^{low}), and regulatory B cells ($CD5^+$, $CD19^{hi}$, $CD1d^{hi}$, $CD23^{+/-}$, $CD43^-$, IgM^{hi}, $IgD^{low/mid}$). B cells express L-selectin, which support rolling on PNAd or PSGL-1 under low shear stress. Most B cells express both LFA-1 and VLA-4 on their surface, which is critical for B cell recruitment to lymph nodes and tissues.[95] B cells also express low levels of α4β7 integrin.[96]

Monocytes comprise at least two subsets, classical and non-classical. The classical subset ($CD14^{hi}$ in humans, Ly-$6C^{hi}$ in mice) express functional PSGL-1 and can roll on P- and E-selectin. They arrest in response to CXCR2 ligands. Although these monocytes prominently express the chemokine receptor CCR2, its ligand CCL2 does not effectively induce arrest.[97] Classical monocyte adhesion occurs through β_2 and α_4 integrins. Not much is known about the adhesion mechanisms used by non-classical monocytes, but injecting an antibody to LFA-1 into mice detaches patrolling monocytes.[98]

Surprisingly little is known about adhesion and recruitment of NK cells.

Eosinophil arrest and recruitment to the airway in asthma are mediated, at least in part, by integrins, including $\alpha_4\beta_1$, $\alpha_6\beta_1$, $\alpha_L\beta_2$, $\alpha_M\beta_2$, $\alpha_X\beta_2$, $\alpha_D\beta_2$, and $\alpha_4\beta_7$.[99]

Basophils express $\alpha_2\beta_1$, $\alpha_4\beta_1$, $\alpha_5\beta_1$, $\alpha_L\beta_2$, $\alpha_M\beta_2$, and $\alpha_X\beta_2$.[100]

5. Leukocyte adhesion in lymphatics

Leukocyte adhesion is not only relevant in blood vessels, but also in lymphatics. Dendritic cells enter into terminal lymphatics and migrate along the lymphatic endothelium to the next lymph node, where they present antigens. The chemokine CCL21, expressed by lymphatic endothelial cells, is important for this process.[101] ICAM-1 and VCAM-1 are involved in the dendritic cell migration to draining lymph nodes,[102] indicating that integrin may be involved.

6. Leukocyte adhesion to thrombi

Monocytes and neutrophils adhere to thrombi. The molecular mechanisms include adhesion to fibrin (by αMβ2 integrin), to von

Willebrand factor, and to platelets by P-selectin interaction with platelet GPIbα and by Mac1 binding to fibrinogen which in turn binds to platelet αIIbβ3 integrin in a process called the fibrinogen bridge.[103] Also, platelet ICAM-2 can bind LFA-1 on leukocytes and leukocyte PSGL-1 binds platelet P-selectin. Monocyte interactions with thrombi are promoted by the chemokines CCL5 and CXCL4, which are highly expressed in platelets.[104] Monocyte and neutrophil recruitment to thrombi is normally important in resolving thrombi, but can also cause inflammation (thrombophlebitis). Activated monocytes express tissue factor, the initiator of the coagulation cascade, and therefore can have pro-thrombotic effects.[105,106]

7. Defects in leukocyte adhesion

There are four known leukocyte adhesion defect syndromes in humans, known as Leukocyte Adhesion Deficiencies (LAD). LAD-I is caused be defective (low or absent) expression of β_2 integrins[107,108] and has also been observed in many other species including dogs and cattle. LAD-II is caused by a defect in fucose transport, resulting in insufficient biosynthesis of selectin ligands.[109] LAD-III is caused by null mutations in kindlin-3, an adapter molecule that is involved in integrin activation.[110] LAD-IV only affects monocyte recruitment and is caused by mutations in CF, the gene that is defective in cystic fibrosis.[111,112] All LAD syndromes are autosomal recessive, meaning that the disease manifests only if both alleles are defective.

LAD-I affects hundreds of patients around the world. If β_2 integrin is completely absent (due to a deleterious mutation in the ITGB2 gene), the syndrome is severe. LAD-I babies present with a failure of the umbilical cord to separate and heal. In LAD-I, expression of ITGB2 ranges from 0% to 10% of normal; people with more than 10% ITGB2 have no clinical symptoms. One diagnostic finding is elevated neutrophil counts, probably due to the compensatory mechanisms mentioned above. Lymphocyte and monocyte counts are not elevated, likely because they express α4 integrins and thus are not as dependent on β_2 integrins as neutrophils.

LAD-II is extremely rare (~10 cases known). A null mutation in the fucose transporter[113,114] causes an almost complete absence of all functional selectin ligands. The clinical phenotype is dominated by mental developmental defects. LAD-II can be overcome by adding excess fucose to the diet, allowing a salvage pathway to transport enough fucose into cells to allow the fucosyl transferases to synthesize selectin ligands.

LAD-III is caused by an absence of kindlin-3 due to premature stops or missense mutations in the FERMT3 gene encoding kindlin-3. LAD-III affects neutrophils and platelets, so the clinical presentation is dominated by bleeding and susceptibility to bacterial and fungal infections. It seems that LFA-1 ($\alpha_L\beta_2$) and $\alpha_{IIb}\beta_3$ are particularly sensitive and cannot become activated in the absence of kindlin-3. Why other integrins are less affected or perhaps not affected at all is currently unknown.

LAD-IV was recently described in a single report.[111,112] Cystic fibrosis patients have a significant defect in monocyte recruitment to the lung and airways. This appears to be caused by an inability to activate $\alpha_4\beta_1$ integrin. Why $\alpha_4\beta_1$ is dependent on this ion channel is not known. If LAD-IV is present in all CF patients, this would be the most common leukocyte adhesion deficiency.

References

1. Ley K, Laudanna C, Cybulsky MI, Nourshargh S. (2007). Getting to the site of inflammation: the leukocyte adhesion cascade updated. *Nat Rev Immunol.* 7:678–689.
2. Kolaczkowska E, Kubes P. (2013). Neutrophil recruitment and function in health and inflammation. *Nat Rev Immunol.* **13**:159–175.
3. Nourshargh S, Alon R. (2014). Leukocyte migration into inflamed tissues. *Immunity.* **41**:694–707.
4. Alon R, Ley K. (2008). Cells on the run: shear-regulated integrin activation in leukocyte rolling and arrest on endothelial cells. *Curr Opin Cell Biol.* **20**:525–532.
5. Luo BH, Carman CV, Springer TA. (2007). Structural basis of integrin regulation and signaling. *Annu Rev Immunol.* **25**:619–647.
6. Arnaout MA, Goodman SL, Xiong JP. (2007). Structure and mechanics of integrin-based cell adhesion. *Curr Opin Cell Biol.* **19**:495–507.
7. Fan Z, Ley K. (2015). Leukocyte arrest: Biomechanics and molecular mechanisms of beta2 integrin activation. *Biorheology.*

8. Ostermann G, Weber KS, Zernecke A, Schroder A, Weber C. (2002). JAM-1 is a ligand of the beta(2) integrin LFA-1 involved in transendothelial migration of leukocytes. *Nat Immunol.* **3**:151–158.
9. Wojcikiewicz EP *et al.* (2009). LFA-1 binding destabilizes the JAM-A homophilic interaction during leukocyte transmigration. *Biophys J.* **96**:285–293.
10. Shimaoka M *et al.* (2003). Structures of the alpha L I domain and its complex with ICAM-1 reveal a shape-shifting pathway for integrin regulation. *Cell.* **112**:99–111.
11. Fan Z *et al.* (2016). Neutrophil recruitment limited by high affinity bent β2 integrin binding ligand in cis. *The Journal of Immunology.* **196**:119.115.
12. Arnaout MA, Mahalingam B, Xiong JP. (2005). Integrin structure, allostery, and bidirectional signaling. *Annu Rev Cell Dev Biol.* **21**:381–410.
13. Davis GE. (1992). The Mac-1 and p150,95 beta 2 integrins bind denatured proteins to mediate leukocyte cell-substrate adhesion. *Exp Cell Res.* **200**:242–252.
14. Wu H *et al.* (2004). Deficiency of CD11b or CD11d results in reduced staphylococcal enterotoxin-induced T cell response and T cell phenotypic changes. *J Immunol.* **173**:297–306.
15. de Azevedo-Quintanilha IG *et al.* (2016). Integrin alphaDbeta2 (CD11d/CD18) mediates experimental malaria-associated acute respiratory distress syndrome (MA-ARDS). *Malar J.* **15**:393.
16. Ley K, Rivera-Nieves J, Sandborn WJ, Shattil S. (2016). Integrin-based therapeutics: biological basis, clinical use and new drugs. *Nat Rev Drug Discov.* **15**:173–183.
17. Brown EJ, Goodwin JL. (1988). Fibronectin receptors of phagocytes. Characterization of the Arg-Gly-Asp binding proteins of human monocytes and polymorphonuclear leukocytes. *J Exp Med.* **167**:777–793.
18. Gresham HD, Adams SP, Brown EJ. (1992). Ligand binding specificity of the leukocyte response integrin expressed by human neutrophils. *J Biol Chem.* **267**:13895–13902.
19. Hemler ME, Jacobson JG, Brenner MB, Mann D, Strominger JL. (1985). VLA-1: A T cell surface antigen which defines a novel late stage of human T cell activation. *Eur J Immunol.* **15**:502–508.
20. Dangerfield J, Larbi KY, Huang MT, Dewar A, Nourshargh S. (2002). PECAM-1 (CD31) homophilic interaction up-regulates alpha6beta1 on transmigrated neutrophils in vivo and plays a functional role in the ability of alpha6 integrins to mediate leukocyte migration through the perivascular basement membrane. *J Exp Med.* **196**:1201–1211.
21. Dangerfield JP, Wang S, Nourshargh S. (2005). Blockade of alpha6 integrin inhibits IL-1beta- but not TNF-alpha-induced neutrophil transmigration in vivo. *J Leukoc Biol.* **77**:159–165.

22. Cox MA, Barnum SR, Bullard DC, Zajac AJ. (2013). ICAM-1-dependent tuning of memory CD8 T-cell responses following acute infection. *Proc Natl Acad Sci USA*. **110**:1416–1421.
23. Most J, Schwaeble W, Drach J, Sommerauer A, Dierich MP. (1992). Regulation of the expression of ICAM-1 on human monocytes and monocytic tumor cell lines. *J Immunol*. **148**:1635–1642.
24. Hubbard AK, Giardina C. (2000). Regulation of ICAM-1 expression in mouse macrophages. *Inflammation*. **24**:115–125.
25. Cumberbatch M, Peters SW, Gould SJ, Kimber I. (1992). Intercellular adhesion molecule-1 (ICAM-1) expression by lymph node dendritic cells: comparison with epidermal Langerhans cells. *Immunol Lett*. **32**:105–110.
26. Woodfin A *et al.* (2016). ICAM-1-expressing neutrophils exhibit enhanced effector functions in murine models of endotoxemia. *Blood*. **127**:898–907.
27. Springer TA, Dustin ML. (2012). Integrin inside-out signaling and the immunological synapse. *Curr Opin Cell Biol*. **24**:107–115.
28. Bullard DC *et al.* (2007). Intercellular adhesion molecule-1 expression is required on multiple cell types for the development of experimental autoimmune encephalomyelitis. *J Immunol*. **178**:851–857.
29. Sundd P *et al.* (2012). 'Slings' enable neutrophil rolling at high shear. *Nature*. **488**:399–403.
30. Bailly P *et al.* (1994). The LW blood group glycoprotein is homologous to intercellular adhesion molecules. *Proc Natl Acad Sci USA*. **91**:5306–5310.
31. Ihanus E, Uotila LM, Toivanen A, Varis M, Gahmberg CG. (2007). *Red-cell ICAM-4 is a ligand for the monocyte/macrophage integrin CD11c/CD18: characterization of the binding sites on ICAM-4*. Vol. 109.
32. Spring FA *et al.* (2001). Intercellular adhesion molecule-4 binds alpha(4) beta(1) and alpha(V)-family integrins through novel integrin-binding mechanisms. *Blood*. **98**:458–466.
33. Kilgannon P, Turner T, Meyer J, Wisdom W, Gallatin WM. (1998). Mapping of the ICAM-5 (telencephalin) gene, a neuronal member of the ICAM family, to a location between ICAM-1 and ICAM-3 on human chromosome 19p13.2. *Genomics*. **54**:328–330.
34. Mestas J, Ley K. (2008). Monocyte-endothelial cell interactions in the development of atherosclerosis. *Trends Cardiovasc Med*. **18**:228–232.
35. Sixt M, Hallmann R, Wendler O, Scharffetter-Kochanek K, Sorokin LM. (2001). Cell adhesion and migration properties of beta 2-integrin negative polymorphonuclear granulocytes on defined extracellular matrix molecules. Relevance for leukocyte extravasation. *J Biol Chem*. **276**:18878–18887.
36. Lu P, Takai K, Weaver VM, Werb Z. (2011). Extracellular matrix degradation and remodeling in development and disease. *Cold Spring Harb Perspect Biol*. **3**.

37. Ley K. (2003). The role of selectins in inflammation and disease. *Trends Mol Med.* **9**:263–268.
38. Sundd P, Pospieszalska MK, Cheung LS, Konstantopoulos K, Ley K. (2011). Biomechanics of leukocyte rolling. *Biorheology.* **48**:1–35.
39. Ley K, Miller YI, Hedrick CC. (2011). Monocyte and macrophage dynamics during atherogenesis. *Arterioscler Thromb Vasc Biol.* **31**:1506–1516.
40. Gerhardt T, Ley K. (2015). Monocyte trafficking across the vessel wall. *Cardiovasc Res.* **107**:321–330.
41. Quintar AA, Hedrick CC, Ley K. (2015). Monocyte phenotypes: when local education counts. *J Exp Med.* **212**:432.
42. Arbones ML. *et al.* (1994). Lymphocyte homing and leukocyte rolling and migration are impaired in L-selectin-deficient mice. *Immunity.* **1**:247–260.
43. Rosen SD. (2004). Ligands for L-selectin: homing, inflammation, and beyond. *Annu Rev Immunol.* **22**:129–156.
44. Hemmerich S, Rosen SD. (2000). Carbohydrate sulfotransferases in lymphocyte homing. *Glycobiology.* **10**:849–856.
45. Stadtmann A *et al.* (2013). The PSGL-1-L-selectin signaling complex regulates neutrophil adhesion under flow. *J Exp Med.* **210**:2171–2180.
46. Kuwano Y, Spelten O, Zhang H, Ley K, Zarbock A. (2010). Rolling on E- or P-selectin induces the extended but not high-affinity conformation of LFA-1 in neutrophils. *Blood.* **116**:617–624.
47. Zarbock A *et al.* (2008). PSGL-1 engagement by E-selectin signals through Src kinase Fgr and ITAM adapters DAP12 and FcR gamma to induce slow leukocyte rolling. *J Exp Med.* **205**:2339–2347.
48. Zarbock A, Lowell, CA, Ley, K. (2007). Spleen tyrosine kinase Syk is necessary for E-selectin-induced alpha(L)beta(2) integrin-mediated rolling on intercellular adhesion molecule-1. *Immunity.* **26**:773–783.
49. Zarbock A, Ley, K, McEver, RP, Hidalgo, A. (2011). Leukocyte ligands for endothelial selectins: specialized glycoconjugates that mediate rolling and signaling under flow. *Blood.* **118**:6743–6751.
50. McEver RP. (1997). Selectin-carbohydrate interactions during inflammation and metastasis. *Glycoconjugate Journal.* **14**:585–591.
51. Singbartl K, Ley K. (2000). Protection from ischemia-reperfusion induced severe acute renal failure by blocking E-selectin. *Critical Care Medicine.* **28**:2507–2514.
52. Veerman KM *et al.* (2007). Interaction of the selectin ligand PSGL-1 with chemokines CCL21 and CCL19 facilitates efficient homing of T cells to secondary lymphoid organs. *Nat Immunol.* **8**:532–539.
53. Bestebroer J *et al.* (2007). Staphylococcal superantigen-like 5 binds PSGL-1 and inhibits P-selectin-mediated neutrophil rolling. *Blood.* **109**: 2936–2943.

54. Hirata T *et al.* (2004). Human P-selectin glycoprotein ligand-1 (PSGL-1) interacts with the skin-associated chemokine CCL27 via sulfated tyrosines at the PSGL-1 amino terminus. *J Biol Chem.* **279**:51775–51782.
55. Zarbock A, Muller H, Kuwano Y, Ley K. (2009). PSGL-1-dependent myeloid leukocyte activation. *J Leukoc Biol.* **86**:1119–1124.
56. Mueller H *et al.* (2010). Tyrosine kinase Btk regulates E-selectin-mediated integrin activation and neutrophil recruitment by controlling phospholipase C (PLC) gamma2 and PI3Kgamma pathways. *Blood.* **115**: 3118–3127.
57. Stadtmann A *et al.* (2011). Rap1a activation by CalDAG-GEFI and p38 MAPK is involved in E-selectin-dependent slow leukocyte rolling. *Eur J Immunol.* **41**:2074–2085.
58. Block H *et al.* (2015). Gnb isoforms orchestrate a signaling pathway comprising Rac1 and Plcbeta2/3 leading to LFA-1 activation and neutrophil arrest in vivo. *Blood.* 2015: blood-2015-06-651034.
59. Herter JM, Rossaint J, Block H, Welch H, Zarbock A. (2013). Integrin activation by P-Rex1 is required for selectin-mediated slow leukocyte rolling and intravascular crawling. *Blood.* **121**:2301–2310.
60. Lefort CT *et al.* (2012). Distinct roles for talin-1 and kindlin-3 in LFA-1 extension and affinity regulation. *Blood.* **119**:4275–4282.
61. Herter J, Zarbock A. (2013). Integrin Regulation during Leukocyte Recruitment. *J Immunol.* **190**:4451–4457.
62. Angiari S *et al.* (2014). TIM-1 glycoprotein binds the adhesion receptor P-selectin and mediates T cell trafficking during inflammation and autoimmunity. *Immunity.* **40**:542–553.
63. Santoso S *et al.* (2002). The junctional adhesion molecule 3 (JAM-3) on human platelets is a counterreceptor for the leukocyte integrin Mac-1. *J Exp Med.* **196**:679–691.
64. Lamagna C *et al.* (2005). Dual interaction of JAM-C with JAM-B and alpha(M)beta2 integrin: function in junctional complexes and leukocyte adhesion. *Mol Biol Cell.* **16**:4992–5003.
65. Bradfield PF, Nourshargh S, Aurrand-Lions M, Imhof BA. (2007). JAM family and related proteins in leukocyte migration (Vestweber series). *Arterioscler Thromb Vasc Biol.* **27**:2104–2112.
66. Muller WA. (1995). The role of PECAM-1 (CD31) in leukocyte emigration: Studies in vitro and in vivo. *J Leukocyte Biol.* **57**:523–528.
67. Schenkel AR, Chew TW, Chlipala E, Harbord MW, Muller WA. (2006). Different susceptibilities of PECAM-deficient mouse strains to spontaneous idiopathic pneumonitis. *Exp Mol Pathol.* **81**:23–30.
68. Bixel MG *et al.* (2010). CD99 and CD99L2 act at the same site as, but independently of, PECAM-1 during leukocyte diapedesis. *Blood.* **116**: 1172–1184.

69. Jung U, Ley K. (1997). Regulation of E-selectin, P-selectin and ICAM-1 expression in mouse cremaster muscle vasculature. *Microcirculation.* **4**:311–319.
70. Tozeren A, Ley K. (1992). How do selectins mediate leukocyte rolling in venules? *Biophys J.* **63**:700–709.
71. Schmidtke DW, Diamond SL. (2000). Direct observation of membrane tethers formed during neutrophil attachment to platelets or P-selectin under physiological flow. *J Cell Biol.* **149**:719–730.
72. Sundd P, Pospieszalska MK, Ley K. (2012). Neutrophil rolling at high shear: Flattening, catch bond behavior, tethers and slings. *Mol Immunol.* 10.
73. Collins RG *et al.* (1999). Viable phenotype but impaired leukocyte rolling and peritoneal emigration in triple selectin (E, L and P) null mice. *Keystone Symposia.* **C4**:39.
74. Fan Z, Ley K. (2015). Leukocyte arrest: Biomechanics and molecular mechanisms of β2 integrin activation. *Biorheology.* In press.
75. Laudanna C, Alon R. (2006). Right on the spot. Chemokine triggering of integrin-mediated arrest of rolling leukocytes. *Thromb Haemost.* **95**:5–11.
76. Harding MG, Zhang K, Conly J, Kubes P. (2014). Neutrophil crawling in capillaries; a novel immune response to Staphylococcus aureus. *PLoS Pathog.* **10**:e1004379.
77. Phillipson M *et al.* (2006). Intraluminal crawling of neutrophils to emigration sites: a molecularly distinct process from adhesion in the recruitment cascade. *J Exp Med.* **203**:2569–2575.
78. Gamrekelashvili J *et al.* (2016). Regulation of monocyte cell fate by blood vessels mediated by Notch signalling. *Nat Commun.* **7**:12597.
79. Carlin LM *et al.* (2013). Nr4a1-Dependent Ly6C(low) Monocytes Monitor Endothelial Cells and Orchestrate Their Disposal. *Cell.* **153**:362–375.
80. Feng D, Nagy JA, Pyne K, Dvorak HF, Dvorak AM. (1998). Neutrophils emigrate from venules by a transendothelial cell pathway in response to fMLP. *J Exp Med.* **187**:903–915.
81. Galkina E *et al.* (2003). L-selectin shedding does not regulate constitutive T cell trafficking but controls the migration pathways of antigen-activated T lymphocytes. *J Exp Med.* **198**:1323–1335.
82. Stark MA *et al.* (2005). Phagocytosis of apoptotic neutrophils regulates granulopoiesis via IL-23 and IL-17. *Immunity.* **22**:285–294.
83. Forlow SB, Rose CE, Ley K. (2002). In *Interactions of Blood and the Pulmonary Circulation.* (eds E.K. Weir, H.L. Reeve, & J.T. Reeves) Ch. **16**, (Futura) pp. 255–275.
84. Zarbock A, Singbartl K, Ley K. (2006). Complete reversal of acid-induced acute lung injury by blocking of platelet-neutrophil aggregation. *J Clin Invest.* **116**:3211–3219.

85. McDonald B *et al.* (2010). Intravascular danger signals guide neutrophils to sites of sterile inflammation. *Science.* **330**:362–366.
86. Phillipson M, Kubes P. (2011). The neutrophil in vascular inflammation. *Nat Med.* **17**:1381–1390.
87. Slaba I *et al.* (2015). Imaging the dynamic platelet-neutrophil response in sterile liver injury and repair in mice. *Hepatology.* **62**:1593–1605.
88. Kolaczkowska E *et al.* (2015). Molecular mechanisms of NET formation and degradation revealed by intravital imaging in the liver vasculature. *Nat Commun.* **6**:6673.
89. Engelhardt B, Wolburg H. (2004). Mini-review: Transendothelial migration of leukocytes: Through the front door or around the side of the house? *Eur J Immunol.* **34**:2955–2963.
90. Engelhardt B *et al.* (2016). Vascular, glial, and lymphatic immune gateways of the central nervous system. *Acta Neuropathol.* **132**:317–338.
91. Sperandio M *et al.* (2003). P-selectin glycoprotein ligand-1 mediates L-selectin-dependent leukocyte rolling in venules. *J Exp Med.* **197**:1355–1363.
92. Moser M, Legate KR, Zent R, Fassler R. (2009). The tail of integrins, talin, and kindlins. *Science.* **324**:895–899.
93. Werr J *et al.* (2000). Integrin alpha(2)beta(1) (VLA-2) is a principal receptor used by neutrophils for locomotion in extravascular tissue. *Blood.* **95**:1804–1809.
94. Baumgarth N. (2011). The double life of a B-1 cell: self-reactivity selects for protective effector functions. *Nat Rev Immunol.* **11**:34–46.
95. Manevich-Mendelson E *et al.* (2010). Talin1 is required for integrin-dependent B lymphocyte homing to lymph nodes and the bone marrow but not for follicular B-cell maturation in the spleen. *Blood.* **116**:5907–5918.
96. Gorfu G *et al.* (2010). Beta7 integrin deficiency suppresses B cell homing and attenuates chronic ileitis in SAMP1/YitFc mice. *J Immunol.* **185**:5561–5568.
97. Huo Y *et al.* (2001). The chemokine KC, but not monocyte chemoattractant protein-**1**:triggers monocyte arrest on early atherosclerotic endothelium. *J Clin Invest.* **108**:1307–1314.
98. Auffray C *et al.* (2007). Monitoring of blood vessels and tissues by a population of monocytes with patrolling behavior. *Science.* **317**:666–670.
99. Johansson MW, Mosher DF. (2013). Integrin activation States and eosinophil recruitment in asthma. *Front Pharmacol.* **4**:33.
100. Sperr WR *et al.* (1992). Differential expression of cell surface integrins on human mast cells and human basophils. *Ann Hematol.* **65**:10–16.
101. Russo E, Nitschke M, Halin C. (2013). Dendritic cell interactions with lymphatic endothelium. *Lymphat Res Biol.* **11**:172–182.
102. Johnson LA *et al.* (2006). An inflammation-induced mechanism for leukocyte transmigration across lymphatic vessel endothelium. *J Exp Med.* **203**:2763–2777.

103. Ley K. (2006). in *Hemostasis and Thrombosis* (eds R.W. Colman *et al.*) Ch. **45**:691–706. Lippincott Williams & Wilkins.
104. Massberg S *et al.* (2002). A critical role of platelet adhesion in the initiation of atherosclerotic lesion formation. *J Exp Med.* **196**:887–896.
105. Owens AP 3rd, Mackman N. (2012). Role of tissue factor in atherothrombosis. *Curr Atheroscler Rep.* **14**:394–401.
106. Tatsumi K, Mackman N. (2015). Tissue Factor and Atherothrombosis. *J Atheroscler Thromb.* **22**:543–549.
107. Crowley CA *et al.* (1980). An inherited abnormality of neutrophil adhesion. Its genetic transmission and its association with a missing protein. *N Engl J Med.* **302**:1163–1168.
108. Etzioni A, Doerschuk CM, Harlan JM. (1999). Of man and mouse: leukocyte and endothelial adhesion molecule deficiencies [review]. *Blood.* **94**: 3281–3288.
109. Wild MK, Luhn K, Marquardt T, Vestweber D. (2002). Leukocyte Adhesion Deficiency II: Therapy and Genetic Defect. *Cells Tissues Organs.* **172**:161–173.
110. Alon R, Etzioni A. (2003). LAD-III, a novel group of leukocyte integrin activation deficiencies. *Trends Immunol.* **24**:561–566.
111. Fan Z, Ley K. (2016). Leukocyte Adhesion Deficiency IV. Monocyte Integrin Activation Deficiency in Cystic Fibrosis. *Am J Respir Crit Care Med.* **193**:1075–1077.
112. Sorio C *et al.* (2016). Mutations of cystic fibrosis transmembrane conductance regulator (CFTR) gene cause a monocyte-selective adhesion deficiency. *Am J Respir Crit Care Med.*
113. Lubke T *et al.* (2001). Complementation cloning identifies CDG-IIc, a new type of congenital disorders of glycosylation, as a GDP-fucose transporter deficiency. *Nat Genet.* **28**:73–76.
114. Etzioni A *et al.* (1993). Leukocyte adhesion deficiency (LAD) II: A new adhesion defect due to absence of sialyl Lewis X, the ligand for selectins. *Immunodeficiency.* **4**:307–308.
115. Fisher KL *et al.* (1997). Identification of the binding site in intercellular adhesion molecule 1 for its receptor, leukocyte function-associated antigen 1. *Mol Biol Cell.* **8**:501–515.
116. Lahti M, Heino J, Kapyla J. (2013). Leukocyte integrins alphaLbeta2, alphaMbeta2 and alphaXbeta2 as collagen receptors — receptor activation and recognition of GFOGER motif. *Int J Biochem Cell Biol.* **45**:1204–1211.
117. Rothlein R, Dustin ML, Marlin SD, Springer TA. (1986). A human intercellular adhesion molecule (ICAM-1) distinct from LFA-1. *J Immunol.* **137**:1270–1274.
118. Stanley P, Hogg N. (1998). The I Domain of Integrin LFA-1 Interacts with ICAM-1 Domain 1 at Residue Glu-34 but Not Gln-73. *Journal of Biological Chemistry.* **273**:3358–3362.

119. Makgoba MW *et al.* (1988). ICAM-1 a ligand for LFA-1-dependent adhesion of B, T and myeloid cells. *Nature.* **331**:86–88.
120. Staunton DE, Dustin ML, Springer TA. (1989). Functional cloning of ICAM-2,a cell adhesion ligand for LFA-1 homologous to ICAM-1. *Nature.* **339**:61–64.
121. Klickstein LB, York MR, Fougerolles AR, Springer TA. (1996). Localization of the binding site on intercellular adhesion molecule-3 (ICAM-3) for lymphocyte function-associated antigen 1 (LFA-1). *J Biol Chem.* **271**: 23920–23927.
122. Ihanus E *et al.* (2003). Characterization of ICAM-4 binding to the I domains of the CD11a/CD18 and CD11b/CD18 leukocyte integrins. *Eur J Biochem.* **270**:1710–1723.
123. Bailly P, Tontti E, Hermand P, Cartron J-P, Gahmberg CG (1995). The red cell LW blood group protein is an intercellular adhesion molecule which binds to CD11/CD18 leukocyte integrins. *European Journal of Immunology.* **25**:3316–3320.
124. Tian L *et al.* (2000). Binding of T lymphocytes to hippocampal neurons through ICAM-5 (telencephalin) and characterization of its interaction with the leukocyte integrin CD11a/CD18. *European Journal of Immunology.* **30**:810–818.
125. Tian L *et al.* (2008). Shedded neuronal ICAM-5 suppresses T-cell activation. *Blood.* **111**:3615–3625.
126. Bechard D *et al.* (2001). Human endothelial-cell specific molecule-1 binds directly to the integrin CD11a/CD18 (LFA-1) and blocks binding to intercellular adhesion molecule-1. *J Immunol.* **167**:3099–3106.
127. Tian L, Yoshihara Y, Mizuno T, Mori K, Gahmberg CG. (1997). The neuronal glycoprotein telencephalin is a cellular ligand for the CD11a/CD18 leukocyte integrin. *J Immunol.* **158**:928–936.
128. Parkos CA *et al.* (1996). Expression and polarization of intercellular adhesion molecule-1 on human intestinal epithelia: consequences for CD11b/CD18-mediated interactions with neutrophils. *Mol Med.* **2**:489–505.
129. Diamond MS *et al.* (1990). ICAM-1 (CD54): a counter-receptor for Mac-1 (CD11b/CD18). *J Cell Biol.* **111**:3129–3139.
130. Diamond MS, Staunton DE, Marlin SD, Springer TA. (1991). Binding of the integrin Mac-1 (CD11b/CD18) to the third immunoglobulin-like domain of ICAM-1 (CD54) and its regulation by glycosylation. *Cell.* **65**:961–971.
131. Xie J *et al.* (1995). Intercellular adhesion molecule-2 (CD102) binds to the leukocyte integrin CD11b/CD18 through the A domain. *J Immunol.* **155**:3619–3628.
132. Kim HY, Skokos EA, Myer DJ, Agaba P, Gonzalez AL. (2014). Alphabeta Integrin Regulation of Respiratory Burst in Fibrinogen Adherent Human Neutrophils. *Cell Mol Bioeng.* **7**:231–242.

133. Altieri DC, Bader R, Mannucci PM, Edgington TS. (1988). Oligospecificity of the cellular adhesion receptor Mac-1 encompasses an inducible recognition specificity for fibrinogen. *J Cell Biol.* **107**:1893–1900.
134. Wright SD *et al.* (1988). Complement receptor type three (CD11b/CD18) of human polymorphonuclear leukocytes recognizes fibrinogen. *Proc Natl Acad Sci USA.* **85**:7734–7738.
135. Plescia J, Altieri DC. (1996). Activation of Mac-1 (CD11b/CD18)-bound factor X by released cathepsin G defines an alternative pathway of leucocyte initiation of coagulation. *Biochem J.* **319(Pt 3)**:873–879.
136. Beller DI, Springer TA, Schreiber RD. (1982). Anti-Mac-1 selectively inhibits the mouse and human type three complement receptor. *J Exp Med.* **156**:1000–1009.
137. Diamond MS, Alon R, Parkos CA, Quinn MT, Springer TA. (1995). Heparin is an adhesive ligand for the leukocyte integrin Mac-1 (CD11b/CD18). *J Cell Biol.* **130**:1473–1482.
138. Simon DI *et al.* (2000). Platelet glycoprotein ibalpha is a counterreceptor for the leukocyte integrin Mac-1 (CD11b/CD18). *J Exp Med.* **192**:193–204.
139. Wetzel A *et al.* (2004). Human Thy-1 (CD90) on activated endothelial cells is a counterreceptor for the leukocyte integrin Mac-1 (CD11b/CD18). *J Immunol.* **172**:3850–3859.
140. Lishko VK, Novokhatny VV, Yakubenko VP, Skomorovska-Prokvolit HV, Ugarova TP. (2004). *Characterization of Plasminogen as an Adhesive Ligand for Integrins αMβ2 (Mac-1) and α5β1 (VLA-5).* Vol. 104.
141. Fink K *et al.* (2013). Mac-1 directly binds to the endothelial protein C-receptor: a link between the protein C anticoagulant pathway and inflammation? *PLoS One.* **8**:e53103.
142. Cai TQ, Wright SD. (1996). Human leukocyte elastase is an endogenous ligand for the integrin CR3 (CD11b/CD**18**,Mac-**1**,alpha M beta 2) and modulates polymorphonuclear leukocyte adhesion. *J Exp Med.* **184**:1213–1223.
143. Schober JM. *et al.* (2002). Identification of integrin alpha(M)beta(2) as an adhesion receptor on peripheral blood monocytes for Cyr61 (CCN1) and connective tissue growth factor (CCN2): immediate-early gene products expressed in atherosclerotic lesions. *Blood.* **99**:4457–4465.
144. Schober JM, Lau LF, Ugarova TP, Lam SC. (2003). Identification of a novel integrin alphaMbeta2 binding site in CCN1 (CYR61), a matricellular protein expressed in healing wounds and atherosclerotic lesions. *J Biol Chem.* **278**:25808–25815.
145. Zhang L, Plow EF. (1997). Identification and reconstruction of the binding site within alphaMbeta2 for a specific and high affinity ligand, NIF. *J Biol Chem.* **272**:17558–17564.

146. Zirlik A *et al.* (2007). CD40 ligand mediates inflammation independently of CD40 by interaction with Mac-1. *Circulation.* **115**:1571–1580.
147. Johansson MW, Patarroyo M, Oberg F, Siegbahn A, Nilsson K. (1997). Myeloperoxidase mediates cell adhesion via the alpha M beta 2 integrin (Mac-1:CD11b/CD18). *J Cell Sci.* **110**(Pt 9):1133–1139.
148. Podolnikova NP, Podolnikov AV, Haas TA, Lishko VK, Ugarova TP. (2015). Ligand recognition specificity of leukocyte integrin alphaMbeta2 (Mac-1,CD11b/CD18) and its functional consequences. *Biochemistry.* **54**:1408–1420.
149. Benimetskaya L *et al.* (1997). Mac-1 (CD11b/CD18) is an oligodeoxynucleotide-binding protein. *Nat Med.* **3**:414–420.
150. Frick C *et al.* (2005). Interaction of ICAM-1 with β2-integrin CD11c/CD18: Characterization of a peptide ligand that mimics a putative binding site on domain D4 of ICAM-1. *Eur J Immunol.* **35**:3610–3621.
151. Choi J, Choi J, Nham S-U. (2010). Characterization of the residues of αX I-domain and ICAM-1 mediating their interactions. *Molecules Cells.* **30**:227–234.
152. Sadhu C *et al.* (2007). CD11c/CD18: novel ligands and a role in delayed-type hypersensitivity. *J Leukoc Biol.* **81**:1395–1403.
153. Loike JD *et al.* (1991). CD11c/CD18 on neutrophils recognizes a domain at the N terminus of the A alpha chain of fibrinogen. *Proce Nat Acad Sci.* **88**:1044–1048.
154. Postigo AA, Corbí AL, Sánchez-Madrid F, de Landázuri MO. (1991). Regulated expression and function of CD11c/CD18 integrin on human B lymphocytes. Relation between attachment to fibrinogen and triggering of proliferation through CD11c/CD18. *The J Exp Med.* **174**:1313–1322.
155. Sen M, Yuki K, Springer TA. (2013). An internal ligand-bound, metastable state of a leukocyte integrin, alphaXbeta2. *J Cell Biol.* **203**:629–642.
156. Myones BL, Dalzell JG, Hogg N, Ross GD. (1988). Neutrophil and monocyte cell surface p150,95 has iC3b-receptor (CR4) activity resembling CR3. *The J Clin Invest.* **82**:640–651.
157. Vorup-Jensen T *et al.* (2007). Binding between the Integrin αXβ2 (CD11c/CD18) and Heparin. *J Biol Chem.* **282**:30869–30877.
158. Yakubenko VP *et al.* (2013). *Platelet-Leukocyte Conjugation Mediated By GPIbα-αXβ2 (CD11c/CD18) Interaction.* Vol. 122.
159. Choi J, Leyton L, Nham S-U. (2005). Characterization of αX I-domain binding to Thy-1. *Biochem Biophys Res Commun.* **331**:557–561.
160. Jongyun G, Jeongsuk C, Joo Hee L, Sang-Uk N. (2007). Identification of Critical Residues for Plasminogen Binding by the αX I-domain of the β2 integrin, αXβ2. *Mol Cells.* **24**:240–246.
161. Van der Vieren M *et al.* (1995) A novel leukointegrin, αdβ2,binds preferentially to ICAM-3. *Immunity.* **3**:683–690.

162. Grayson MH *et al.* (1998). alphadbeta2 integrin is expressed on human eosinophils and functions as an alternative ligand for vascular cell adhesion molecule 1 (VCAM-1). *J Exp Med.* **188**:2187–2191.
163. Van der Vieren M *et al.* (1999). The leukocyte integrin alpha D beta 2 binds VCAM-1: evidence for a binding interface between I domain and VCAM-1. *J Immunol.* **163**:1984–1990.
164. Yakubenko VP, Yadav SP, Ugarova TP. (2006). Integrin alphaDbeta**2**, an adhesion receptor up-regulated on macrophage foam cells, exhibits multiligand-binding properties. *Blood.* **107**:1643–1650.
165. Mamdouh Z, Chen X, Pierini LM, Maxfield FR, Muller WA. (2003). Targeted recycling of PECAM from endothelial surface-connected compartments during diapedesis. *Nature* **421**:748–753.

Chapter 6

Neutrophil Extracellular Traps

Tobias A. Fuchs*, Abdul Hakkim† and Constantin F. Urban‡

1. Introduction

Neutrophils release DNA filaments to form extracellular lattices known as neutrophil extracellular traps (NETs, Fig. 1). NETs were first described in 2004 as a measure to trap and kill bacteria during infection.[1] Today, NETs are fundamentally integrated in infectious or sterile inflammatory conditions. Here, we summarize the major findings of basic and translational research on NETs in the past decade. We provide an overview of the architecture and composition of NETs, the biology of NET formation and clearance, as well as how NETs contribute to infection, tissue injury, thrombosis, and autoimmunity.

*University Medical Center Hamburg-Eppendorf. E-mail: t.fuchs@uke.de
†Massachusetts General Hospital and Harvard Medical School. E-mail: hakkim@molbio.mgh.harvard.edu
‡Umeå University. E-mail: constantin.urban@umu.se

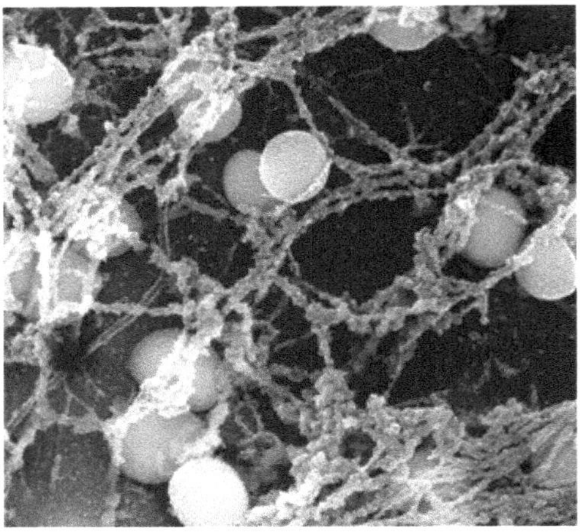

Fig. 1. Neutrophil extracellular traps. Electron micrograph of Neutrophil Extracellular Traps with entangled *Staphylococcus aureus*. Cover art from © Brinkmann *et al.*[1] Reproduced with permission.

1.1. *Introduction of neutrophils*

The life of a neutrophil begins in the bone marrow with the commitment of a hematopoietic stem cell to the myeloid linage.[2,3] During the development of a myeloblast to a mature neutrophil, the cytoplasm fills with storage granules, which carry ready-made enzymes and peptides. Prominent examples of granular proteins are the serine protease neutrophil elastase (NE) and components of the NAPDH oxidase, a reactive oxygen species (ROS)-producing enzyme. Further in neutrophil development, euchromatin shifts progressively to highly condensed and transcriptionally inactive heterochromatin, which is stored in a multi-lobulated nucleus in mature cells. Neutrophils entering the sinus of the bone marrow are short lived and terminally differentiated cells. In blood, neutrophils are not capable of cell division or differentiation, but are fully equipped to promptly take part in the inflammatory response. Indeed, neutrophils are the first leukocytes which are recruited to sites of inflammation.[4,5] This immediate response is ensured by constant surveillance of neutrophils for inflammatory markers expressed on the vascular endothelium.[6] After binding the inflamed endothelium, neutrophils leave the bloodstream and migrate to sites of infection or sterile inflammation. During their passage through tissue, some granules fuse with the plasma membrane to release NE into the extracellular environment. Extracellular NE is immobilized and concentrated on the cell surface to enable an efficient degradation of the extracellular matrix and thus increase the mobility of neutrophils.[7] At the site of inflammation, neutrophils become fully activated and internalize microbes or sterile particles into a phagosome.[8] Along with macrophages, neutrophils are considered professional phagocytes. The phagocytic uptake is a specialized and well-orchestrated mechanism, which allows only traces of external medium to enter the cell, while granules are intensively discharged into the phagosome. Within the phagosomal compartment, granular proteins as well as ROS produced by NADPH oxidase reach locally high concentrations, which allow the efficient destruction of the internalized material.

1.2. *Discovery of NETs*

Pathogenic bacteria have evolved mechanisms to evade phagocytic killing. *Shigella flexneri*, the causative agent of bacterial dysentery, can escape from the phagosome in macrophages. This process is mediated by Ipa (invasion plasmid antigens), virulence proteins secreted by *S. flexneri*. Dr. Arturo Zychlinsky and colleagues uncovered that *S. flexneri* is entrapped and subsequently killed within the neutrophil phagosome due to the degradation of Ipa proteins by NE.[9] The antimicrobial activity of NE is not restricted to *S. flexneri*. Instead NE selectively degrades virulence factors of multiple bacterial pathogens. Microscopic analysis of extracellular NE on stimulated neutrophils by Dr. Volker Brinkmann revealed that NE in part localizes in unconventional extracellular structures comprising DNA and histones (Fig. 2, Box 1).[1] These structures were termed Neutrophil

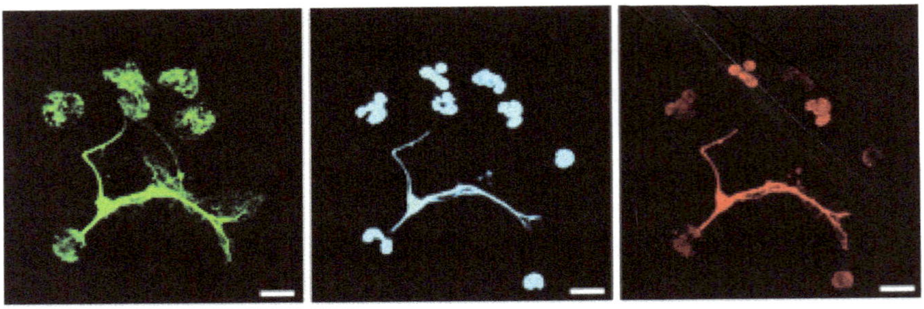

Fig. 2. Definition of Neutrophil Extracellular Traps. Activated neutrophils release extracellular fibers composed of granular components like elastase (a), DNA (b), and histones (c). Bars equal 10 μm. Reproduced with permission from © Brinkmann *et al.*[1]

Box 1. Definition of neutrophil extracellular traps (NETs)

- NETs are released by stimulated neutrophils
- DNA builds the structural backbone of NETs
- NET-DNA is associated with histones and granular proteins

Extracellular Traps (NETs) due to their ability to immobilize bacteria and disarm virulence factors in the extracellular environment.

2. Architecture and composition of NETs

Scanning electron microscopy illustrated the fine architecture of NETs. The main structural component of NETs are smooth filaments with interspersed globules, which resemble "beads-on-a-string" (Fig. 3).[1,10] The smooth stretches measure approximately 5 nm in width and 10 nm in depth, while globular domains are about 25–50 nm in diameter. Multiple strings can be combined to from thicker fibers, which likely provide a stable scaffold for the thinner elements. The overall structure appears like delicate webs, which inspired the acronym "NETs". The lattice-like appearance is often used to reference NETs as neutrophil "spider webs" or "fishing nets".

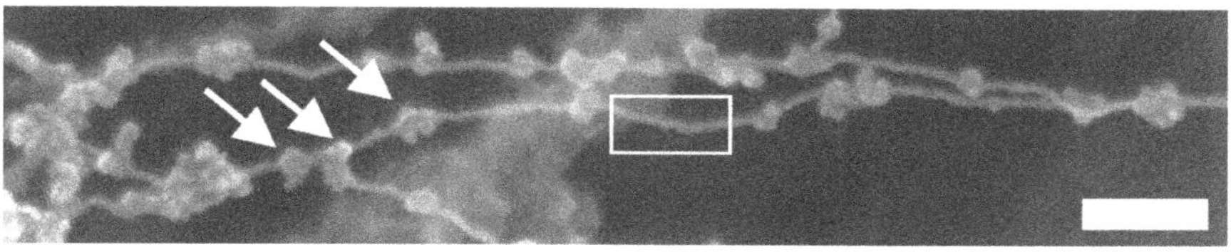

Fig. 3. Fine architecture of NETs. Scanning electron microscopy of NETs revealed a delicate beads-on-a-string morphology. Globular domains (arrows) are connected thin and smooth stretches (box). Scale bar = 100 nm. Reproduced with permission from © Urban CF *et al.*[10]

DNA is the major component of NETs.[1] It is organized as double-stranded DNA because several DNA-intercalating dyes label NETs. Furthermore, the integrity of NETs is efficiently destroyed by deoxyribonuclease1 (DNase1), which preferentially degrades double-stranded DNA. Proteases and phosphatases do not compromise the structure of NETs, supporting the concept of NETs as a DNA scaffold. Histones are the second major element of NETs. Histones are proteins that fold DNA strands into nucleosomes and higher-order structures of chromatin. Nucleosomes, the basic building blocks of chromatin, comprise approximately 180 base pairs of DNA wrapped around a core of double represented histone proteins H2A, H2B, H3, and H4. A linker DNA of 10 to 100 bp connects nucleosomes. Quantitative and qualitative analysis identified that core histones account for up to 70% of all proteins in NETs (Box 2).[10] Histones and DNA in NETs are likely organized in nucleosomal structure given that smooth threads in NETs have the dimensions of unfolded strings of nucleosomes. Histone H1 is present in NETs but only in trace amounts.[1] Histone H1 binds to the linker DNA and is important for additional chromatin folding. Consequently, the low abundance of histone H1 explains the highly unfolded nature of DNA in NETs. Micrococcal nuclease (MNase) is a bacterial DNase which cleaves the linker DNA between nucleosomes. MNase does not act upon folded DNA because histone H1 bound to linker DNA inhibits its action. MNase efficiently cleaves NETs into DNA fragments of 180 base pairs and multiples thereof,

Box 2. Most abundant neutrophil proteins in NETs

- Nuclear Proteins: Histones (H2A, H2B, H3, H4)
- Granular Proteins: Neutrophil elastase, Lactoferrin, Azurocidin, Cathepsin G, Myeloperoxidase, Proteinase 3
- Cytosolic Proteins: MRP8/14 (Calprotectin)

confirming that unfolded strings of nucleosomes are the backbone of NETs.[11]

Granular enzymes and peptides are second in abundance to histones and account for up to 20% of NET-proteins.[10] Neutrophils contain three types of granules with distinct protein loads, which are named according to their appearance in neutrophil development. NETs contain proteins from primary granules (also known as azurophilic granules) e.g., neutrophil serine proteases (NE, Cathepsin G and Proteinase 3), myeloperoxidase (MPO), bactericidal/permeability-increasing protein and azurocidin; from secondary granules (specific granules) e.g., lactoferrin, lysozyme, the antimicrobial peptide hCAP-18/LL-37, and pentraxin 3.[12] Gelatinase from tertiary granules was also identified in NETs.[1] Therefore, NETs contain proteins from all types of neutrophil granules. Importantly, neutrophil granular enzymes such as NE and MPO retain their catalytic activity within NETs and contribute to NET functions.[1,13]

NETs exclude almost all cytosolic proteins.[1,10] However, calprotectin (MRP8/14), a heterocomplex with zinc chelating and potent antifungal activity, is present in NETs. In addition, traces of actin are found in NETs as well. Membrane proteins are absent in NETs.[1,10] Indeed, transmission electron microscopy showed that NET-filaments are not surrounded by membranes.[1] In summation, NETs are a filamentous scaffold of unfolded DNA strands which are wrapped around a histone core and are associated with a small number of different neutrophil proteins. Importantly, more than 95% of the proteins in NETs, including histones,[14] are known to exhibit antimicrobial functions.

3. Formation of NETs

Neutrophils form NETs by distinct cellular mechanisms which share the requirement for neutrophil stimulation, but differ in the origin of NET-DNA, the composition of NETs, and the fate of netting neutrophils.[15–17] NET formation was first introduced as an active cell death program which culminates in the extrusion of chromatin-derived NETs.[11] This process of NET formation was termed NETosis in analogy to cell death by apoptosis or necrosis.[18] More recent discoveries illustrate that viable neutrophils actively release chromatin or mitochondrial DNA to form NETs.[19,20] The prepositions *suicidal* and *vital* are used to distinguish the different mechanisms of NETosis.[17]

3.1. *Suicidal NETosis*

Suicidal NETosis encompasses different stages with characteristic granular and nuclear morphologies (Fig. 4).[11,21] Suicidal NETosis is initiated by the activation of a naïve neutrophil. Briefly after stimulation, granules are still dispersed in the cytoplasm and the lobulated nucleus is rich in heterochromatin (Fig. 5). Prolonged stimulation leads to the delobulation of the nucleus, while chromatin remains condensed and the nuclear and granular membranes are intact. Further stimulation causes the disintegration of granules and releases their content into the cytoplasm. Granular proteins translocate from the cytoplasm to the nucleus, followed by the breakdown of the

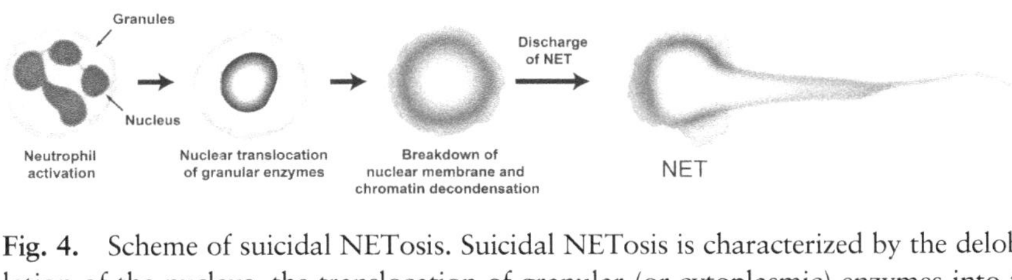

Fig. 4. Scheme of suicidal NETosis. Suicidal NETosis is characterized by the delobulation of the nucleus, the translocation of granular (or cytoplasmic) enzymes into the nucleus, the breakdown of the nuclear envelope, the decondensation of chromatin, and the disintegration of the plasma membrane to discharge NETs. Reproduced with permission from Fuchs *et al.* © Arterioscler Thromb Vasc Biol. 2012. 32(8): 1777–83.

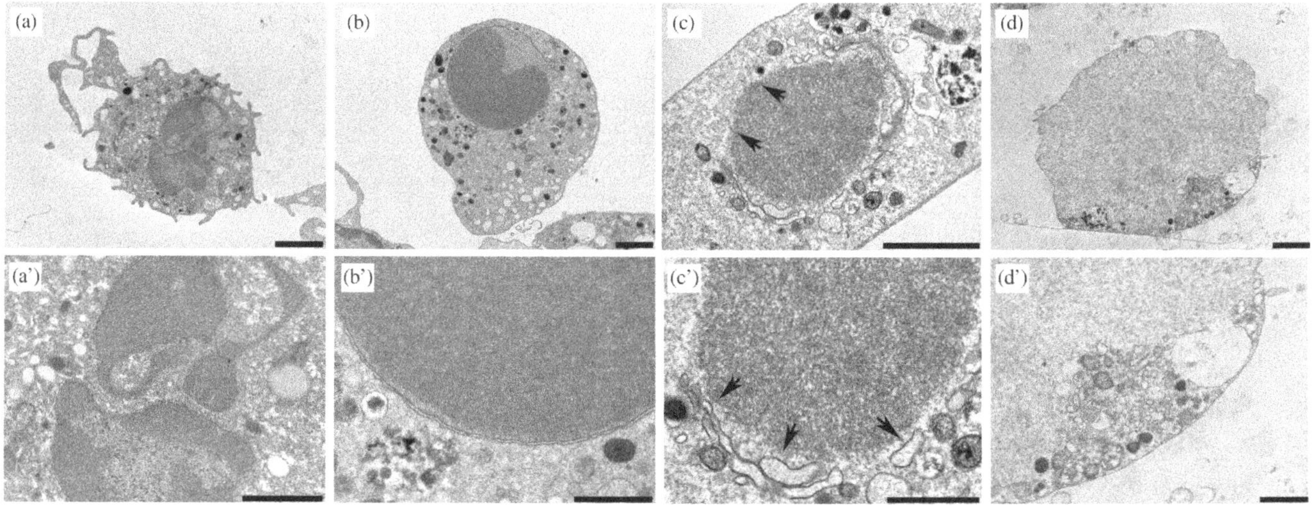

Fig. 5. Hallmarks of suicidal NETosis. Electron micrographs of (a, a′) a naïve neutrophil; (b, b′) a stimulated meutrophil with a delobulated nucleus, (c) nuclear envelope breakdown, (c′) arrows point toward vesicles from the nuclear membrane and (d) an anucleated neutrophil with decondensed chromatin, and (d′) reminiscent organelles. Time from A to D: approximately 4 hours. Scale Bars = 2 μm. Reproduced with permission from © Fuchs *et al.*[11]

nuclear envelope and the unfolding of chromatin. In the absence of internal membranes, chromatin and granular content is distributed homogenously over the entire cell. The plasma membrane appears intact and prevents the diffusion of proteins into the extracellular environment. At this stage, unfolded chromatin is selectively loaded with granular and cytoplasmic content to assemble NET components intracellularly.

How NETs are released into the extracellular space is best illustrated by filming individual neutrophils during NETosis in the presence of a cell-impermeable fluorescent DNA dye (Fig. 6).[11,22] After stimulation, neutrophils flatten and appear like "fried eggs" with abundant cytoplasmic vacuoles. Further stimulation leads to the abovementioned delobulation and breakdown of the nucleus as well as chromatin decondensation. DNA is not exposed at this point. In the final stages of NETosis, neutrophils detach from the surface and the plasma membrane ruptures to liberate NETs as evidenced by fluorescent dye staining the DNA. Furthermore, these movies show the difference between NETosis and apoptosis and necrosis.[23] Necrosis is an uncontrolled cell death which is provoked by external stimuli. Necrosis is characterized by the disintegration of the plasma membrane and the exposure of intracellular components, features which are also present in NETosis.

Apoptosis is a silent form of cell death which is designed to limit the exposure of intracellular components to the extracellular environment. A hallmark of apoptosis is the exposure of phosphatidylserine (PS) on the cell surface of intact cells. PS is usually localized to the inner leaflet of the cell membrane, but flips to the outer leaflet in apoptotic cells. PS acts as an "eat-me-signal" and mediates the phagocytosis of apoptotic cells by macrophages. However in the absence of phagocytic clearance, the plasma membrane of apoptotic cells becomes corrupted and releases intracellular contents in a process termed secondary necrosis. To discriminate NETosis from apoptosis and necrosis, the imaging of neutrophils includes an extracellular fluorescent ligand of PS. Using this setup, senescent neutrophils undergoing apoptosis are visualized due to exposure of PS on intact plasma membranes. Necrosis in these cells is illustrated

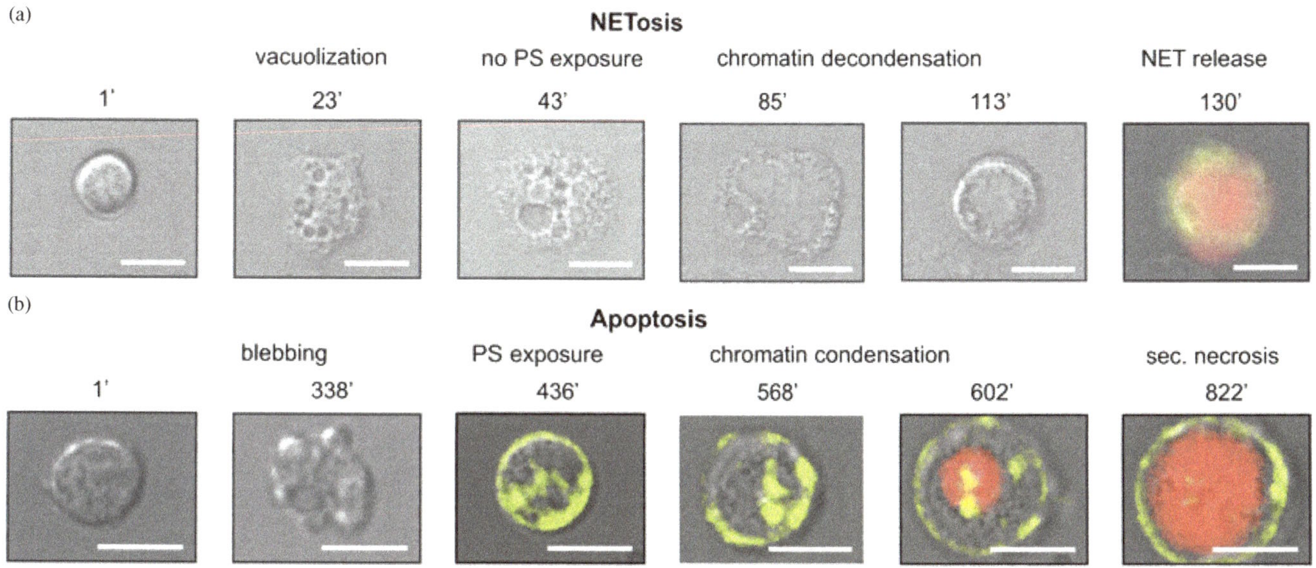

Fig. 6. Live cell imaging of NETosis and apoptosis: (a) NETosis is characterized by chromatin decondensation within viable activated neutrophils as evidenced by absent propidium iodide (PI; red) and PS exposure (AnnexinV, green) staining. NETs are released upon rupture of the plasma membrane indicated by a simultaneous staining for PI and Annexin V (130'). (b) Apoptosis leads to PS exposure (Annexin V staining at 436') prior to the loss of the plasma membrane integrity (PI staining at 602'). Chromatin decondensation occurs after cell death in secondary necrotic neutrophils (822'). Scale bars = 10 μm. Reproduced with permission from © Remijsen *et al.*[23]

by a perforated plasma membrane leading to a staining of DNA in the nucleus. At this stage, the nucleus is delobulated and chromatin is compact despite the broken plasma membrane. The chromatin eventually unfolds leading to a morphology that appears similar to neutrophils post NETosis. However, important differences between necrotic and NETotic neutrophils exist. In NETosis, chromatin decondensation occurs in viable neutrophils with an intact plasma membrane, which may be required for the intracellular assembly of NETs. In necrosis (following apoptosis), the unfolding of chromatin occurs after the perforation of the plasma membrane. Granular and cytoplasmic components may diffuse into the extracellular environment not allowing association with unfolded chromatin.

Importantly, comparison of the subcellular structure of apoptotic, necrotic, and NETotic neutrophils revealed that the breakdown of the nuclear envelope in intact neutrophils is a hallmark of NETosis (Fig. 7). Electron micrographs of apoptotic neutrophils illustrate delobulated nuclei with intact nuclear membranes and highly condensed heterochromatin. Intact envelopes are also observed in nuclei of necrotic neutrophils with decondensed chromatin. NETotic neutrophils instead are characterized by an absent nucleus as a consequence of the nuclear envelope disintegration and a cytoplasm filled with unfolded chromatin. NETosis is, unlike apoptosis, not

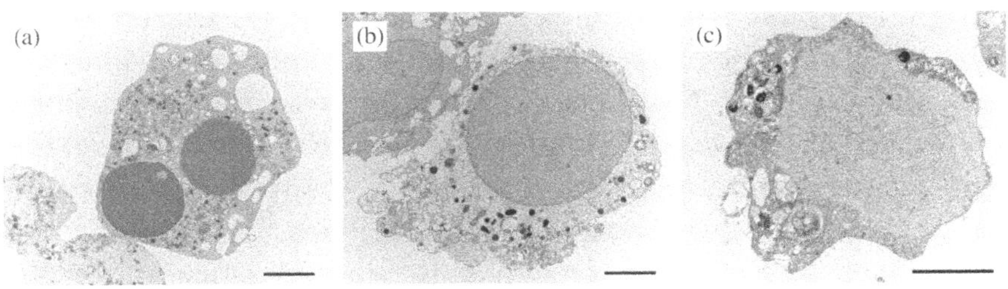

Fig. 7. NETosis is distinct from apoptosis and necrosis. The nuclear envelope remains intact in (a) apoptosis and (b) necrosis. The breakdown of the nucleus including the dissolution of the nuclear membrane is a hallmark of (c) NETosis. Bars = 2 μm. Reproduced with permission from © Fuchs *et al.*[11]

dependent on caspases. Caspases are key proteases in the apoptotic cell death program. Pharmacological inhibition of caspases prevents apoptosis, but has no effect on NETosis or necrosis. In summary, suicidal NETosis is characterized by sequential changes in neutrophil granular and nuclear morphologies, which are distinct from apoptosis and necrosis. This cellular program may prove especially useful if vital functions of neutrophils are not sufficient or are impaired.[24] In such scenarios, suicidal NETosis enables neutrophils to participate in inflammation even beyond their life span.

3.2. *Vital NETosis*

The initial discovery of NETs suggested that viable neutrophils engage an active and fast release mechanism to liberate NETs.[1] However this hypothesis was later rejected because imaging of NET formation *in vitro* revealed suicidal NETosis.[11] More recent studies following individual neutrophils *in vivo* show that neutrophils are indeed capable of releasing NETs without facing cell death.[17] In vital NETosis, the nuclear envelope remains intact, while DNA is released via a vesicular mechanism comparable to degranulation.[25] Vesicles filled with nuclear material are budding of the nuclear envelope and are transported to the plasma membrane. Fusion of the DNA-filled vesicles with the plasma membrane releases NETs into the extracellular environment without disintegration of the plasma membrane. This process eventually continues until the nucleus is entirely exteriorized and an anuclear cytoplast remains.[20] Importantly, anuclear neutrophils remain functional.[26] Vital NETosis therefore allows neutrophils to release NETs while retaining their capacity for migration, degranulation, and phagocytosis.[20] Mitochondria-derived NETs are released by a subtype of vital NETosis.[16] Here mitochondrial DNA but not nuclear DNA is released from stimulated neutrophils.[19] Consequently, mitochondria-derived NETs lack histones and have a different composition. Originally observed in eosinophils,[27] this form of DNA release and was later expanded to neutrophils.[19] Mitochondria-derived NETs are released in rapid catapult-like fashion without compromising cell viability, a process which is completed within seconds post stimulation. Multitasking of neutrophils following the formation of mitochondria-derived NETs therefore seems possible.

It is conceivable that different mechanisms of NETosis co-exist and cooperate. Interestingly, mitochondrial functions disappear early in suicidal NETosis,[22] and NETs released by this mechanism also contain fractions of mitochondrial DNA.[28] However, it is currently not clear how granular components assemble with DNA in vital forms of NETosis. NET components could be assembled in the extracellular space, if DNA is released via vesicles or mitochondria, while granular content is liberated using classical degranulation. Vital forms of NETosis may occur in conjunction with degranulation and phagocytosis, whereas suicidal NETosis might be engaged when all other neutrophil functions have been exhausted.

4. Induction of NETosis

NETosis can be triggered by numerous stimuli (Box 3). Neutrophils release NETs upon encountering gram-positive and -negative bacteria, fungi, protozoa, and viruses. Additionally, microbial compounds such as elements of the bacterial or fungal cell wall stimulate NETosis. The abundance of microbial inducers of NETs is sensible because NETs exhibit potent antimicrobial activity. However, NETs are also involved in sterile inflammatory conditions. Consequently, multiple non-infectious stimuli induce NETs including inflammatory molecules, ROS and reactive nitrogen species (RNS), complement factors, and autoantibodies or immune complexes. Many stimuli require cell surface receptors to be recognized by neutrophils. This implicates toll-like receptors (TLRs) as sensors of microbes or microbial compounds, as well as Fc-receptors of immunoglobulins, and complement or cytokines receptors in the induction of NETosis.[29–31] Furthermore, certain stimuli act synergistically, which adds to the complexity of triggers of NETosis.

Box 3. Selected stimuli of NETosis

- Microbes: var. viruses, bacteria, fungi, protozoa[32–34]
- Microbial compounds: LPS, LTA, fMLP, beta-glucan, Leukocidin[1,11,35,36]
- Inflammatory mediators: TNFα, INFs, IL-8, PAF, HMGB1[1,37–40]
- ROS, RNS: Superoxide, H_2O_2, HOCL, NO[11,41–44]
- Plasma proteins: Complement factor C5a, autoantibodies, immune complexes, heme, uric acid[31,37,38,45,46]
- Cellular interactions: Neutrophil binding to endothelium, platelets[29,47]
- Non-physiological stimuli: PMA, calcium ionophore, statins, aluminum adjuvants[1,48–50]

Despite the abundance of sterile or infectious triggers of NETs release, the underlying type of NETosis is not known for the majority of stimuli. The most commonly used stimulus of NETosis is phorbol-myristate-acetate (PMA). PMA is a non-physiological compound which mimics diacylglycerol and is a potent physiological activator of neutrophils. PMA along with ROS and certain microbes induces suicidal NETosis.[11,21,24] Suicidal NETosis is a relatively slow process (30–240 min); however, the kinetics and extent vary with the concentration, size, and type of the stimulus. Vital NETosis, in contrast, is a rapid mechanism (<30 min). The rapid release of mitochondria to from NETs is triggered by a combination of stimuli (e.g., GM-CSF + LPS).[19] Vital NETosis releasing DNA vesicles occurs in response to infections with Gram-negative or-positive bacteria. Cell–cell interactions are critical for vital NETosis. Platelets expressing TLR type 4 sense lipopolysaccharides (LPS),[29,30] a component of the cell wall of gram-negative cell bacteria which is shed into circulation in infections. LPS-stimulated platelets interact with neutrophils and trigger vital NETosis. Vital NETosis can also be induced by Gram-positive bacteria including Staphylococci and Streptococci.[20,25,30] In these infections, TLR type 2, which senses lipoteichoic acids (LTA) of the gram-positive bacterial cell wall, is a requirement for vital NETosis.

5. Regulation of NETosis

Due to its early discovery, intracellular regulatory mechanisms are best understood for suicidal NETosis. Three main regulatory mechanisms have been identified: reactive oxygen species, NE, and peptidylarginine deminase 4 (PAD4).

5.1. *Reactive oxygen species*

Endogenous or exogenous ROS are potent inducers of NETosis. ROS are produced in neutrophils by the cooperation of NADPH oxidase and MPO. NADPH oxidase is a multi-component enzyme which assembles into its active state upon stimulation with PMA or microbes. NADPH oxidase produces superoxide, which converts to hydrogen peroxide. MPO uses hydrogen peroxide for the production of hypochlorous acid, a type of ROS with potent antimicrobial activity. NETosis is severely impaired in neutrophils from patients with mutations in these enzymes.[11,51] Consequently, defects in signal pathways leading to NADPH oxidase activation, including Raf/MEK/Erk, PKC,[28,52] and Rac2,[53] interfere with ROS production and NETosis. The involvement of NADPH oxidase and ROS in NETosis is best illustrated by neutrophils from patients with chronic granulomatous disease (CGD), which carry mutations in components of the NADPH oxidase. Activation of CGD neutrophils with PMA or microbes does not cause NETosis due to a defect in nuclear envelope breakdown and chromatin decondensation.[11,54] Reconstitution of neutrophil NADPH oxidase in CGD patients by gene therapy restored this defect.[54] Importantly, impaired NETosis in CGD neutrophils is also rescued by stimulation with hydrogen peroxide. These experiments show a requirement of ROS, but not NADPH oxidase, for NETosis. The activation of the ROS production pathway may be required to inhibit caspase activity and to upregulate anti-apoptotic proteins, guiding neutrophils toward NETosis.[55] However, ROS are not sufficient to induce NETs in neutrophils from neonates,[39] indicating that additional factors are required.

5.2. *Neutrophil elastase*

A crucial step of suicidal NETosis is the unfolding of chromatin within viable neutrophils. Histones, in particular linker histone H1, are critical for the condensation state of chromatin. During NETosis, the enzymatic modification of histones by NE drives the generation decondensed DNA filaments.[21] The production of ROS by NADPH oxidase and MPO trigger the release of granular content into the neutrophil cytoplasm.[56] Cytoplasmic NE is then selectively translocated into the nucleus, where it cleaves histone H1 and core histones to facilitate the unfolding of chromatin to strings of nucleosomes. Therefore, histones are smaller in NETs than in nuclei.[10] The fragmentation of histones is facilitated by MPO, independent of its enzymatic activity.[21] Histones are potent mediators of NET functions, but fully fragmented histones lose their activity.[57] Therefore histone degradation is controlled in NETosis. The interaction of NE with DNA leads to reduced enzymatic activity. Furthermore, an endogenous inhibitor of NE, serpinB1, locates to the nucleus during NETosis.[58] DNA and SerpinB1 limit NE activity and thus likely preserve the functionality of NETs.

5.3. *Peptidylarginine deminase 4*

Peptidylarginine demininases (PAD) modify proteins posttranslationally by converting arginine residues to citrulline. This conversion reduces the positive charge in proteins. Out of five known PADs, PAD2 and PAD4 are expressed in the cytosol of neutrophils. PAD4 contains a nuclear localization signal and is required for NETosis. PAD4 translocates to nucleus upon neutrophil activation and citrullinates the linker histone H1 as well as core histones.[50,59,60] The reduced positive charge in citrullinated histones results in a weaker interaction with negatively charged DNA, ultimately leading to the unfolding of chromatin. PADs, including PAD4, are calcium-dependent enzymes, and PAD4 is activated by increasing concentrations of calcium ions in the cytosol. Consequently, calcium ionophores are potent stimuli of PAD4-driven chromatin decondensation and NETosis.

Regulation of NE and PAD4 activity provides a key mechanism to control NETosis. NADPH oxidase activates NE through the generation of endogenous ROS, but is not required for NETosis. It is conceivable that alternative mechanisms for NE activation exist because several stimuli induce NETs independent of NAPDH oxidase.[52] Moreover, mechanisms operating independently of NADPH such as autophagy[22,61] or transcriptional regulation by HIF1a[62] control NETosis. PAD4 activity is regulated by calcium, and is thus independent of ROS. Importantly, recent studies suggest that NE and PAD4-driven chromatin condensation are not synergistic but rather are independent processes.[52] Nevertheless, the requirement of NE and PAD4 for NETosis was confirmed in murine infection models. Therefore, NE- and PAD4-deficient mice are currently used as models for genetically impaired NETosis.[21,59] In addition, targeting the enzymatic activity of NE and PAD4 by pharmacological inhibitors is commonly used to address the role of NETs in animal models.[24,63,64] Considering the large variety of stimuli of NETs and different mechanism of NETosis, it is rational that different cellular pathways trigger NET formation.

6. Clearance of NETs

Pus formation is a common mechanism to resolve inflammation. Pus is a greenish-yellowish exudate mainly comprising dead neutrophils. Indeed, neutrophil MPO gives pus its characteristic color. A fraction of the neutrophils in pus display morphologies characteristic of suicidal NETosis, namely an anucleated cytoplasm with dispersed intracellular chromatin and granular proteins.[15] If pus is formed superficially, it may leave the body by drainage. Therefore, pus formation represents a major route for NET clearance.

Pus formation in tissues commonly leads to the formation of an abscess. How NETs are cleared in inflamed internal tissues is poorly understood. The clearance mechanism likely involves the opsonization, fragmentation, and phagocytosis of NETs. Fragmentation of NET-DNA is required because NETs are insoluble and too large for internalization. DNase1 is the main enzyme in circulation responsible for degradation of extracellular DNA. Indeed, DNase1 in plasma or serum degrades NETs efficiently *in vitro*.[65,66] Complement factors may opsonize NET fragments and thus facilitate the internalization by macrophages.[67] As we will discuss below, NET degradation is defective in autoimmune and thrombotic diseases[65,66] and can be manipulated by bacterial pathogens.[68]

7. General Functions of NETs

In order to function optimally, the neutrophil granular proteins need to be locally concentrated when they meet their targets (e.g., bacteria or ECM). The phagosome is a prototypic compartment that enriches granular proteins along with their targets. Immobilization of granular proteins on the cell surface upon degranulation is another mechanism of concentration. NETs feature three main properties to support the activity of neutrophil proteins in the extracellular space.

(1) **NETs form a large and stable scaffold.** NETs exceed the size of a single cell by several magnitudes. The precise dimensions of a NET derived from a single neutrophil are not known. The length of DNA in chromosomes is at least 2 cm, 2000 times the diameter of a neutrophil. Bundles of NETs exposed to a laminar flow form multi-cm long fibers that can withstand high shear forces.[69]

(2) **NETs have a reactive surface.** DNA, histones, and neutrophil proteins are firmly bound in NETs, while retaining their activity. This stable interaction keeps NET proteins locally concentrated and prevents their diffusion into the extracellular environment. Consequently, NETs are means for the extracellular operation of neutrophil proteins. Furthermore, neutrophil proteins can function at a distance of or independent from neutrophil bodies in contrast to enzymes immobilized on the cell surface upon degranulation.

(3) **NETs immobilize soluble and insoluble material.** The binding of bacteria led to the term "Neutrophil Extracellular Traps". Currently, multiple cellular binding partners of NETs are known. Cells or particles may be passively entrapped in the dense meshwork of DNA fibers. "Neutrophils cast nets" is a commonly used catchphrase to describe this principle. Importantly, NETs provide a sticky surface facilitating the adhesion of insoluble or soluble compounds. DNA is negatively charged due to phosphate groups in its sugar backbone. The majority of proteins in NETs, including most granular proteins, are highly positively charged. Therefore, soluble or insoluble compounds can bind to NETs based on strong electrostatic interactions. Additionally, several proteins are known to comprise specific binding domains for NETs or its components (e.g., DNA-binding domains). Selective binding to NETs further enriches targets of neutrophil proteins in NETs.

In conclusion, NETs enrich molecules or cells within a stable extracellular DNA-scaffold for processing by concentrated neutrophil proteins.

8. Functions of NETs in disease

NETs take action in diverse inflammatory responses during infection, autoimmunity, thrombosis, tissue damage, or cancer. The list of NET-binding partners includes microbes, components of the immune system, host tissue, and blood (Box 4). NET-binding partners face the

Box 4. NET functions in inflammatory diseases

- Antimicrobial function through interaction with microbes or microbial compounds in infectious diseases.
- Cytotoxic activity through binding to host cells during inflammatory tissue damage.
- Pro-thrombotic properties through interaction with vascular endothelium, blood cells, and plasma proteins.
- Immunogenic functions via interaction with the adaptive immune system in autoimmune diseases.
- Anti-inflammatory properties through interaction with chemokines and cytokines during acute inflammation.

action of neutrophil proteins, in particular proteases and histones. Consequently, NETs exhibit antimicrobial, cytotoxic, prothrombotic, immunogenic, and anti-inflammatory properties depending on the type of interaction partner and disease. Importantly, NET-binding partners often have reciprocal functions and also act as inducers of NETs or neutralize NET functions. How NETs contribute to different inflammatory diseases will be discussed in the second part of this chapter.

9. Antimicrobial NETs

NETs were originally discovered upon *in vitro* infection with *Shigella flexneri*.[1] Early on, the ensnaring and inhibiting effect of NETs has been shown and it seemed appealing that NETs are an extracellular mechanism of neutrophils to control spread of invading microbes in addition to phagocytosis and ROS-mediated intoxication. While following studies revealed the broad effectiveness of NETs against parasites, fungi, bacteria, and viruses, the features determining pathogen-induced stimulation of NETs and involved intracellular signaling cascades are less well understood. The differential implications for relevance of NETs during different viral and microbial infections will be discussed (Box 5).

Box 5

Antimicrobial NETs	NET induction *in vitro*	NET induction *in vivo*	ROS-dependent	ROS-independent	Inhibited killed by NETs	Escape mechanism from NETs	Ref.
Viruses							
HIV-1	+	+	nd	nd	+	Induction of IL-10	70
Hantavirus	+	+ β2 integrin receptors	nd	nd	+	Hyper-induction of NETs	71
Influenza A	+ via lung epithelium	+	+	nd	resistant	unknown	72
Bacteria							
Shigella flexneri	+	nd	+	nd	+	nd	1
Escherichia coli	+ gluthatione reductase	nd	+	nd	+	nd	73, 32
Pseudomonas aeruginosa	+ flagella / pyocyanin	+	+	nd	resistant	mucoid strains	74,75
Klebsellia pneumoniae	–	+ Co-stimulus?	nd	nd	+ Partly via calprotectin		76
Vibrio cholerae	+	nd	nd	nd	+	Ex. nucleases	

(*Continued*)

(*Continued*)

Box 5

Antimicrobial NETs	NET induction in vitro	NET induction in vivo	ROS-dependent	ROS-independent	Inhibited killed by NETs	Escape mechanism from NETs	Ref.
Staphylococcus aureus	+	+	Via plasma membrane disruption	extruded by living PMNs	+	Ex. nucleases, cytolysin, catalase	11, 32, 25
Streptococci *S. pneumoniae* *S. pyogenes* *S. suis*	+ surface-localized M1 or α-enolase	+	+	nd	+	Ex. nucleases, M1 inhibits LL37	77, 78, 79, 80
Mycobacterium tuberculosis	+	nd	+	nd	nd	nd	81
Fungi							
Candida spp.	+	+	+	+ co-stimulation with EM[36]	+ calprotectin	nd	
C. albicans							33
C. dubliniensis							82
C. glabrata							83

(*Continued*)

(*Continued*)

Box 5

Antimicrobial NETs	NET induction in vitro	NET induction in vivo	ROS-dependent	ROS-independent	Inhibited killed by NETs	Escape mechanism from NETs	Ref.
Aspergillus spp	+	+	+	nd	+	*RodA* reduces	
A. fumigatus					calprotectin	NET	84
A. nidulans						formation	54
Parasites							
Leishmania spp.	+	+	–	+	+ hsitones	3'-nucleotidase	
L. amozonensis, L. major, L. donovani, L. chagasi L. infantum		subcutaneous infection				activity	85, 34
Toxoplasma gondii	+	+	+ via ERK signaling	nd	+	nd	86
Eimeria spp.	+	nd	+	nd	resistant	nd	87
E. bovis							88
E. arloingi							
Plasmodium falciparum	+	+ In circulation	nd	nd	nd	nd	89

Notes: The cell surface protein M1 from *S. pyogenes* is such a virulence factor that can modulate NET release and protect against NET killing, EM = extracellular matrix, nd = not determined.

9.1. *Viral infections*

Neutrophils are traditionally considered irrelevant for viral infections. Their classical antimicrobial defenses, most of all phagocytosis, are inefficient against viruses, since they are too small. Viral particles tend to fail inducing measurable neutrophil activation. However, a few recent studies have investigated the role of NET formation in response to viral infection. Interestingly, human immunodeficiency virus (HIV)-1 induces release of NETs,[70] but the mechanisms of viral NET induction remains unknown. NETs ensnare and neutralize HIV virions and, in doing so, considerably decrease HIV infectivity. A role of NETs in combating HIV may therefore be plausible. Additionally, HIV triggers IL-10 release by dendritic cells (DCs).[70] Anti-inflammatory IL-10 in turn suppresses NET formation. Thus, NETs were shown to be involved in antiviral defense, which is supported by the finding that HIV has adapted to this potential defense by evading NET killing. Another example for viral evasion from NETs is the Feline leukemia virus (FeLV), which can repress neutrophil activation by inhibiting NADPH oxidase stimulation to reduce ROS production.[90]

Remarkably, hantaviruses strongly induce NET release.[71] Hantaviruses are rodent-borne human pathogens causing severe disease with increasing frequency. As hantaviruses replicate in endothelial and epithelial cells in the absence of significant cytopathic effects, mechanisms of immunopathology remain largely unknown. Hantaviruses induce high systemic levels of NETs in circulation of infected patients.[71] This systemic NET overproduction triggers increased titers of autoantibodies to nuclear antigens. Downstream analyses revealed that β2 integrin receptors were crucial for hantavirus-induced NET release and may act as previously unrecognized hantavirus entry receptors. Systemic NET overproduction therefore seems to be a molecular explanation for characteristic aspects of hantavirus-associated immunopathology, such as lung and kidney damage. Medically important influenza A virus (IVA) infections, with yearly 3–5 million severe cases worldwide, were investigated for critical contributions of neutrophils and NETs.

Interestingly, although IVA does not activate neutrophils directly, it induces infected lung epithelium to produce superoxide and H_2O_2.[91] Although this results in NET formation in the infected mouse lung, NET-deficient PAD4 knockout mice are equally susceptible to infection as their wild-type littermates.[72] Studies addressing the role of NETs during viral infection are still scarce. However, strong evidence for powerful neutrophil recruitment and activation by viruses suggests that NETs might have implications in antiviral defense.

9.2. *Bacterial infections*

A considerable number of Gram-negative and Gram-positive bacteria were reported to trigger NET release and to be trapped as well as killed within NET fibers. *S. flexneri* was one of the first examples described, and NET-associated neutrophil elastase is able to degrade virulence factors from *S. flexneri* to additionally disarm the pathogen.[1] Enteropathogenic *Escherichia coli* strain WS2572 induces NET formation *ex vivo* in mouse neutrophils as well.[73] Interestingly, NET formation depended on glutathione reductase (GSR), which contributes to maintain a reducing environment within the cytoplasm. Thus, it seems that NET release is hampered under hyper-oxidative conditions.

The opportunistic bacterial pathogen *Pseudomonas aeruginosa,* which causes a wide variety of infectious diseases, is the prevalent colonizer of cystic fibrosis (CF) patients. CF is caused by a mutation in the cystic fibrosis transmembrane conductance regulator (CFTR). Increased levels of extracellular DNA constitutes a hallmark of CF[92] indicating that it is at least partially derived from NETs. The dominance of *Pseudomonas* as CF colonizer might be explained by its extraordinary pathoadaptability to resist bactericidal immune activities, such as NETs. During colonization in CF patients *P. aeruginosa* mutates from non-mucoid strains toward mucoid strains.[93] Current data indicate that non-mucoid *P. aeruginosa* are efficiently ensnared by NETs.[74,75] Furthermore, the non-mucoid strains induce NET formation more avidly than the mucoid strains. Notably, this suggests, among other non-mutually exclusive explanations, that pathogen entrapment in NET fibers might improve bacterial microcolonization and induce bacterial pathoadaptation by driving mutability, since mechanical clearance of these microcolonies is disabled in CF patients' lungs. In fact, NETs contain LL-37, a protein which is also implicated in mutagenesis of *P. aeruginosa*.[94] In this context, several surface molecules from *P. aeruginosa* are implicated to have NET-inducing capacities, including flagella and pyocyanin.[74,95] Nontheless, the exact contribution of NETs to the pathogenicity of *P. aeruginosa* infections in CF and other patients remains to be determined.

The respiratory pathogen *Klebsellia pneumoniae* induces robust NET formation in a lung infection model of mice.[21,96] A possible contribution of NETs to immune defense against *K. pneumoniae* is further supported by investigations dissecting antimicrobial components of NETs. NETs from neutrophils deficient in myeloid-related protein 14 (MRP14) cannot control *K. pneumoniae in vitro* and MRP14 knockout mice are more susceptible to *K. pneumoniae*, as the bacteria can disseminate in the absence of MRP14.[97] While these findings suggest a role of NETs as barriers against bacterial dissemination, surprisingly *K. pneumoniae* fails to trigger NET release in purified neutrophils *ex vivo*.[24] Therefore, microbial virulence may be one important NET-inducing stimulus which in certain cases needs to be accompanied by co-activating effectors, such as pro-inflammatory cytokines, for complete activation of NET formation.

The gastrointestinal pathogen *Vibrio cholerae*, on the other hand, induces NETs in isolated neutrophils *ex vivo*, whereas the DNA traps could not be directly visualized in a mouse gastrointestinal infection model.[76] Nevertheless, *V. cholerae* expresses two extracellular nucleases which enable the bacterium to evade trapping and killing by NETs (Fig. 8). The nuclease-deficient *V. cholerae* strains were less virulent in gastrointestinal infection. Interestingly, by depletion of neutrophils in mice prior to infection this attenuation is overcome, indicating that the decrease in virulence of nuclease-deficient *V. cholerae* depends on the presence of neutrophils and NETs.[76]

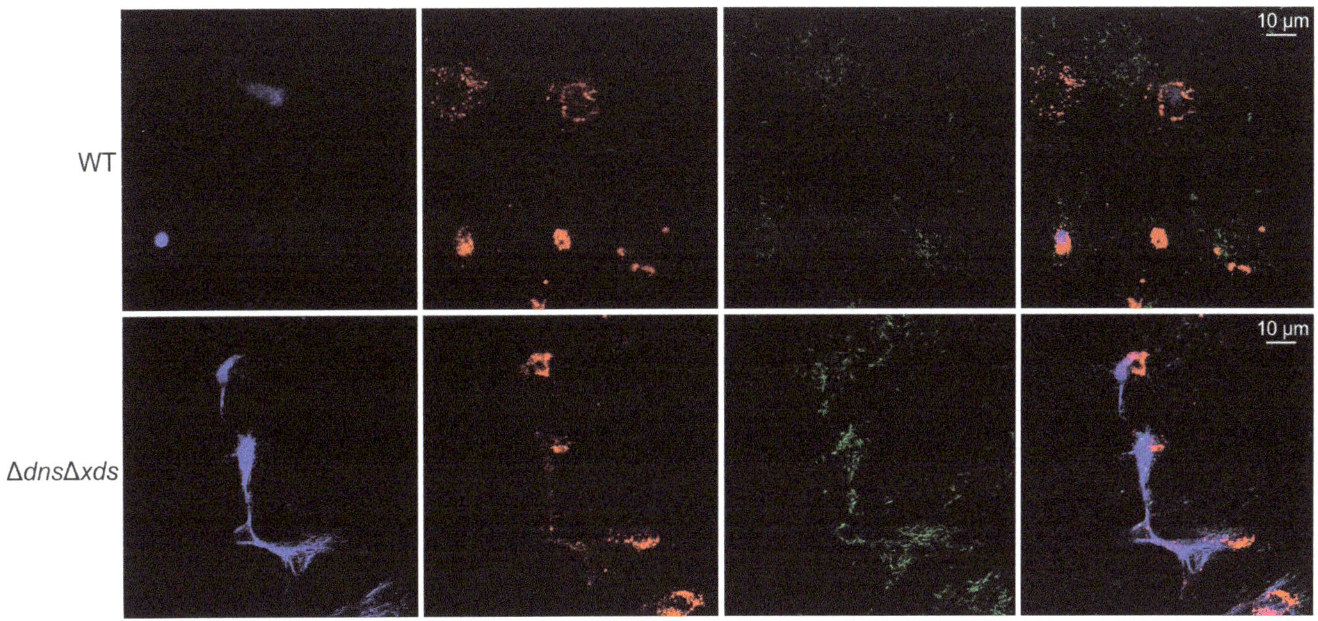

Fig. 8. NET formation induced by *V. cholerae*. Human neutrophils were infected with wild-type *V. cholerae* (upper row) and nuclease mutant strain *ΔdnsΔxds* (lower row) for 6 h. Indirect immunofluorescence micrographs of samples stained for DNA (DAPI, blue), neutrophil elastase (NE, Cy3 conjugated, red), and *V. cholerae* expressing GFP (green). NETs are patchy, web-like structures co-staining for DNA and MPO only present in infection with *ΔdnsΔxds*, since wild-type *V. cholerae* efficiently degrades the DNA traps. Reproduced with permission from © Seper *et al.*[84]

In summary, it seems that Gram-negative pathogenic bacteria induce NET release, which in turn activates evasion strategies, subsequently increasing bacterial virulence and dissemination.

Staphylococcus aureus is a gram-positive opportunistic bacterial pathogen and an efficient stimulator of NET formation.[11] Interestingly, *S. aureus*-induced NETosis in human neutrophils *ex vivo* was dependent on NADPH oxidase and ROS production, while MPO was dispensable for NET release as demonstrated with neutrophils deficient in NADPH oxidase and MPO, respectively.[32] However, MPO is abundant and active in NET-mediating killing of entangled *S. aureus* in the presence of H_2O_2.[13] To evade DNA traps, *S. aureus* seems to have evolved numerous strategies. One of those is the expression of pore-forming peptides that neutralize neutrophils and thus prevent NET formation by destroying the plasma membrane. Furthermore, *S. aureus* catalase efficiently removes H_2O_2 to protect from oxidative damage within the bacteria and potentially blocking ROS functions in NETosis.[11] Given these evasion mechanisms, it seems plausible that neutrophils may have evolved an alternative rapid and ROS-independent NET expulsion mechanism in order to control *S. aureus* or other catalase-positive strains.[25] Methicillin-resistant *S. aureus* (MRSA) express, like *V. cholerae*, extracellular nucleases, which promote biofilm dispersal and dismantle NETs.[98] MRSA-infected mice are more susceptible than controls infected with a strain deficient in nuclease, which is also more sensitive to extracellular killing by neutrophils. Nuclease inhibitors could therefore serve as new treatment of certain bacterial infections.

Different species of Gram-positive *Streptococci* interact with NETs. *Streptococcus* spp. includes non-pathogenic commensal strains, zoonotic, and highly virulent human-specific pathogens. *S. pneumoniae* causes community-acquired pneumonia. Not uncommon complications in children or elderly are meningitis or bacteraemia. *S. pyogenes*, a group A *Streptococcus* (GAS) can cause severe soft tissue or systemic infections.[99,100] A large number of streptococcal virulence factors have been described that allow the bacteria to evade immune attack and to establish infection. Several of these virulence factors are implicated in the interaction with and neutralization of NETs. The cell surface protein M1 from *S. pyogenes* is such a virulence factor that can modulate NET release and protect against NET killing. *S. pyogenes* appears to induce NETosis via complexes which are formed by bacterial M1 protein and tissue-derived fibrinogen. Interestingly, despite the NET-inducing activity of M1, it also protects the bacteria from NET killing by neutralizing the antimicrobial NET component cathelicidin LL-37. This is confirmed by M1 deletion mutants of invasive serotypes which became more susceptible to killing by NETs.[79] *S. pneumonia* α-enolase, a glycolytic enzyme additionally transported to the cell wall of the bacteria, is able to induce NET formation by direct binding to the neutrophil myoblast antigen 241D5.[77] Moreover, *Streptococci* escape NETs. They were the first bacteria described to express extracellular nucleases capable of degrading NETs. Invasive *S. pneumoniae* strain TIGR4 expresses the DNase endA[78] and *S. pyogenes* the nuclease Sda1.[101,102] Mutant strains lacking endA or Sda1, likewise, are less virulent in mouse infection models and are unable to digest DNA traps. In invasive GAS strain M1T1, the importance for evasion from NETs is illustrated by expression of the SpeB protease. SpeB degrades Sda1 and thus eliminates nuclease-mediated NET evasion of MIT1. In infected mice, however, disseminated bacteria accumulate mutations that inactivate SpeB and thus maintain Sda1 activity and NET escape.[103] More recently, *S. suis*, a zoonotic strain prevalent in pigs, was demonstrated to express the cell surface localized nuclease SsnA which similarly allowed for NET degradation and escape.[80] These observations strongly indicate that NETs act as antimicrobial barriers to prevent dissemination of bacteria. The barriers subsequently create selective pressure on microorganisms to evolve strategies for NET neutralization in order to spread beyond the initial site of infection. Sda1 was also shown to degrade bacterial DNA, which in turn prevents recognition and immune activation via Toll-like receptor 9 (TLR9).[104] Thus, virulence attributed to Sda1 does not entirely depend on NET evasion, but very likely involves additional immune evasion mechanisms. To this end, in coinfection with influenza *S. pneumoniae* frequently causes otitis media in children. IVA infection promotes outgrowth of *S. pneumoniae* within the middle ear by inducing local inflammation. Interestingly, antibody-dependent NET formation in the middle ear actually facilitated pneumococcal replication.[105] Instead of clearing pneumococcal infection, NETs allowed the bacteria to grow and in accordance, and DNase treatment reduced bacterial load. This suggests that NETs exert hazardous effects to the host not only in sterile inflammatory disorders but also in acute infections by creating a hyper-inflammatory milieu which allows for microbial replication.

Mycobacterium tuberculosis, the causative agent of tuberculosis, can successfully evade host immunity by a facultative intracellular lifestyle. Macrophages are key players during tuberculosis; however, accumulating evidence indicates that neutrophils also contribute to control of the infection.[106] Like other pathogenic bacteria, *M. tuberculosis* is able to activate neutrophils to produce ROS and to release NETs.[81] Remarkably, NETs efficiently ensnared *M. tuberculosis*, whereas they were unable to kill the bacteria. Whether entrapping of *M. tuberculosis* in NETs indeed contributes to infection containment needs to be determined in further studies.

9.3. *Fungal infections*

Neutropenia — low numbers in neutrophils — is an established risk factor for the development of invasive fungal infections. This is apparent particularly in hematologic patients who often are neutropenic due to chemotherapy or just after bone marrow transplantation. These patients frequently acquire severe mycoses caused by *Candida spp.*, *Aspergillus spp.* or newly emerging zygomycetes.[107] A common denominator of these fungal pathogens is the ability to form long filaments, the so-called hyphae, which are too large to be phagocytozed by individual neutrophils. NETs are therefore likely to play a crucial role in the containment and removal of these pathogens that cannot be compensated for by other phagocytes than neutrophils, rendering neutropenic patients susceptible to these mycoses. The importance of NETs in controlling filamentous *Candida* and *Aspergillus* spp. has been recently demonstrated.[24]

Dectin-1, a pattern recognition receptor widely expressed on phagocytes and other immune cells specifically binding β-glucans, seems to play a crucial role. As it induces phagocytosis, hyphae, too large to be engulfed, prevent activation via Dectin-1. Instead, a NETosis program is launched in order to initiate a defense mechanism that appears to be more suitable to control extracellular filaments.[24] Thus, neutrophils seem to selectively release NETs in response to large pathogens. This pathway can similarly be triggered by blockage of phagocytosis.

Candida albicans is the most frequent human fungal pathogen causing different types of infections ranging from localized superficial infections, such as vulvovaginitis, to life-threatening systemic infections in immunocompromised patients, as in individuals with hematologic disorders mentioned above.[108] Similar to bacterial opportunists, *C. albicans* colonizes a large percentage of the worldwide population as a commensal of the mucosae and thus does not need to be transmitted from one individual to the other. The ability to reversibly switch between yeast form and filamentous growth is inevitably correlated to virulence of *C. albicans*. The yeast form enables fast proliferation for systemic dissemination, while hyphae promote tissue invasion and persistence as well as biofilm formation.[109] The first study to demonstrate that a fungal pathogen can induce NETs and be ensnared and killed by these NETs was in fact performed with *C. albicans* yeasts and hyphae.[33] Among other human-pathogenic *Candida* species *C. dubliniensis*[82] and *C. glabrata*[83] were shown to induce NETs. *C. dubliniensis* is also trapped and killed by NETs.[82]

Apart from yeasts, molds have been investigated for their interaction with NETs. Induction of NETosis by *Aspergillus fumigatus* does not depend on viability of the mold, as inactivated conidia and hyphae suffice to trigger release of NETs.[84] Conidia are small roundish asexual spores of *Aspergilli* that are easily dispersed by air, and hyphae germinate out of these spores when they are carried to growth-promoting environments. As mentioned above, *Aspergillus* spp often cause invase mycoses in hematologic patients. Aspergilli are not commensal; however, they are ubiquitous fungi. Inhalation of *Aspergillus* condiia is therefore very common. An intact immune system can prevent germination and spread of these spores. Both conidia and hyphae from *A. fumigatus*[110] and *A. nidulans*[54] can be killed via NETs, albeit conidia less efficiently than hyphae. Interestingly, different fungal morphotypes seem to induce NETs, which depends on exposure of different fungal surface molecules. Conidia induce fewer NETs than hyphae. This is because conidia express hydrophobin RodA, a cell surface protein rendering conidia, the inhaled form of Aspergilli, immunologically inert.[84] RodA probably masks NET activating surface molecules. This is reasonable, since in healthy individuals inhaled spores are prevented from germination and removed before they can form hyphae, most probably by phagocytosis. Only when conidia escape and build hyphae are neutrophils triggered to release NETs. If neutrophils are absent, such as in neutropenic patients, the fungus can disseminate and spread. Still, little is known about upstream recognition receptors on neutrophils and their corresponding fungal surface ligands which regulate NET formation in response to fungi. A recent study presented Dectin-1 as a major pattern recognition receptor responsible for NET induction by fungi. β-glucan-covered particles were sufficient to induce NETosis. Downstream Src kinases were shown to be important for intracellular signaling events that eventually led to release of NETs.[111] This study challenges the size-selective induction of NETs which could be induced by Dectin-1 blockage.[24] However, the latter study demonstrates increased NET formation in fungus-infected Dectin-1-deficient mice as compared to wild-type littermates. Whether Dectin-1 is NET-activating or NET-blocking might therefore depend on the milieu.

Attempts to characterize antifungal components in NETs resulted in the identification of MRP8/14 (calprotectin) as major antifungal agent upon challenge with *C. albicans*.[10] Calprotectin is a cytoplasmic protein complex formed by two subunits MRP8 and MRP14 (also referred to as S100A8 and S100A9). Both components are required for full antimicrobial activity, as only the complex forms binding sites for Zn^{2+} and Mn^{2+} ions. These metal ions are firmly bound by calprotectin, and similar to iron-binding by lactoferrin, microbial growth in turn is prevented when these trace elements are unavailable. This antimicrobial defense mechanism has therefore been termed nutritional immunity. Fungi are particularly susceptible to Zn^{2+} deprivation, as many essential proteins are dependent on Zn^{2+} as cofactor, such as transcription factors and ROS-detoxifying enzymes. Neutrophils release calprotectin via NETosis,[10] both as a soluble molecule and bound to NETs, highlighting NET formation as a major route for secretion of NET-bound antimicrobials as well as soluble factors. The importance of calprotectin in antifungal defense is reflected by a high susceptibility of calprotectin-deficient mice toward candidiasis.[10] The role of calprotectin in antifungal defense is broad. It is also an important NET-associated factor in the defense against *A. nidulans*. At low doses, calprotectin is reversibly fungistatic, whereas high doses lead to starvation and irreversible killing of the fungus.[112] CGD patients frequently suffer from *Aspergillus* infections due to absence of ROS production, insufficient activation of neutrophil proteases, as well as absence of extracellular killing via NETosis. Neutrophils from patients who received gene therapy to reinstall NADPH oxidase function and consequently NET release cleared *A. nidulans* in a NET- and calprotectin-dependent manner.[54,112] CGD patients additionally suffer from exacerbated inflammation. Interestingly, a recent study revealed that NADPH oxidase is not only essential for NETosis, but also for induction of a proper apoptotic program in recruited neutrophils during pulmonary aspergillosis[113] (Fig. 9). Thus, this indicates that in addition to impaired antimicrobial activity of neutrophils, the improper regulation of neutrophil apoptosis contributes to an extreme phenotype in CGD.

Human and animal fungal pathogens constitute a diverse group of microbes against which NET formation is likely to play differential roles. Further studies are needed to dissect the contribution of NETs in antifungal immunity. The effectiveness of NETs against large fungal growth forms such as hyphae, which are difficult to phagocytose, strongly suggest that NETs are an essential immune strategy to defeat fungal pathogens (Fig. 10).

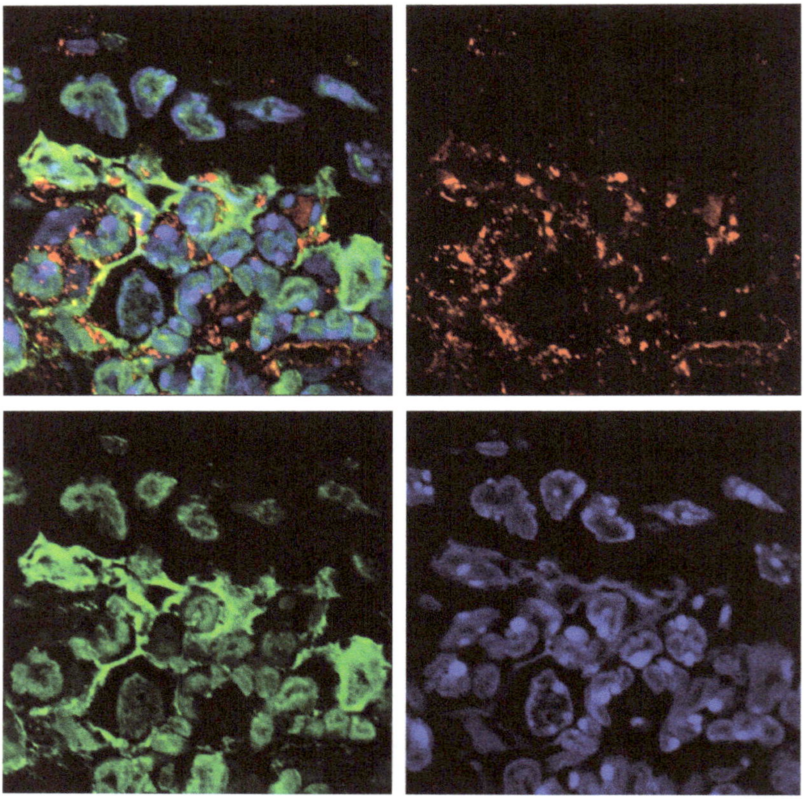

Fig. 9. Tissue section from mice with pulmonary aspergillosis displayed using indirect immunofluorescence. Shown are neutrophil infiltrates in the bronchi (lower parts of panels) close to epithelial layer (upper parts of panels). The sections have been stained with DAPI (4′,6-diamidino-2-phenylindole) for DNA (blue), with anti-histone H1 antibody to stain histone in NETs and cell nuclei (green), and with anti-myeloperoxidase (MPO) antibody to stain MPO within neutrophils and NETs (red). The upper left panel is a merge of all channels. NETs are patchy, web-like structures close to the epithelial layer with colocalization of DNA, histone, and MPO. Images were captured with a C1 confocal microscope (Nikon Instruments) at ×100 magnification. Reproduced with permission from © Infection and Immunity, May 2014, volume 82, issue 5, issue cover illustration.

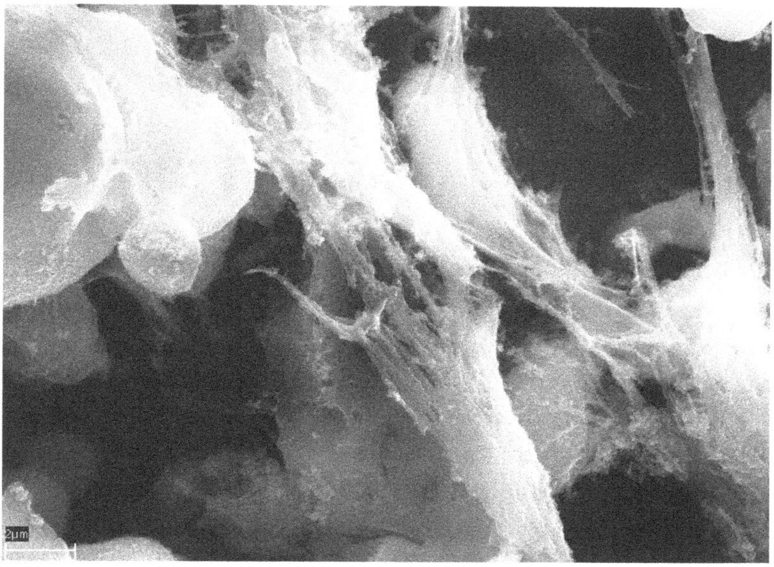

Fig. 10. Fine structure of NETs in pulmonary *C. albicans* infection. SEM section from mouse lungs infected with *C. albicans*. A bronchiole colonized with *C. albicans* and infiltrated by host immune cells is shown with NETs covering fungal surfaces (arrow). Scale bar = 2 μm. Reproduced with permission from Urban CF *et al.*[10]

9.4. *Parasitic infections*

The potential role of NETs in immune defense against protozoan parasites has been investigated in a number of different studies. *Leishmania* parasites are the causative agents of several types of leishmaniasis diseases. The phenotype of leishmaniasis is dependent on the species and ranges from mild cutaneous or subcutaneous lesions to potentially lethal visceral leishmaniasis, also known as black fever, responsible for up to 500,000 infections each year worldwide.[114] The life cycle of *Leishmania* parasites is complex, but can be divided into two major parasite stages: promiastigotes, the form that colonizes the insect vector sandfly, and amastogites, the type found in the mammalian host. The promastigote morphology is defined by an anterior flagellum allowing free extracellular movement, whereas amastigotes are nonflagellated, intracytoplasmic leishmanial forms residing predominantly within macrophages. Both forms are able to trigger NET formation in purified neutrophils, as observed with promastigotes from *Leishmania amozonensis, L. major, L. donovani, L. chagasi*, and *L. infantum* as well as with amastigotes from *L. amozonensis*. The broad NET induction activity of several *Leishmania* spp. suggests that NETs might be an important immune defense mechanism in leishmaniasis. In contrast to many bacterial or fungal inducers, NET release in response to *Leishmania* spp was not dependent on NADPH oxidase activity and ROS production. Additionally, promastigotes of *L. infantum* escaped NET-mediated killing by expressing 3'-nucleotidase/nuclease activity and subsequent dismantling of DNA traps. Due to a low efficiency of NETs to inhibit growth of *Leishmania*, different studies account for the functionality of NETs during leishmaniasis which is entrapment of parasites which contribute to the containment of the infection.[34,85,115]

Surface molecules on promastigotes involved in the induction of NETs were identified. Glycolipid lipophosphoglycan (LPG) was sufficient to trigger NET formation in a dose-dependent manner.[34] However, Gabriel et al. observed LPG-independent NET induction, whereas the surface molecule protected the parasite from NET-mediated killing.[85] Interestingly, histones mediated anti-parasitic activity of NETs as demonstrated with blocking of NET killing using anti-histone antibodies or addition of recombinant histone H2B which destroys the parasite efficiently.[34,116] Thus, it is likely that LPG protects the parasite against NET-associated histones.

NETs seem to additionally be implicated in infections with *Toxoplasma gondii*, an obligate intracellular parasite. *T. gondii* can infect numerous warm-blooded animals and causes, in correlation with the host immune status, either asymptomatic disease in otherwise healthy individuals or severe infections in immunosuppressed hosts. Many different *T. gondii* strains were shown to induce NET formation.[86] Elicitation of NET release was promoted by intracellular signaling cascades involving extracellular signal-regulated kinases 1/2 (ERK1/2), which previously have been demonstrated to be important for NET formation.[55] However, inhibition of ERK1/2 did not entirely abrogate NET formation.[86] Invasion of the intracellular parasite into neutrophils was not required for NET release, as inhibition of the cytoskeleton preventing parasite entry had no effect on NET formation.[86] On the contrary, NETs could only kill approximately 25% of ensnared parasites, again suggesting the primary trapping function of NETs during parasitic infection. In mice, experimental pulmonary infection with *Toxoplasma* induces strong neutrophil influx and high amounts of extracellular DNA in bronchoalveolar fluids, indicating the presence of NETs.[86]

Parasites of hoofed animals *Eimeria bovis*[87] and *E. arloingi*[88] are strong inducers of NETs in purified neutrophils from cattle or the goat apicomplexan, respectively. Notably, NET formation induced by *E. bovis*, was more efficient than by strong pharmacological triggering using PMA.[87] NET formation was dependent on NADPH oxidase and ROS production for both parasite species. *E. arloingi* sporozoites were trapped but not killed in NET fibers.[88]

Finally, NET fibers are present in circulation of *Plasmodium falciparum*-infected children with uncomplicated malaria. NETs were able to ensnare infected erythrocytes containing residing parasites and trophozoites alone. Interestingly, in infected individuals, increased titers of antinuclear antibodies (ANAs) were observed which could even exceed titers associated with autoimmune disease.[89] It is therefore plausible that NETs and accumulation of ANAs could promote development of malaria and accompanying autoimmune phenotypes in children, but at the same time may induce gradual immune protection in adults.[89]

In conclusion, these investigations indicate that NETs may be crucial contributors to immune defense against protozoan parasites. While NETs only show moderate anti-parasitic activity, they seem to be more important to physically restrict the entangled pathogens.

10. Cytotoxic NETs

The inflammatory response to infections accidentally injures host tissue and organs.[117,118] The damage to host cells during inflammation is in part ascribed to the antimicrobial arsenal of neutrophils. Release of granular content and ROS into the extracellular environment counteracts microbial pathogens. The toxicity is not specifically directed toward microbes, but also causes collateral damage to the surrounding host tissue. Neutrophil-mediated tissue destruction in sterile conditions is furthermore a major contributor to inflammatory pathologies. Neutrophil proteases, antimicrobial peptides, and ROS produced by NADPH oxidase and MPO damage the host cells. Neutrophil proteases degrade multiple substrates including the ECM and tight junctions, destabilizing tissue and blood vessels. The antimicrobial peptide LL37 and ROS target host cell viability directly and induce apoptosis and cytotoxicity. NETs contribute to this neutrophil-mediated tissue damage in sterile and infectious conditions.

10.1. *Cytotoxic activity of NETs*

NETs are neither specifically released in infections nor do NETs exclusive bind microbes. However, NETs contain the injurious proteins of neutrophil granules. Consequently, NETs contribute to the collateral damage during infection as well as sterile inflammation. Cell culture experiments provided the first evidence for the cytotoxic activity of NETs. NETs compromised the integrity of the plasma membrane of endothelial or epithelial cells *in vitro*.[29,119] Importantly, the cytotoxicity of NETs was not fully dependent on granular proteins in NETs, but was rather mediated by histones. Histones, the predominant proteins in NETs, exhibit remarkable cytotoxic properties *in vitro*. The precise cytotoxic action of histones is not identified. Early studies of the interaction purified histones with epithelial cells revealed that these highly cationic proteins have a strong affinity for phospholipids. Interaction of histones with the plasma membrane causes the disruption of the membrane potential and the influx of ions from the extracellular milieu into the cell.[120,121] The *in vivo* relevance of these findings remained unrecognized until the discovery of the cytotoxic potential of histones in sepsis.[57] Sepsis is a blood-borne bacterial infection, which triggers a systemic inflammatory response leading to multi-organ failure and death. Cytotoxicity and tissue damage in sepsis is greatly affected by extracellular histones. Neutralization of histones ameliorates organ failure and increases survival of septic animals. Despite sharing a similar structure and charge, not all histones are equally cytotoxic. Histone H4 from the core complex displays the highest cytotoxic potential, whereas the linker histone H1 is not harmful to cells. Future studies may identify molecular mechanism behind this phenotype. Intravenous infusion of purified histones into mice leads to organ damage and death, which illustrates the importance of histones as executers of tissue damage. Extracellular histones may be released in NETs, while necrotic tissue is a rich source of histones as well.[122–124] Importantly, neutralizing histones renders NETs non-cytotoxic to host cells *in vitro*.[119] Taken together, the cytotoxic activity of NETs may aggravate tissue damage during infection or sterile conditions.

10.2. *Infection*

The *in vivo* contribution of NETs to tissue damage during infections is best illustrated in the liver. The vascular bed of the liver filters bacteria in blood-borne infections through phagocytosis by Kupffer cells. When infections become overwhelming to Kupffer cells, neutrophils facilitate the bacterial clearance process in the liver through the generation of NETs.[20,29,30] Platelets, stimulated by circulating bacteria, bind to neutrophils and trigger vital NETosis. Within the hepatic sinusoids, NETs enhance the trapping of bacteria several fold and thus decrease the amount of circulating bacteria. However, trapping of bacteria by NETs is accompanied by collateral damage to hepatocytes. Indeed, preventing NET production by blocking platelets or by degrading NETs through infusion of DNases ameliorates the hepatic damage while aggravating bacteremia in circulation.

CF is another example of infection-induced tissue damage. CF is a severe infection-mediated airway inflammation characterized by dehydration and increased mucus viscosity. This environment facilitates the development of chronic bacterial infections, which precipitate inflammation and tissue damage. Neutrophils, in particular neutrophil proteases, contribute to airway damage by degrading ECM in these patients.[125] Furthermore, large amounts of extracellular DNA accumulate in the sputum of CF patients. This fact linked CF to NETs soon after their discovery.[126] Indeed, NETs contribute to sputum DNA and increase sputum viscosity.[127] CF patients are commonly treated with inhalations of aerosolized recombinant human DNase1. DNase1 cleaves sputum DNA into smaller fragments and reduces the sputum viscosity. Degradation of NETs in CF sputum by DNase1 may explain this beneficial effect. However, degradation of NETs activates the injurious activity of NE, which is in part inhibited by DNA.[127,128] Future studies may address the clinical benefit of NET degradation in CF-patients. It is conceivable that neutrophils of CF patients release NETs to combat airway infection, but NETs increases sputum viscosity and NE-mediated tissue injury may aggravate the disease during therapy.

10.3. *Sterile inflammation*

NETs contribute to tissue injury in sterile inflammatory conditions as well. Acute lung injury (ALI) is commonly caused by bacterial or viral infections, but can also be precipitated by sterile triggers such mechanical ventilation or blood transfusions. The role of NETs in transfusion-related ALI (TRALI) exemplifies NET-mediated tissue injury under sterile conditions.[129,130] In animal models of TRALI, NETs appear as a fibrous meshwork in the alveolar space (Fig. 11). Treating mice with DNase1 or antibodies against histone H4 improved the lung functions as evidenced by increased blood oxygenation and survival of the animals. NETs are generated during prolonged storage of blood transfusions and could therefore be infused into patients directly.[131] However, blood transfusions are commonly depleted of leukocytes before storage, eliminating NETs as a potential hazard. A severe form of TRALI was found in patients who received blood transfusions containing antibodies against a human neutrophil antigen (HNA-3).[132] Stimulation of

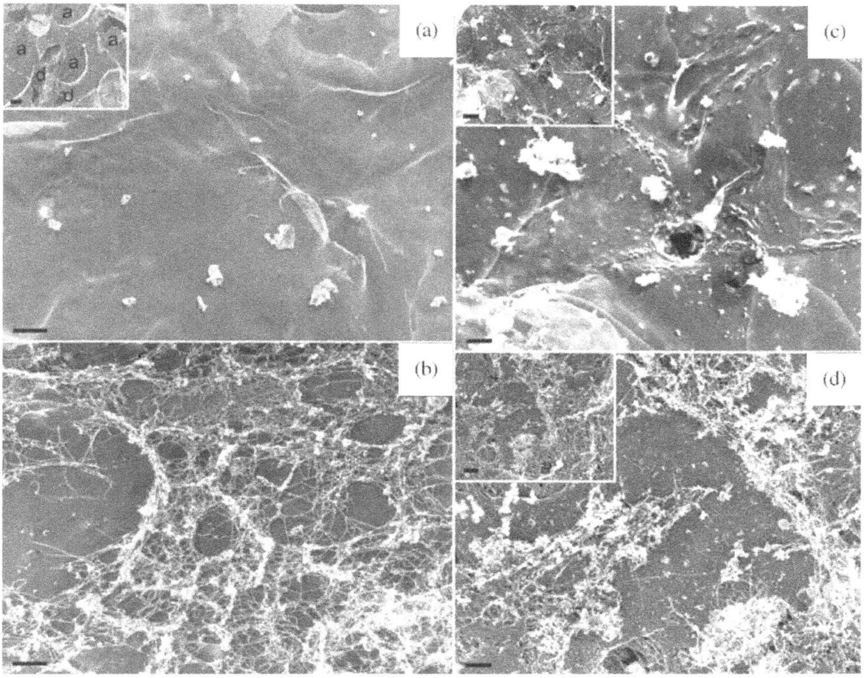

Fig. 11. NETs in lungs from mice with TRALI. (a-d) Transmission electron micrographs of the lung epithelial surface of control mice (a) and mice with TRALI (b,d). The abundant fibrous meshwork in TRALI lungs represents NETs because these structures are absent in mice treated with DNase1 before the induction of TRALI (c). Scale bar = 1 μm. The insets show low magnification views of the lung surface revealing alveolar sacs (a) and ducts (d); inset scale bars = 2 μm. Reproduced with permission from © Thomas *et al.*[130]

human neutrophils with HNA-3 antibodies caused the release of NETs *in vitro* and may stimulate NETosis in transfusion recipients.[130] TRALI is only one example of NET-mediated tissue injury under sterile conditions. Anti-neutrophil-antibody mediated NETosis may also trigger destruction of blood vessels in autoimmune vasculitis,[37] whereas heme-induced NETs may contribute to organ failure in hemolytic disorders.[45]

Ischemia–perfusion injury is a type of inflammation-fuelled tissue damage and a common cause of organ infarction or transplant-related injury.[133] The obstruction of blood flow to organs causes tissue ischemia due to a lack of oxygen. Several inflammatory stimuli, expressed by ischemic tissue and blood vessels, initiate the recruitment and activation of neutrophils after the re-establishment of blood flow. The tissue damage experienced in the course of ischemia–perfusion is usually regarded as a combination of ischemic damage and inflammatory damage. Neutrophils mediate the inflammatory tissue damage and NETs may contribute to this damage. Animal models of ischemia–reperfusion injury of the heart, brain, kidney, or liver are commonly used to mimic myocardial infarction, stroke, acute kidney failure, or hepatic shock in patients, respectively. Targeting PAD4, infusion of DNase1 or anti-histone H4 antibodies ameliorates the ischemia–perfusion injury of these organs in animal models.[122,134–136] However, the ischemic injury of tissue liberates DNA as well as histones into circulation, and it is conceivable that the beneficial effects of DNase1 and anti-histone-antibodies are only in part due to the neutralization of NETs.

Considering the spectrum of sterile inducers of NETs, NET-meditated tissue damage may be a common byproduct of inflammation.

11. Prothrombotic NETs

NETs contribute to blood clotting, the underlying processes of hemostasis and thrombosis. Hemostasis enables the rapid formation of a blood clot at the site of vascular injury to prevent excessive hemorrhage.

Thrombosis is the formation of blood clots within intact blood vessels and the pathologic counterpart to hemostasis. Thrombosis and hemostasis are both driven by the formation of platelet aggregates and tissue factor (TF)-driven fibrin generation. Thrombosis additionally engages the intrinsic arm the of the coagulation cascade, which triggers fibrin formation through contact activation of the plasma protease Factor XII. Thrombosis occurs largely in the absence of injured endothelium. Its primary triggers are stasis or turbulent blood flow, endothelial dysfunction, and hypercoagulability of the blood. Inflammation strongly cooperates with thrombosis

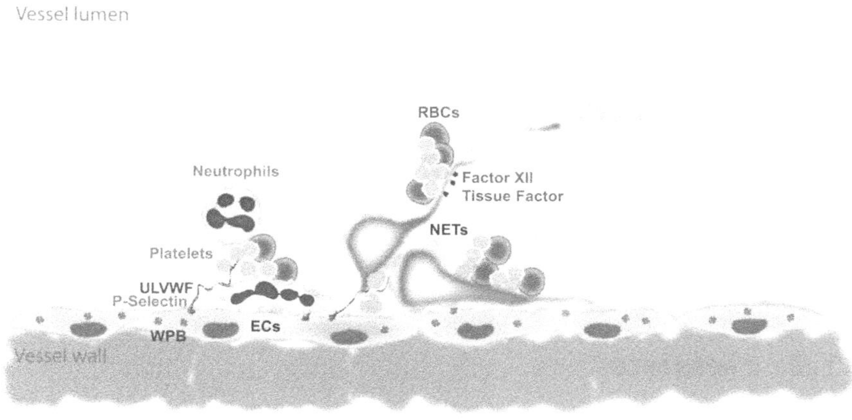

Fig. 12. Prothrombotic activity of NETs. Thrombosis is triggered by endothelial activation and adhesion of platelets and neutrophils. NETs potentially promote thrombosis through interaction with endothelium, platelets, RBCs, and clotting factors (Factor XII and Tissue Factor).

Source: Reproduced with permission from © Fuchs *et al.*

through altering endothelial functions and increasing the coagulability of blood.[137–139] NETs contribute to this linkage by binding to endothelial cells, immobilizing platelets, RBCs, and plasma component to expose them to locally high concentrations of neutrophil proteases and histones (Fig. 12).

11.1. *Endothelium*

Inflammatory stimuli or alterations of blood flow initiate thrombosis through the activation of vascular endothelium. Activated endothelium discharges Weibel–Palade bodies (WBP) to expose ultra-large von Willebrand factor (ULVWF) and P-selectin, which bind circulating platelets and neutrophils, respectively. Adherent neutrophils can be induced to release NETs through interaction with platelets and endothelium. Co-cultures of activated endothelial cells and neutrophils promote NET formation, which is dependent on platelets or IL-8 released from endothelium.[29,140] Importantly, endothelial vWF interacts with DNA and histones and thus potentially immobilizes NETs onto the vascular endothelium.[141,142] The interaction of the vessel wall with NETs may enable the action of histones on the endothelial cells. Histones perforate membranes,[143–145] and an increase in membrane permeability leads to an influx of calcium ions into the cytosol, which in turn triggers the discharge of WBP. It is therefore plausible that the interaction of NETs with endothelium could promote thrombosis by exacerbating endothelial activation and WBP release through an increase of intracellular calcium levels.[146]

11.2. *Platelets*

Platelet adhesion and activation leading to the formation of platelet aggregates is critical for thrombosis. NETs facilitate the formation of platelet aggregates by immobilizing platelets. When perfused with blood, NETs bind platelets and support their aggregation.[147] Whether the adhesion of platelets to NETs is mediated by entrapment, electrostatic affinity, or via a receptor–ligand interaction is not clear. Naïve platelets measure 2–3 μm in diameter and could be entangled in the meshwork of NETs. Nucleosomes, the building blocks of the chromatin fibers in NETs, could interact with Toll-like receptors on platelets.[148] Platelets can bind directly to histones under flow conditions.[149] Therefore, an electrostatic interaction between phospholipids[143] or carbohydrates[150] on the platelet surface and positively charged histones in NETs is possible. This interaction also enables the action of histones on platelets. Here, histones act also as triggers of calcium influx into platelets. Increased cytosolic calcium levels rapidly activate platelets leading to the exposure of pro-coagulant phosphatidylserine, the release of pro-coagulant polyphosphates from platelet granules,[148,151] and the formation platelet aggregates.[69,149] Infusion of histones into animals causes platelet activation and promotes thrombosis,[149,152] illustrating the prothrombotic activity of histones *in vivo*.

11.3. *Red blood cells*

When perfused with blood, NETs bind RBCs in addition to platelets. Unlike platelets, the role of RBCs in thrombus formation is not well defined and they are considered to be passively entrapped in the fibrin meshwork. More recently, RBCs have been shown to be actively recruited to sites of thrombus formation.[153] RBCs may promote coagulation by exposing phosphatidylserine and altering blood viscosity.[154] The interaction of RBCs with NETs is likely similar to platelets. In RBCs and platelets, the histone-induced calcium influx triggers the exposure of PS on the cell surface. Exposed PS assembles the prothrombinase complex, a critical step in the generation of thrombin.[155] Consequently, NET binding of RBCs may increase the coagulability of blood.

11.4. *Coagulation*

Coagulation requires the sequential activation of plasma proteases of the extrinsic or intrinsic pathway. In thrombosis, NETs stimulate the extrinsic pathway through activation of TF from monocytes.[156,157] NE is known to cleave TFPI and enhance thrombin activity.[158] NETs bind TFPI and facilitate proteolytic inactivation of TFPI by NE.[157] In addition to neutrophil proteases, DNA and histones in NETs may play an important role in stimulating coagulation. The intrinsic coagulation pathway is initiated by contact activation of FXII on negatively charged surfaces. NETs also bind Factor XII and NET-DNA may provide a negatively charged structure to activate FXII.[156] Indeed, nucleic acids enhance the activity of several coagulation proteases.[159] In addition, histones inhibit anticoagulants in plasma. Histones interact with thrombomodulin (TM) and protein C and prevent TM-mediated protein C activation.[160] As a consequence, histones dose-dependently increase plasma thrombin generation *in vitro*. NET generation in blood may therefore contribute to hypercoagulability.

11.5. *Thrombolysis*

Thrombolysis is mediated by the proteolytic degradation of fibrin by plasmin, which requires activation of its zymogen by tPA to gain activity. Blood clots with NETs are partially resistant to tPA-induced thrombolysis.[147] Instead, NETs provide an alternative scaffold to fibrin for the adhesion of blood cells. NETs interact with fibrin and increase its mechanical stability, while making it less susceptible to plasmin degradation.[161] Efficient thrombolysis may require the combination of NET- and fibrin degradation. Indeed, *in vitro* blood clots with NETs could be efficiently degraded by tPA in combination with DNase1.[147] DNase1 is the predominant DNA-degrading enzyme in plasma. The plasminogen system cooperates with DNase1 during chromatin degradation.[162] DNase1 has only limited activity against chromatin as it preferentially degrades protein-free DNA. Plasminogen, activated by either tPA or urokinase-type plasminogen activator (uPA), degrades histones and therefore allows for degradation of DNA by DNase1.[162] Interestingly, plasma DNA[147] follows similar kinetics as the fibrin degradation product D-dimer.[163] It is therefore conceivable that NET- and fibrin degradation cooperate during thrombolysis.

11.6. *Animal models of thrombosis*

The pro-thrombotic activity of NETs has been documented in several animal models of thrombosis including arterial and venous thrombosis, atherosclerosis, and microvascular thrombosis. To analyze the function of NETs, either the production of NETs was inhibited by interfering with PAD4 activity or animals were treated with infusion of DNase1 or anti-DNA antibodies to dismantle or block NETs, respectively. In arterial thrombosis, triggered by a dysfunctional endothelium, which is a fast and strongly platelet-dependent processes, inhibiting NETosis or NETs blocked the formation of a stable and occlusive thrombus.[64,164] In venous thrombosis in response to disturbances in blood flow, which is a rather slow process mainly driven by fibrin formation, DNase1 infusions or PAD4 deficiency reduced the frequency of thrombus formation.[152,165,166] In mice prone to develop atherosclerosis, chronic inhibition of PAD4 activity reduced the atherosclerotic lesion and the thrombosis in atherosclerotic vessels.[167] In a murine model of cancer-induced thrombosis, which is characterized by systemic microvascular thrombosis, infusion of DNase1-mediated degradation of NETs reduced the hypercoagulability of blood.[168] In summation, targeting NETs or NET components ameliorates thrombosis *in vivo*.

11.7. *Patients with thrombosis*

The association of NETs with thrombosis in patients is mostly established via illustrating NETs in tissue biopsies or via quantification of NET components in plasma samples. NETs have been identified in thrombi from patients with venous thromboembolism[169] and atherosclerosis,[170] or in plasma samples from patients with deep vein thrombosis,[171,172] coronary artery disease,[173] or thrombotic microangiopathies.[174] Furthermore, NET degradation was compromised in patients with thrombotic microangiopathies due to a deficiency in plasma DNase1.[66] Impaired NET degradation may contribute to the severe microvascular thrombosis in these patients.

In summary, NETs contribute to thrombosis by several means. NETs provide scaffolding for thrombus stability, alone or through fortifying the fibrin framework. NETs also serve as an adhesive surface to immobilize RBCs, platelets, and clotting factors, which in turn are rendered prothrombotic by the action of histones or neutrophil proteases. It is noteworthy that despite the well-documented antithrombotic effect of DNase1 infusion and PAD4 inhibition, neither measure interferes with hemostasis. It is conceivable that inflammation promotes blood clotting under pathological conditions. Cooperation of inflammation and blood clotting may have its origin in protecting against infections.[137] Indeed, interfering with inflammation or blood clotting promotes the dissemination of bacterial pathogens from sites of infection.[164] Inflammation and blood clotting together constrain pathogens at the site of entry. This cooperation of inflammation and thrombosis leads to the term "immunothrombosis".[137]

12. Immunogenic NETs

Neutrophils have long been viewed as specialized innate immune effectors with limited contribution to adaptive immunity.[175] However, recent studies suggest novel roles for neutrophils in the pathogenesis of a wide range of diseases, including autoimmune disorders,[65] chronic inflammation,[175] and cancer.[176] The discovery of NETosis has bridged gaps between innate and adaptive immunity and autoimmunity.[177,178] The various autoantigens associated with several autoimmune disorders are integral components of NETs (Box 6). This strongly advocates for a role of NETs in the pathogenesis and progression of autoimmune disorders. Apart from being immunogenic, NETs have detrimental roles in several autoimmune disorders: Recent studies provide insight into how NETs are beneficial in resolving inflammation.[179] In the following subsections, the role of NETosis in systemic lupus erythematous, vasculitis, rheumatoid arthritis, and other autoimmune diseases will be discussed.

Box 6. Autoantibodies against NET components in various autoimmune diseases

NET Antigen	*Autoimmune Disease*	
• Actin	RA, SLE nephritis	180,181
• Annexin	SLE	182
• Azurocidin	Vasculitis	183
• Catalase	SLE, RA	184
• Cathepsin G	Vasculitis	185
• Neutrophil defensins (HNP)	SLE	186
• dsDNA/chromatin	SLE nephritis	187
• Elastase	SLE, Vasculitis	188,189
• Enolase	RA	190
• Glyceraldehyde 3-phospate dehydrogenase	Multiple sclerosis, SLE	191,192
• Histones	SLE, RA, Felty's syndrome	193–196
• Histone-H4 (Citrullinated)	RA	197
• LL37	SLE	186
• Lysozyme	Vasculitis	185
• Myeloperoxidase	Vasculitis, SLE	185
• Proteinase 3	Vasculitis, SLE	185

The box is based on the NET-proteomic data from Urban et al,[10] *and the review by Darrah et al.*[198]

12.1. NETs in systemic lupus erythematosus and vasculitis

Systemic lupus erythematous (SLE) is a systemic, multifaceted, chronic autoimmune disorder[199] with severe pathological effects. The etiology of the disease is poorly understood. The disease course is unpredictable with periods of illness (flares) and remissions.[200] Immunosuppressants are virtually the only choice of therapy. However, this expectedly increases the susceptibility to infection, causing high mortality in all stages of SLE.[201,202] The hallmark of SLE is the production of circulating auto-antibodies against various tissues and cellular components, such as DNA,[187] nucleosomes,[193,194] complement proteins,[203,204] and granulocyte proteins such as MPO or proteinase 3 (PR3). Some of these antigens are neutrophil-specific, and hence the auto-antibodies against these antigens are collectively referred to as anti-neutrophil cytoplasmic antibodies (ANCA).[205] These antibodies are predominantly present in SLE and other autoimmune diseases such as vasculitis, a systemic autoimmune disease that causes inflammation of blood vessels.[206] Small-vessel vasculitis (SVV) affects the post-capillary venules and it is associated with PR3-ANCAs. However, the role of these antibodies in the progression of disease has been a point of debate because it is not clear how and why these antibodies are generated against intracellular proteins of neutrophils. Abnormalities in function and phenotypes have long been observed in SLE patients' neutrophils.[207] However, the characterization of NETs brought new insights into the understanding of how these antigens are exposed to the immune system and thus bridges the long-standing association between infection, neutrophils, and autoimmunity.

Interestingly, sera from SLE patients contain undigested NETs with self-DNA and antimicrobial peptide LL-37, which facilitate the activation of plasmacytoid dendritic cells (pDCs) in a TLR9-dependent fashion. This in turn results in the production of INF-α, which promotes the generation of LL-37 and dsDNA antibodies. LL-37 release and dsDNA antibody generation further activate circulating neutrophils to produce even more NETs. The culmination of events leads to a chronic activation of pDC, exacerbating the disease.[186] In addition to LL-37, SLE NETs contain alarmins such as HMGB1. This renders the NETs highly immunogenic and activates pDCs to produce IFN-α. This is evident from type I interferon (IFN)-primed mature neutrophils from pediatric SLE patients which undergo NETosis upon stimulation with sera containing anti-ribonucleoprotein antibodies.[208] Furthermore, a subset of circulating neutrophils from SLE patients, termed low-density granulocytes, can undergo spontaneous NET formation. This type of NET formation causes vascular damage and generates increased amounts of IFNs, which can potentiate SLE pathogenesis.[209] Interestingly, ANCA-IgG trigger neutrophils to undergo NETosis, prompting NET-mediated tissue damage in SVV. NET debris in the microvasculature of SVV patients suggests the pathogenic nature of NETs in vasculitis.[37] Additionally, NETs were identified in biopsies from inflamed skin vessels of a patient diagnosed with SVV.[210] Furthermore, propythiouracil (PTU), a drug used to manage hyperthyroidism is known to induce ANCA-associated vasculitis in a rodent model. Interestingly, treatment with PTU along with PMA results in abnormal conformation of NETs that are resistant to NET degradation by DNase I, suggesting that ANCA-associated NETs may be resistant to degradation, and thus this contributes to the pathogenesis of MPO ANCA-associated vasculitis.[211] Similarly, vasculitis can be triggered by adoptively transferring NET-activated myeloid DCs to naïve mice. NETs are immunogenic and trigger the production of ANCAs in mice, which can be abrogated with DNase1 infusion.[212]

Lupus is a disease of clearance deficiency. The debris from dying cells has been suggested to be the major source of auto-antigens contributing to the pathology of SLE.[213] NETs are composed of DNA, histones, antimicrobial peptides, and other granule proteins. Interestingly, 84% of NET components are reported in patients with autoimmunity. Among them, 74% have been reported to be associated with systemic autoimmune diseases, including SLE, RA, and vasculitis.[198] Thus, an efficient degradation and clearance of NETs is essential to prevent the immune system from processing components of NETs as antigens. NETosis, unlike apoptosis, lacks caspase activation, and therefore the caspase-activated DNase (CAD)[214,215] does not degrade NETs. However, serum DNase1 degrades NETs efficiently.[65] The crucial link between NETs and SLE is that subsets of SLE patients (around 40%) have impaired NET degradation (non-degraders) compared to healthy donors. This is because the patients have DNase1 inhibitors in the serum that prevent NET degradation or they have anti-NET-antibodies that protect the NETs from serum DNase1 or both.[65] This was independent of the DNase1 mutation that was reported in a small cohort from Japan.[216]

SLE affects almost any part of the body that can exhibit inflammation. Blood vessel anomalies include bland vasculopathy, vasculitis, and deposition of immune complexes. Several organs and tissues are targeted during the progression and the end stage of SLE.[217] Lupus nephritis is an inflammation of the kidney that is characterized by high levels of protein (proteinurea) in the urine, which is an indirect measure of the function of filtration by the glomeruli. Additionally, monitoring kidney biopsies over the course of the disease show abnormalities in basement membrane and immune complex depositions. Interestingly, the patients who do not degrade NETs (SLE-non-degraders) are prone to more severe forms of lupus nephritis compared to the degraders, and also show evidence for NET–immune complexes in kidney biopsies, suggesting that impairment in NET degradation contributes to the severity of the SLE.[65]

Impaired NET degradation in SVV is also attributed to the pathogenic NET deposition in the microvasculature.[37] A plausible therapeutic intervention could be to complement patients with recombinant DNase1 to degrade the NETs. For patients who have inhibitors of DNase1 in their sera, a therapeutically compatible alternative nuclease or an engineered DNase1 that is resistant to inhibitors of DNase1 could be administered. For those patients who have anti-NET antibodies, an immune depletion of anti-NET antibodies may restore the serum DNase1 activity. Additionally, NET degradation efficiency correlates with severity of lupus nephritis, and this may be used as a novel diagnostic tool for assessing the severity of lupus nephritis.

12.2. *NETs in rheumatoid arthritis*

Rheumatoid arthritis (RA) is a systemic autoimmune disease characterized by synovial inflammation causing swelling and destruction of cartilages and bones, leading to deformity. RA patients often present with elevated levels of citrullinated proteins and high titers of anticitrullinated peptide antibodies (ACPA's).[218,219] However, the underlying mechanism of the disease is obscure. Like SLE, infection, pathobionts, or their effectors[220–225] have long been thought to be the trigger for RA progression. However, there are no unifying mechanisms that may explain this phenomenon.

NETs are abundant in the synovial fluids (SF), rheumatoid nodules, and skin. The serum containing ACPAs in the presence of SF is sufficient to initiate NET formation. Furthermore, NET formation is also spontaneous in neutrophils isolated from RA patients.[226] The SF has elevated levels of proinflammatory cytokines such as IL17A and TNF-α. However, IL-17A and TNF-α alone do not prompt NET formation in RA patient's neutrophils, whereas LPS-primed neutrophils undergo NETosis. Citrullinated vimentin is exposed during NET formation and anticitrullinated vimetin antibodies from RA patients can trigger NETosis. This potentiates a vicious cycle leading to aberrant NET formation in RA patients.[227] In line with this, metalloprotease-8 (MMP-8), an inactive pro-protein, is activated only by cleavage by extracellular proteinases. Interestingly, MMP-8 is predominant in NETs triggered by RA antibodies. Since NETs release proteinases, this may cleave and activate the MMP-8, which may degrade the extracellular matrix contributing to tissue damage in arthritis.

12.3. *NETs in other autoimmune diseases*

NETs have also been associated with other autoimmune diseases, which are less prevalent compared to SLE and RA. Felty's syndrome is one such disease which shows symptoms similar to RA, along with splenomegaly (enlarged spleen) and neutropenia. Patients with Felty syndrome have autoantibodies against PAD-4-deiminated histones which bind to NETs.[196] However, further studies will aid in understanding if NETs are produced in Felty syndrome patients and if those NETs have pro- or anti-inflammatory activity during the disease progression.

Another autoimmune disorder associated with NETs is type 1 diabetes (T1D). The disease results from autoimmune-mediated destruction of insulin-producing beta cells in the pancreas. Here again, the cause of T1D is unclear. In T1D patients, the neutrophil proteins PR3 and NE positively correlated with the autoantibodies against beta-cell antigens. Furthermore, T1D patients have elevated levels of NETs and decreased levels of alpha1-antitrypsin, an inhibitor of neutrophil serine proteases, suggesting a role for NETs in the pathogenesis of T1D.[228]

Taken together, it is plausible to assume that infection or inflammatory responses trigger NETosis. Impaired NET degradation or aberrant NET formation may contribute to immunogenic NETs that activate pDCs to produce inflammatory molecules. This in turn may initiate a feed-forward autoimmune cycle resulting in the progression of SLE, RA, vasculitis, and other autoimmune diseases. A timely intervention of this vicious cycle by either regulating aberrant NET formation using inhibitors of NETosis[55] or by aiding the degradation of NETs by therapeutically administering recombinant DNase1 might open new avenues in autoimmune therapy for diseases such as SLE. Recent studies have also identified specific targets for inhibition of NET formation. For example, inhibitors of peptidylarginine deiminases effectively block NET formation *in vitro* and also in mouse models of lupus.[64] The compound GSK106 is a novel inhibitor for PAD4 which has the potential to treat NET associated diseases.[229]

13. Anti-inflammatory NETs

Analysis of gout revealed anti-inflammatory properties of NETs.[179] Gout is an acute inflammatory disease of the joints, which resolves within a few days and leaves patients with characteristic gouty tophi.

Gout is precipitated by the deposition of MSU crystals in the synovial fluid, which triggers a strong inflammatory response characterized by a massive invasion of neutrophils. MSU crystals stimulate neutrophils to release NETs in the synovial space. Upon binding to NETs, synovial cytokines and chemokines are proteolytically inactivated by neutrophil serine proteases. Through the inactivation of pro-inflammatory stimuli, NETs diminish further neutrophil recruitment and limit inflammation in gout. Importantly, NETs also exhibit anti-inflammatory properties when induced by stimuli other than MSU crystals, indicating a prominent role for NETs the resolution of inflammation.

14. Conclusions

The original discovery of NETs in 2004 led almost 2000 follow-up studies published in the last decade. Antimicrobial activity and cytotoxic, pro-thrombotic, immunogenic, and anti-inflammatory properties have been attributed to NETs. Consequently, NETs ameliorate infections and limit acute inflammatory reactions while aggravating disease activity in cardiovascular or autoimmune conditions. The broad spectrum of NET-associated conditions will likely be further expanded. NETs have recently been identified in the periphery of tumors[230] and linked to metastasis,[176] associating NETs with cancer. The broad spectrum of NET-associated diseases indicates that NETs are a fundamental part of the acute inflammatory response. However, NETs are a challenging field of study due to limitations in the specificity of available techniques. Scanning electron microscopy, commonly used to illustrate the fine architecture of NETs, cannot distinguish the NETs from the fibrin scaffold.[231] Targeting NE- or PAD4-mediated chromatin decondensation in NETosis blocks NET release in murine disease models. Importantly, NE is also required for neutrophil functions mediated by phagocytosis or degranulation, while unfolding of chromatin by PAD4 controls gene expression in stem cells and hematopoietic development.[232,233] Promoting NET degradation by infusions of DNase1 is another commonly used method to address NET functions *in vivo*. DNase1 is not specific against NETs, but targets extracellular DNA in general. Considering that collateral tissue necrosis is commonly observed in inflammation, it conceivable that DNase1-mediated effects are in part to due to the degradation of DNA released from necrotic cells. Alternatively, DNase1 may target extracellular traps release by cells other than neutrophils. Indeed, extracellular trap (ET) formation is not limited to neutrophils and has been documented for mast cells,[234] eosinophils,[27,235] and monocytes.[48] ET is not restricted to humans[1] or mice,[236] but is also found in cats,[90] rabbits,[1] birds,[237] fish,[238] insects,[239] and even plants.[240] The omnipresence of ETs may be due to the fact that the majority of ET functions are mediated by DNA and histones. DNA and histones are highly conserved molecules, which themselves display antimicrobial, cytotoxic, and pro-thrombotic activities. In conclusion, the release of DNA and histones in the form of ET may be an evolutionarily conserved mechanism to fight microbes in the extracellular space.

Acknowledgments

This work was supported by a Marie Curie Fellowship to T.A.F. (ESR 628264) and by funding from Åke Wiberg Foundation to C.F.U. (M14-0076). We thank Brent Cezairliyan for critical reading of the manuscript.

References

1. Brinkmann V *et al.* (2004). Neutrophil extracellular traps kill bacteria. *Science*. 303:1532–1535.
2. Borregaard N. (2010). Neutrophils, from marrow to microbes. *Immunity*. 33:657–670.
3. Borregaard N, Cowland JB. (1997). Granules of the human neutrophilic polymorphonuclear leukocyte. *Blood*. 89:3503–3521.
4. Amulic B, Cazalet C, Hayes GL, Metzler KD, Zychlinsky A. (2012). Neutrophil function: from mechanisms to disease. *Ann Rev Immunol*. 30:459–489.

5. Nauseef WM, Borregaard N. (2014). Neutrophils at work. *Nat Immunol.* **15**:602–611.
6. Frenette PS, Wagner DD. (1996). Adhesion molecules — Part II: Blood vessels and blood cells. *The New England J Med.* **335**:43–45.
7. Owen CA, Campbell MA, Sannes PL, Boukedes SS, Campbell EJ. (1995). Cell surface-bound elastase and cathepsin G on human neutrophils: a novel, non-oxidative mechanism by which neutrophils focus and preserve catalytic activity of serine proteinases. *The J Cell Biol.* **131**:775–789.
8. Hampton MB, Kettle AJ, Winterbourn CC. (1998). Inside the neutrophil phagosome: oxidants, myeloperoxidase, and bacterial killing. *Blood.* **92**:3007–3017.
9. Weinrauch Y, Drujan D, Shapiro SD, Weiss J, Zychlinsky A. (2002). Neutrophil elastase targets virulence factors of enterobacteria. *Nature.* **417**:91–94.
10. Urban CF *et al.* (2009). Neutrophil extracellular traps contain calprotectin, a cytosolic protein complex involved in host defense against Candida albicans. *PLoS pathogens.* **5**:e1000639.
11. Fuchs TA *et al.*(2007). Novel cell death program leads to neutrophil extracellular traps. *The J Cell Biol.* **176**:231–241.
12. Jaillon S *et al.* (2007). The humoral pattern recognition receptor PTX3 is stored in neutrophil granules and localizes in extracellular traps. *The J Expe Medi.* **204**:793–804.
13. Parker H, Albrett AM, Kettle AJ, Winterbourn CC. (2012). Myeloperoxidase associated with neutrophil extracellular traps is active and mediates bacterial killing in the presence of hydrogen peroxide. *J Leukocyte Biol.* **91**:369–376.
14. Hirsch JG. (1958). Bactericidal action of histone. *The J Expe Medi.* **108**:925–944.
15. Brinkmann V, Zychlinsky A. (2012). Neutrophil extracellular traps: is immunity the second function of chromatin? *The J Cell Biol.* **198**:773–783.
16. Simon D, Simon HU, Yousefi S. (2013). Extracellular DNA traps in allergic, infectious, and autoimmune diseases. *Allergy.* **68**:409–416.
17. Yipp BG, Kubes P. (2013). NETosis: how vital is it? *Blood.* **122**:2784–2794.
18. Steinberg BE, Grinstein S. (2007). Unconventional roles of the NADPH oxidase: signaling, ion homeostasis, and cell death. *Science's STKE: Signal Trans. Knowledge Environ.* **2007**:pe11.
19. Yousefi S, Mihalache C, Kozlowski E, Schmid I, Simon HU. (2009). Viable neutrophils release mitochondrial DNA to form neutrophil extracellular traps. *Cell Death Diffe.* **16**:1438–1444.
20. Yipp BG *et al.* (2012). Infection-induced NETosis is a dynamic process involving neutrophil multitasking *in vivo*. *Nat Medi.* **18**:1386–1393.

21. Papayannopoulos V, Metzler KD, Hakkim A, Zychlinsky A. (2010). Neutrophil elastase and myeloperoxidase regulate the formation of neutrophil extracellular traps. *The J Cell Biol.* **191**:677–691.
22. Remijsen Q *et al.* (2011). Neutrophil extracellular trap cell death requires both autophagy and superoxide generation. *Cell Res.* **21**:290–304.
23. Remijsen Q *et al.* (2011). Dying for a cause: NETosis, mechanisms behind an antimicrobial cell death modality. *Cell Death Diffe.* **18**:581–588.
24. Branzk N *et al.* (2014). Neutrophils sense microbe size and selectively release neutrophil extracellular traps in response to large pathogens. *Nat Immunol.* **15**:1017–1025.
25. Pilsczek FH *et al.* (2010). A novel mechanism of rapid nuclear neutrophil extracellular trap formation in response to Staphylococcus aureus. *J Immunol.* **185**:7413–7425.
26. Malawista SE, De Boisfleury Chevance A. (1982). The cytokineplast: purified, stable, and functional motile machinery from human blood polymorphonuclear leukocytes. *The J Cell Biol.* **95**:960–973.
27. Yousefi S *et al.* (2008). Catapult-like release of mitochondrial DNA by eosinophils contributes to antibacterial defense. *Nat Medi.* **14**:949–953.
28. Keshari RS *et al.* (2012). Cytokines induced neutrophil extracellular traps formation: implication for the inflammatory disease condition. *PloS One.* 7:e48111.
29. Clark SR *et al.* (2007). Platelet TLR4 activates neutrophil extracellular traps to ensnare bacteria in septic blood. *Nat Medi.* **13**:463–469.
30. McDonald B, Urrutia R, Yipp BG, Jenne CN, Kubes P. (2012). Intravascular neutrophil extracellular traps capture bacteria from the bloodstream during sepsis. *Cell Host Microbe.* **12**:324–333.
31. Chen K *et al.* (2012). Endocytosis of soluble immune complexes leads to their clearance by FcgammaRIIIB but induces neutrophil extracellular traps via FcgammaRIIA *in vivo*. *Blood.* **120**:4421–4431.
32. Parker H, Dragunow M, Hampton MB, Kettle AJ, Winterbourn CC. (2012). Requirements for NADPH oxidase and myeloperoxidase in neutrophil extracellular trap formation differ depending on the stimulus. *J Leukocyte Biol.* **92**:841–849.
33. Urban CF, Reichard U, Brinkmann V, Zychlinsky A. (2006). Neutrophil extracellular traps capture and kill Candida albicans yeast and hyphal forms. *Cellular Microbiol.* **8**:668–676.
34. Guimaraes-Costa AB *et al.* (2009). Leishmania amazonensis promastigotes induce and are killed by neutrophil extracellular traps. *Proc Nat Acade Sci USA.* **106**:6748–6753.
35. Neeli I, Dwivedi N, Khan S, Radic M. (2009). Regulation of extracellular chromatin release from neutrophils. *J Innate Immunity.* **1**:194–201.

36. Byrd AS, O'Brien XM, Johnson CM, Lavigne LM, Reichner JS. (2013). An extracellular matrix-based mechanism of rapid neutrophil extracellular trap formation in response to Candida albicans. *J Immunol.* **190**:4136–4148.
37. Kessenbrock K *et al.* (2009). Netting neutrophils in autoimmune small-vessel vasculitis. *Nat Medi.* **15**:623–625.
38. Martinelli S *et al.* (2004). Induction of genes mediating interferon-dependent extracellular trap formation during neutrophil differentiation. *The J Biol Chem.* **279**:44123–44132.
39. Yost CC *et al.* (2009). Impaired neutrophil extracellular trap (NET) formation: a novel innate immune deficiency of human neonates. *Blood.* **113**:6419–6427.
40. Tadie JM *et al.* (2013). HMGB1 promotes neutrophil extracellular trap formation through interactions with Toll-like receptor 4. *American Journal of physiology. Lung Cell Molecular Physiol.* **304**:L342–349.
41. Patel S *et al.* (2010). Nitric oxide donors release extracellular traps from human neutrophils by augmenting free radical generation. *Nitric Oxide: Biol. Chem/Offi. J Nitric Oxide Soci.* **22**:226–234.
42. Palmer LJ *et al.* (2012). Hypochlorous acid regulates neutrophil extracellular trap release in humans. *Clin Exp Immunol.* **167**:261–268.
43. Kirchner T *et al.* (2012). The impact of various reactive oxygen species on the formation of neutrophil extracellular traps. *Medi Inflamm.* **2012**:849136.
44. Akong-Moore K, Chow OA, von Kockritz-Blickwede M, Nizet V. (2012). Influences of chloride and hypochlorite on neutrophil extracellular trap formation. *PloS One.* **7**:e42984.
45. Chen G *et al.* (2014). Heme-induced neutrophil extracellular traps contribute to the pathogenesis of sickle cell disease. *Blood.* **123**:3818–3827.
46. Schorn C *et al.* (2012). Monosodium urate crystals induce extracellular DNA traps in neutrophils, eosinophils, and basophils but not in mononuclear cells. *Front Immunol.* **3**:277.
47. Gupta AK *et al.* (2010). Activated endothelial cells induce neutrophil extracellular traps and are susceptible to NETosis-mediated cell death. *FEBS Lett.* **584**:3193–3197.
48. Chow OA *et al.* (2010). Statins enhance formation of phagocyte extracellular traps. *Cell Host Microbe.* **8**:445–454.
49. Munks MW *et al.* (2010). Aluminum adjuvants elicit fibrin-dependent extracellular traps *in vivo*. *Blood.* **116**:5191–5199.
50. Neeli I, Khan SN, Radic M. (2008). Histone deimination as a response to inflammatory stimuli in neutrophils. *J Immunol.* **180**:1895–1902.
51. Metzler KD *et al.* (2011). Myeloperoxidase is required for neutrophil extracellular trap formation: implications for innate immunity. *Blood.* **117**:953–959.
52. Neeli I, Radic M. (2013). Opposition between PKC isoforms regulates histone deimination and neutrophil extracellular chromatin release. *Fronti Immunol.* **4**:38.

53. Lim MB, Kuiper JW, Katchky A, Goldberg H, Glogauer M. (2011). Rac2 is required for the formation of neutrophil extracellular traps. *J Leukocyte Biol.* **90**:771–776.
54. Bianchi M *et al.* (2009). Restoration of NET formation by gene therapy in CGD controls aspergillosis. *Blood.* **114**:2619–2622.
55. Hakkim A *et al.* (2011). Activation of the Raf-MEK-ERK pathway is required for neutrophil extracellular trap formation. *Nat Chem Biol.* **7**:75–77.
56. Metzler KD, Goosmann, C, Lubojemska, A, Zychlinsky, A, Papayannopoulos, V. (2014). A myeloperoxidase-containing complex regulates neutrophil elastase release and actin dynamics during NETosis. *Cell Rep.* **8**:883–896.
57. Xu J *et al.* (2009). Extracellular histones are major mediators of death in sepsis. *Nat Medi.* **15**:1318–1321.
58. Farley K, Stolley JM, Zhao P, Cooley J, Remold-O'Donnell E. (2012). A serpinB1 regulatory mechanism is essential for restricting neutrophil extracellular trap generation. *J Immunol.* **189**:4574–4581.
59. Li P *et al.* (2010). PAD4 is essential for antibacterial innate immunity mediated by neutrophil extracellular traps. *The J Exp Medi.* **207**:1853–1862.
60. Wang Y *et al.* (2009). Histone hypercitrullination mediates chromatin decondensation and neutrophil extracellular trap formation. *The J Cell Biol.* **184**:205–213.
61. Kambas K *et al.* (2012). Autophagy mediates the delivery of thrombogenic tissue factor to neutrophil extracellular traps in human sepsis. *PloS One.* **7**:e45427.
62. McInturff AM *et al.* (2012). Mammalian target of rapamycin regulates neutrophil extracellular trap formation via induction of hypoxia-inducible factor 1 alpha. *Blood.* **120**:3118–3125.
63. Willis VC *et al.* (2011). N-alpha-benzoyl-N5-(2-chloro-1-iminoethyl)-L-ornithine amide, a protein arginine deiminase inhibitor, reduces the severity of murine collagen-induced arthritis. *J Immunol.* **186**:4396–4404.
64. Knight JS *et al.* (2013). Peptidylarginine deiminase inhibition is immunomodulatory and vasculoprotective in murine lupus. *The J Clin Invest.* **123**:2981–2993.
65. Hakkim A *et al.* (2010). Impairment of neutrophil extracellular trap degradation is associated with lupus nephritis. *Proc Nat Acad Sci USA.* **107**:9813–9818.
66. Jimenez-Alcazar M *et al.* (2014). Impaired DNase1-mediated degradation of neutrophil extracellular traps is associated with acute thrombotic microangiopathies. *J Thrombosis Haemostasis.*
67. Farrera C, Fadeel B. (2013). Macrophage clearance of neutrophil extracellular traps is a silent process. *J Immunol.* **191**:2647–2656.
68. Thammavongsa V, Missiakas DM, Schneewind O. (2013). Staphylococcus aureus degrades neutrophil extracellular traps to promote immune cell death. *Science.* **342**:863–866.

69. Fuchs TA *et al.* (2010). Extracellular DNA traps promote thrombosis. *Proc Nat Acade Scie USA.* **107**:15880–15885.
70. Saitoh T *et al.* (2012). Neutrophil extracellular traps mediate a host defense response to human immunodeficiency virus-1. *Cell Host & Microbe.* **12**:109–116.
71. Raftery MJ *et al.* (2014). beta2 integrin mediates hantavirus-induced release of neutrophil extracellular traps. *The J Expe Medi.* **211**:1485–1497.
72. Hemmers S, Teijaro JR, Arandjelovic S, Mowen KA. (2011). PAD4-mediated neutrophil extracellular trap formation is not required for immunity against influenza infection. *PloS One.* **6**:e22043.
73. Yan J *et al.* (2012). Glutathione reductase facilitates host defense by sustaining phagocytic oxidative burst and promoting the development of neutrophil extracellular traps. *J Immunol.* **188**:2316–2327.
74. Dwyer M *et al.* (2014). Cystic fibrosis sputum DNA has NETosis characteristics and neutrophil extracellular trap release is regulated by macrophage migration-inhibitory factor. *J Innate Immu.* **6**:765–779.
75. Young RL *et al.* (2011). Neutrophil extracellular trap (NET)-mediated killing of Pseudomonas aeruginosa: evidence of acquired resistance within the CF airway, independent of CFTR. *PloS one.* **6**:e23637.
76. Seper A *et al.* (2013). Vibrio cholerae evades neutrophil extracellular traps by the activity of two extracellular nucleases. *PLoS Pathogens.* **9**:e1003614.
77. Mori Y *et al.* (2012). α-Enolase of Streptococcus pneumoniae Induces Formation of Neutrophil Extracellular Traps. *The J Biol Chem.* **287**:10472–10481.
78. Beiter K *et al.* (2006). An Endonuclease Allows Streptococcus pneumoniae to Escape from Neutrophil Extracellular Traps. *Curr Biol.* **16**:401–407.
79. Lauth X *et al.* (2009). M1 protein allows Group A streptococcal survival in phagocyte extracellular traps through cathelicidin inhibition. *J Innate Immu.* **1**:202–214.
80. de Buhr N, Neumann A, Jerjomiceva N, von Kockritz-Blickwede M, Baums CG. (2014). Streptococcus suis DNase SsnA contributes to degradation of neutrophil extracellular traps (NETs) and evasion of NET-mediated antimicrobial activity. *Microbiol.* **160**:385–395.
81. Ramos-Kichik V *et al.* (2009). Neutrophil extracellular traps are induced by Mycobacterium tuberculosis. *Tuberculosis.* **89**:29–37.
82. Svobodova E *et al.* (2012). Differential interaction of the two related fungal species Candida albicans and Candida dubliniensis with human neutrophils. *J Immunol.* **189**:2502–2511.
83. Springer DJ *et al.* (2010). Extracellular fibrils of pathogenic yeast Cryptococcus gattii are important for ecological niche, murine virulence and human neutrophil interactions. *PloS One.* **5**:e10978.

84. Bruns S *et al.* (2010). Production of extracellular traps against Aspergillus fumigatus in vitro and in infected lung tissue is dependent on invading neutrophils and influenced by hydrophobin RodA. *PLoS pathogens.* **6**:e1000873.
85. Gabriel C, McMaster WR, Girard D, Descoteaux A. (2010). Leishmania donovani promastigotes evade the antimicrobial activity of neutrophil extracellular traps. *J Immunol.* **185**:4319–4327.
86. Abi Abdallah DS *et al.* (2012). Toxoplasma gondii triggers release of human and mouse neutrophil extracellular traps. *Infect Immun.* **80**:768–777.
87. Behrendt JH, Ruiz A, Zahner H, Taubert A, Hermosilla C. (2010). Neutrophil extracellular trap formation as innate immune reactions against the apicomplexan parasite Eimeria bovis. *Veterinary Immunol. Immunopathol.* **133**:1–8.
88. Silva LM *et al.* (2014). The apicomplexan parasite Eimeria arloingi induces caprine neutrophil extracellular traps. *Parasitol Res.* **113**:2797–2807.
89. Baker VS *et al.* (2008). Cytokine-associated neutrophil extracellular traps and antinuclear antibodies in Plasmodium falciparum infected children under six years of age. *Malaria J.* **7**:41.
90. Wardini AB *et al.* (2010). Characterization of neutrophil extracellular traps in cats naturally infected with feline leukemia virus. *The J General Virol.* **91**:259–264.
91. Narasaraju T *et al.* (2011). Excessive neutrophils and neutrophil extracellular traps contribute to acute lung injury of influenza pneumonitis. *The Am J Pathol.* **179**:199–210.
92. Brandt T, Breitenstein S, von der Hardt H, Tummler B. (1995). DNA concentration and length in sputum of patients with cystic fibrosis during inhalation with recombinant human DNase. *Thorax.* **50**:880–882.
93. Rahman S, Gadjeva M. (2014). Does NETosis Contribute to the Bacterial Pathoadaptation in Cystic Fibrosis? *Front. Immunol.* **5**:378.
94. Limoli DH *et al.* (2014). Cationic antimicrobial peptides promote microbial mutagenesis and pathoadaptation in chronic infections. *PLoS pathogens.* **10**:e1004083.
95. Rada B *et al.* (2013). Pyocyanin-enhanced neutrophil extracellular trap formation requires the NADPH oxidase. *PloS One.* **8**:e54205.
96. Belaaouaj A *et al.* (1998). Mice lacking neutrophil elastase reveal impaired host defense against gram negative bacterial sepsis. *Nat Medi.* **4**:615–618.
97. Achouiti A *et al.* (2012). Myeloid-related protein-14 contributes to protective immunity in gram-negative pneumonia derived sepsis. *PLoS pathogens.* **8**:e1002987.
98. Berends ET *et al.* (2010). Nuclease expression by Staphylococcus aureus facilitates escape from neutrophil extracellular traps. *J Innate Immu.* **2**:576–586.

99. Henriques-Normark B, Normark S. (2010). Commensal pathogens, with a focus on Streptococcus pneumoniae, and interactions with the human host. *Exp Cell Res.* **316**:1408–1414.
100. O'Loughlin RE *et al.* (2007). The epidemiology of invasive group A streptococcal infection and potential vaccine implications: United States, 2000-2004. *Clinical Infectious Diseases: An Official Publ Inf Diseases Soci of Am.* **45**:853–862.
101. Sumby P *et al.* (2005). Extracellular deoxyribonuclease made by group A Streptococcus assists pathogenesis by enhancing evasion of the innate immune response. *Proc Nat Acad Sci USA.* **102**:1679–1684.
102. Buchanan JT *et al.* (2006). DNase expression allows the pathogen group A Streptococcus to escape killing in neutrophil extracellular traps. *Curr Biol CB.* **16**:396–400.
103. Walker, MJ *et al.* (2007). DNase Sda1 provides selection pressure for a switch to invasive group A streptococcal infection. *Nat Med.* **13**:981–985.
104. Uchiyama S, Andreoni F, Schuepbach RA, Nizet V, Zinkernagel AS. (2012). DNase Sda1 allows invasive M1T1 Group A Streptococcus to prevent TLR9-dependent recognition. *PLoS Pathogens.* **8**:e1002736.
105. Short KR *et al.* (2014). Antibodies Mediate Formation of Neutrophil Extracellular Traps in the Middle Ear and Facilitate Secondary Pneumococcal Otitis Media. *Inf Immu.* **82**:364–370.
106. Nandi B, Behar SM. (2011). Regulation of neutrophils by interferon-gamma limits lung inflammation during tuberculosis infection. *The J Exp Med.* **208**:2251–2262.
107. Hicheri Y, Cook G, Cordonnier C. (2012). Antifungal prophylaxis in haematology patients: the role of voriconazole. *Clinical microbiology and infection: The Official Pub Europ Soc Clin Microbiol Inf Diseases.* **18**(Suppl 2): 1–15.
108. Martins N, Ferreira IC, Barros L, Silva S, Henriques M. (2014). Candidiasis: predisposing factors, prevention, diagnosis and alternative treatment. *Mycopathol.* **177**:223–240.
109. Gow NA, van de Veerdonk FL, Brown AJ, Netea MG. (2012). Candida albicans morphogenesis and host defence: discriminating invasion from colonization. *Nat Rev Microbiol.* **10**:112–122.
110. McCormick A *et al.* (2010). NETs formed by human neutrophils inhibit growth of the pathogenic mold Aspergillus fumigatus. *Microbes and Infection/Institut Pasteur.* **12**:928–936.
111. Nani S *et al.* (2015). Src Family Kinases and Syk Are Required for Neutrophil Extracellular Trap Formation in Response to beta-Glucan Particles. *J Innate Immu.* 7:59–73.
112. Bianchi M, Niemiec MJ, Siler U, Urban CF, Reichenbach J. (2011). Restoration of anti-Aspergillus defense by neutrophil extracellular traps in

human chronic granulomatous disease after gene therapy is calprotectin-dependent. *The J Allergy Clin Immunol.* **127**:1243–1252 e1247.

113. Rohm M *et al.* (2014). NADPH oxidase promotes neutrophil extracellular trap formation in pulmonary aspergillosis. *Infect Immun.* **82**:1766–1777.
114. Kumar R, Engwerda C. (2014). Vaccines to prevent leishmaniasis. *Clin Translational Immunol.* **3**:e13.
115. Guimaraes-Costa AB *et al.* (2014). 3'-nucleotidase/nuclease activity allows Leishmania parasites to escape killing by neutrophil extracellular traps. *Infect Immun.* **82**:1732–1740.
116. Wang Y *et al.* (2011). Differential microbicidal effects of human histone proteins H2A and H2B on Leishmania promastigotes and amastigotes. *Infect Immun.* **79**:1124–1133.
117. Grommes J, Soehnlein O. (2011). Contribution of neutrophils to acute lung injury. *Molecular Medi.* **17**:293–307.
118. Segel GB, Halterman MW Lichtman MA. (2011). The paradox of the neutrophil's role in tissue injury. *J Leukocyte Biol.* **89**:359–372.
119. Saffarzadeh M *et al.* (2012). Neutrophil extracellular traps directly induce epithelial and endothelial cell death: a predominant role of histones. *PloS One.* **7**:e32366.
120. Kleine TJ, Gladfelter A, Lewis PN, Lewis SA. (1995). Histone-induced damage of a mammalian epithelium: the conductive effect. *The Am J Physiol.* **268**:C1114–1125.
121. Kleine TJ, Lewis PN, Lewis SA. (1997). Histone-induced damage of a mammalian epithelium: the role of protein and membrane structure. *The Am J Physiol.* **273**:C1925–1936.
122. De Meyer SF, Suidan GL, Fuchs TA, Monestier M, Wagner D.D. (2012). Extracellular chromatin is an important mediator of ischemic stroke in mice. *Arteriosclerosis, Thrombosis, and Vascular Biol.* **32**:1884–1891.
123. Huang H *et al.* (2011). Endogenous histones function as alarmins in sterile inflammatory liver injury through Toll-like receptor 9 in mice. *Hepatol.* **54**:999–1008.
124. Xu J, Zhang X, Monestier M, Esmon NL, Esmon CT. (2011). Extracellular histones are mediators of death through TLR2 and TLR4 in mouse fatal liver injury. *J Immunol.* **187**:2626–2631.
125. Voynow JA, Fischer BM, Zheng S. (2008). Proteases and cystic fibrosis. *The Inter J Biochem Cell Biol.* **40**:1238–1245.
126. Lee WL, Grinstein S. Immunology. (2004). The tangled webs that neutrophils weave. *Science.* **303**:1477–1478.
127. Papayannopoulos V, Staab D, Zychlinsky A. (2011). Neutrophil elastase enhances sputum solubilization in cystic fibrosis patients receiving DNase therapy. *PloS One.* **6**:e28526.

128. Dubois AV *et al.* (2012). Influence of DNA on the activities and inhibition of neutrophil serine proteases in cystic fibrosis sputum. *Am J Res Cell Molecular Biol.* **47**:80–86.
129. Caudrillier A *et al.* (2012). Platelets induce neutrophil extracellular traps in transfusion-related acute lung injury. *The J Clin Investi.* **122**:2661–2671.
130. Thomas GM *et al.* (2012). Extracellular DNA traps are associated with the pathogenesis of TRALI in humans and mice. *Blood.* **119**:6335–6343.
131. Fuchs TA *et al.* (2013). Neutrophils release extracellular DNA traps during storage of red blood cell units. *Transfusion.* **53**:3210–3216.
132. Shaz BH, Stowell SR, Hillyer CD. (2011). Transfusion-related acute lung injury: from bedside to bench and back. *Blood.* **117**:1463–1471.
133. Carden DL, Granger DN. (2000). Pathophysiology of ischaemia-reperfusion injury. *The J Pathol.* **190**:255–266.
134. Allam R *et al.* (2012). Histones from dying renal cells aggravate kidney injury via TLR2 and TLR4. *J Am Soci Nephrol: JASN.* **23**:1375–1388.
135. Savchenko AS *et al.* (2014). VWF-mediated leukocyte recruitment with chromatin decondensation by PAD4 increases myocardial ischemia/reperfusion injury in mice. *Blood.* **123**:141–148.
136. Huang H *et al.* (2013). Histones activate the NLRP3 inflammasome in Kupffer cells during sterile inflammatory liver injury. *J Immunol.* **191**:2665–2679.
137. Engelmann B, Massberg S. (2013). Thrombosis as an intravascular effector of innate immunity. *Nat Rev Immunol.* **13**:34–45.
138. Libby P, Simon DI. (2001). Inflammation and thrombosis: the clot thickens. *Circulation.* **103**:1718–1720.
139. Esmon CT. (2013). Molecular circuits in thrombosis and inflammation. *Thrombosis and Haemostasis.* **109**:416–420.
140. Gupta AK *et al.* (2010). Activated endothelial cells induce neutrophil extracellular traps and are susceptible to NETosis-mediated cell death. *FEBS Lett.* **584**:3193–3197.
141. Ward CM, Tetaz TJ, Andrews RK, Berndt MC. (1997). Binding of the von Willebrand factor A1 domain to histone. *Thrombosis Res.* **86**:469–477.
142. Grassle S *et al.* (2014). von Willebrand factor directly interacts with DNA from neutrophil extracellular traps. *Arteriosclerosis, Thrombosis Vascular Biol.* **34**:1382–1389.
143. Pereira LF *et al.* (1994). Histones interact with anionic phospholipids with high avidity; its relevance for the binding of histone-antihistone immune complexes. *Clin Exp Immu.* **97**:175–180.
144. Kleine TJ, Gladfelter A, Lewis PN, Lewis SA. (1995). Histone-induced damage of a mammalian epithelium: the conductive effect. *Am J Physiol.* **268**:C1114–1125.

145. Xu J *et al.* (2009). Extracellular histones are major mediators of death in sepsis. *Nat Med.* **15**:1318–1321.
146. Sporn LA Marder VJ, Wagner DD. (1986). Inducible secretion of large, biologically potent von Willebrand factor multimers. *Cell.* **46**:185–190.
147. Fuchs TA *et al.* (2010). Extracellular DNA traps promote thrombosis. *Proc Natl Acad Sci USA.* **107**:15880–15885.
148. Semeraro F *et al.* (2011). Extracellular histones promote thrombin generation through platelet-dependent mechanisms: involvement of platelet TLR2 and TLR4. *Blood.* **118**:1952–1961.
149. Fuchs TA, Bhandari AA, Wagner DD. (2011). Histones induce rapid and profound thrombocytopenia in mice. *Blood.* **118**:3708–3714.
150. Watson K, Gooderham NJ, Davies DS, Edwards RJ. (1999). Nucleosomes bind to cell surface proteoglycans. *J Biol Chem.* **274**:21707–21713.
151. Muller F *et al.* (2009). Platelet polyphosphates are proinflammatory and procoagulant mediators *in vivo*. *Cell.* **139**:1143–1156.
152. Brill A *et al.* (2012). Neutrophil extracellular traps promote deep vein thrombosis in mice. *Journal of thrombosis and haemostasis: JTH.* **10**:136–144.
153. Barr JD, Chauhan AK, Schaeffer GV, Hansen JK, Motto DG. (2013). Red blood cells mediate the onset of thrombosis in the ferric chloride murine model. *Blood.* **121**:3733–3741.
154. Andrews DA, Low PS. (1999). Role of red blood cells in thrombosis. *Curr Opin Hematol.* **6**:76–82.
155. Semeraro F, Ammollo CT, Esmon NL, Esmon CT. (2014). Histones induce phosphatidylserine exposure and a procoagulant phenotype in human red blood cells. *Journal of thrombosis and haemostasis: JTH.* **12**:1697–1702.
156. von Bruhl ML *et al.* (2012). Monocytes, neutrophils, and platelets cooperate to initiate and propagate venous thrombosis in mice *in vivo*. *J Exp Med.* **209**:819–835.
157. Massberg S *et al.* (2010). Reciprocal coupling of coagulation and innate immunity via neutrophil serine proteases. *Nat Med.* **16**:887–896.
158. Higuchi DA, Wun TC, Likert KM, Broze GJ, Jr. (1992). The effect of leukocyte elastase on tissue factor pathway inhibitor. *Blood.* **79**:1712–1719.
159. Kannemeier C *et al.* (2007). Extracellular RNA constitutes a natural procoagulant cofactor in blood coagulation. *Proc Natl Acad Sci USA.* **104**:6388–6393.
160. Ammollo CT, Semeraro F, Xu J, Esmon NL, Esmon CT. (2011). Extracellular histones increase plasma thrombin generation by impairing thrombomodulin-dependent protein C activation. *J Thromb Haemost.* **9**:1795–1803.
161. Longstaff C *et al.* (2013). Mechanical stability and fibrinolytic resistance of clots containing fibrin, DNA, and histones. *The J Biol Chem.* **288**: 6946–6956.

162. Napirei M, Wulf S, Mannherz HG. (2004). Chromatin breakdown during necrosis by serum Dnase1 and the plasminogen system. *Arthritis Rheum.* **50**:1873–1883.
163. Meier TR *et al.* (2008). Prophylactic P-selectin inhibition with PSI-421 promotes resolution of venous thrombosis without anticoagulation. *Thromb Haemost.* **99**:343–351.
164. Massberg S *et al.* (2010). Reciprocal coupling of coagulation and innate immunity via neutrophil serine proteases. *Nat Med.* **16**:887–896.
165. Martinod K *et al.* (2013). Neutrophil histone modification by peptidylarginine deiminase 4 is critical for deep vein thrombosis in mice. *Proc Nat Acad Sci USA.* **110**:8674–8679.
166. von Bruhl, ML *et al.* (2012). Monocytes, neutrophils, and platelets cooperate to initiate and propagate venous thrombosis in mice *in vivo*. *The J Exp Med.* **209**:819–835.
167. Knight JS *et al.* (2014). Peptidylarginine deiminase inhibition reduces vascular damage and modulates innate immune responses in murine models of atherosclerosis. *Circulation. Res.* **114**:947–956.
168. Demers M *et al.* (2012). Cancers predispose neutrophils to release extracellular DNA traps that contribute to cancer-associated thrombosis. *Proc Nat Acad Sci USA.* **109**:13076–13081.
169. Savchenko AS *et al.* (2014). Neutrophil extracellular traps form predominantly during the organizing stage of human venous thromboembolism development. *J. Thrombosis Haemostasis.* **12**:860–870.
170. Megens RT *et al.* (2012). Presence of luminal neutrophil extracellular traps in atherosclerosis. *Thrombosis Haemostasis.* **107**:597–598.
171. Diaz JA *et al.* (2013). Plasma DNA is Elevated in Patients with Deep Vein Thrombosis. *Journal of Vascular Surgery. Venous and Lymphatic Disorders* **1**.
172. van Montfoort ML *et al.* (2013). Circulating nucleosomes and neutrophil activation as risk factors for deep vein thrombosis. *Arteriosclerosis, Thrombosis, Vascular Biol.* **33**:147–151.
173. Borissoff JI *et al.* (2013). Elevated levels of circulating DNA and chromatin are independently associated with severe coronary atherosclerosis and a prothrombotic state. *Arteriosclerosis, Thrombosis, Vascular Biol.* **33**: 2032–2040.
174. Fuchs TA, Kremer Hovinga JA, Schatzberg D, Wagner DD, Lammle B. (2012). Circulating DNA and myeloperoxidase indicate disease activity in patients with thrombotic microangiopathies. *Blood.* **120**:1157–1164.
175. Mantovani A, Cassatella MA, Costantini C, Jaillon S. (2011). Neutrophils in the activation and regulation of innate and adaptive immunity. *Nature Rev Immunol.* **11**:519–531.
176. Cools-Lartigue J *et al.* (2013). Neutrophil extracellular traps sequester circulating tumor cells and promote metastasis. *The J Clin Investi.*

177. Kaplan MJ. (2013). Role of neutrophils in systemic autoimmune diseases. *Arthritis Research Therapy*. **15**:219.
178. Puga I *et al.* (2012). B cell-helper neutrophils stimulate the diversification and production of immunoglobulin in the marginal zone of the spleen. *Nat Immunol*. **13**:170–180.
179. Schauer C *et al.* (2014). Aggregated neutrophil extracellular traps limit inflammation by degrading cytokines and chemokines. *Nat Medi*. **20**:511–517.
180. Darrah E, Rosen A, Giles JT, Andrade F. (2012). Peptidylarginine deiminase 2, 3 and 4 have distinct specificities against cellular substrates: novel insights into autoantigen selection in rheumatoid arthritis. *Ann Rheumatic Diseases*. **71**:92–98.
181. Renaudineau Y *et al.* (2007). Anti-alpha-actinin antibodies: a new marker of lupus nephritis. *Autoimmunity Rev*. **6**:464–468.
182. Iaccarino L *et al.* (2011). Anti-annexins autoantibodies: their role as biomarkers of autoimmune diseases. *Autoimmunity Rev*. **10**:553–558.
183. Zhao MH, Jones SJ, Lockwood CM. (1995). Bactericidal/permeability-increasing protein (BPI) is an important antigen for anti-neutrophil cytoplasmic autoantibodies (ANCA) in vasculitis. *Clin Expe Immunol*. **99**:49–56.
184. Mansour RB *et al.* (2008). Increased levels of autoantibodies against catalase and superoxide dismutase associated with oxidative stress in patients with rheumatoid arthritis and systemic lupus erythematosus. *Scandinavian J Rheumatol*. **37**:103–108.
185. Schultz DR, Tozman EC. (1995). Antineutrophil cytoplasmic antibodies: major autoantigens, pathophysiology, and disease associations. *Seminars in Arthritis Rheumatism*. **25**:143–159.
186. Lande R *et al.* (2011). Neutrophils activate plasmacytoid dendritic cells by releasing self-DNA-peptide complexes in systemic lupus erythematosus. *Science Translational Medi*. **3**:73ra19.
187. Hahn BH. (1998). Antibodies to DNA. *The New England J Medi*. **338**:1359–1368.
188. Nassberger L, Jonsson H, Sjoholm AG, Sturfelt G, Heubner A. (1989). Circulating anti-elastase in systemic lupus erythematosus. *Lancet*. **1**:509.
189. Nassberger L, Sjoholm AG, Jonsson H, Sturfelt G, Akesson A. (1990). Autoantibodies against neutrophil cytoplasm components in systemic lupus erythematosus and in hydralazine-induced lupus. *Clin Expe Immunol*. **81**:380–383.
190. Wegner N *et al.* (2010). Autoimmunity to specific citrullinated proteins gives the first clues to the etiology of rheumatoid arthritis. *Immunol Rev*. **233**:34–54.
191. Kolln J *et al.* (2006). Triosephosphate isomerase- and glyceraldehyde-3-phosphate dehydrogenase-reactive autoantibodies in the cerebrospinal fluid of patients with multiple sclerosis. *J Immunol*. **177**:5652–5658.

192. Takasaki Y *et al.* (2004). Glyceraldehyde 3-phosphate dehydrogenase is a novel autoantigen leading autoimmune responses to proliferating cell nuclear antigen multiprotein complexes in lupus patients. *Int Immunol.* **16**:1295–1304.
193. Rubin RL, Waga S. (1987). Antihistone antibodies in systemic lupus erythematosus. *The Journal of rheumatology. Supplement.* **14**(Suppl 13): 118–126.
194. Burlingame RW, Boey ML, Starkebaum G, Rubin RL. (1994). The central role of chromatin in autoimmune responses to histones and DNA in systemic lupus erythematosus. *The J Clin Investi.* **94**:184–192.
195. Sokolove J, Zhao X, Chandra PE, Robinson WH. (2011). Immune complexes containing citrullinated fibrinogen costimulate macrophages via Toll-like receptor 4 and Fcgamma receptor. *Arthritis Rheumatism.* **63**:53–62.
196. Dwivedi N *et al.* (2012). Felty's syndrome autoantibodies bind to deiminated histones and neutrophil extracellular chromatin traps. *Arthritis Rheumatism.* **64**:982–992.
197. Pratesi F *et al.* (2014) Antibodies from patients with rheumatoid arthritis target citrullinated histone 4 contained in neutrophils extracellular traps. *Ann Rheumatic Diseases.* **73**:1414–1422.
198. Darrah E, Andrade F. (2012). NETs: the missing link between cell death and systemic autoimmune diseases? *Front Immunol.* **3**:428.
199. Kotzin BL. (1996). Systemic lupus erythematosus. *Cell.* **85**:303–306.
200. Ruiz-Irastorza G, Khamashta MA, Castellino G, Hughes GR. (2001). Systemic lupus erythematosus. *Lancet.* **357**:1027–1032.
201. Zandman-Goddard G, Shoenfeld Y. (2005). Infections and SLE. *Autoimmunity.* **38**:473–485.
202. Molina V, Shoenfeld Y. (2005). Infection, vaccines and other environmental triggers of autoimmunity. *Autoimmunity.* **38**:235–245.
203. Shoenfeld Y *et al.* (2007). Autoantibodies against protective molecules — C1q, C-reactive protein, serum amyloid P, mannose-binding lectin, and apolipoprotein A1:prevalence in systemic lupus erythematosus. *Ann NY Acade Scien.* **1108**:227–239.
204. Rahman MA, Isenberg DA. (1994). Autoantibodies in systemic lupus erythematosus. *Curr Opinion Rheumatol.* **6**:468–473.
205. Bosch X, Guilabert A, Font J. (2006). Antineutrophil cytoplasmic antibodies. *Lancet.* **368**:404–418.
206. Jennette JC, Falk RJ. (2014). Pathogenesis of antineutrophil cytoplasmic autoantibody-mediated disease. *Nature Rev Rheumatol.* **10**:463–473.
207. Kaplan MJ. (2011). Neutrophils in the pathogenesis and manifestations of SLE. *Nature Rev Rheumatol.* **7**:691–699.
208. Garcia-Romo GS *et al.* (2011). Netting neutrophils are major inducers of type I IFN production in pediatric systemic lupus erythematosus. *Sci Translational Medi.* **3**:73ra20.

209. Carmona-Rivera C, Zhao W, Yalavarthi S, Kaplan MJ. (2014). Neutrophil extracellular traps induce endothelial dysfunction in systemic lupus erythematosus through the activation of matrix metalloproteinase-2. *Ann Rheumatic Diseases*.
210. Abreu-Velez AM, Smith JG, Jr, Howard MS. (2009). Presence of neutrophil extracellular traps and antineutrophil cytoplasmic antibodies associated with vasculitides. *North Am J Medi Scie*. **1**:309–313.
211. Nakazawa D *et al.* (2012). Abnormal conformation and impaired degradation of propylthiouracil-induced neutrophil extracellular traps: implications of disordered neutrophil extracellular traps in a rat model of myeloperoxidase antineutrophil cytoplasmic antibody-associated vasculitis. *Arthritis and Rheumatism*. **64**:3779–3787.
212. Sangaletti S *et al.* (2012). Neutrophil extracellular traps mediate transfer of cytoplasmic neutrophil antigens to myeloid dendritic cells toward ANCA induction and associated autoimmunity. *Blood*. **120**:3007–3018.
213. Savill J, Dransfield I, Gregory C, Haslett C. (2002). A blast from the past: clearance of apoptotic cells regulates immune responses. *Nature Reviews Immunol*. **2**:965–975.
214. Sakahira H, Enari M, Nagata S. (1998). Cleavage of CAD inhibitor in CAD activation and DNA degradation during apoptosis. *Nat*. **391**:96–99.
215. Enari M *et al.* (1998). A caspase-activated DNase that degrades DNA during apoptosis, and its inhibitor ICAD. *Nat*. **391**:43–50.
216. Yasutomo K *et al.* (2001). Mutation of DNASE1 in people with systemic lupus erythematosus. *Nat Genetics*. **28**:313–314.
217. Rahman A, Isenberg DA. (2008). Systemic lupus erythematosus. *The New England J Medi*. **358**:929–939.
218. Chang X *et al.* (2005). Localization of peptidylarginine deiminase 4 (PADI4) and citrullinated protein in synovial tissue of rheumatoid arthritis. *Rheumatol*. **44**:40–50.
219. McInnes IB, Schett G. (2011). The pathogenesis of rheumatoid arthritis. *The New England J Medi*. **365**:2205–2219.
220. Scher JU *et al.* (2013). Expansion of intestinal Prevotella copri correlates with enhanced susceptibility to arthritis. *eLife*. **2**:e01202.
221. Scher JU *et al.* (2015). Decreased bacterial diversity characterizes the altered gut microbiota in patients with psoriatic arthritis, resembling dysbiosis in inflammatory bowel disease. *Arthritis & Rheumatology*. **67**:128–139.
222. Scher JU *et al.* (2012). Periodontal disease and the oral microbiota in new-onset rheumatoid arthritis. *Arthritis and Rheumatism*. **64**:3083–3094.
223. Kamphuis S *et al.* (2005). Tolerogenic immune responses to novel T-cell epitopes from heat-shock protein 60 in juvenile idiopathic arthritis. *Lancet*. **366**:50–56.

224. Auger I, Roudier J. (1997). A function for the QKRAA amino acid motif: mediating binding of DnaJ to DnaK. Implications for the association of rheumatoid arthritis with HLA-DR4. *The J Clin Investi.* **99**:1818–1822.
225. Wegner N *et al.* (2010). Peptidylarginine deiminase from Porphyromonas gingivalis citrullinates human fibrinogen and alpha-enolase: implications for autoimmunity in rheumatoid arthritis. *Arthritis and Rheumatism.* **62**:2662–2672.
226. Sur Chowdhury C *et al.* (2014). Enhanced neutrophil extracellular trap generation in rheumatoid arthritis: analysis of underlying signal transduction pathways and potential diagnostic utility. *Arthritis Research Therapy.* **16**:R122.
227. Khandpur R *et al.* (2013). NETs are a source of citrullinated autoantigens and stimulate inflammatory responses in rheumatoid arthritis. *Science Translational Medi.* **5**:178ra140.
228. Wang Y *et al.* (2014). Increased Neutrophil Elastase and Proteinase 3 and Augmented NETosis Are Closely Associated With beta-Cell Autoimmunity in Patients With Type 1 Diabetes. *Diabetes.* **63**:4239–4248.
229. Lewis HD *et al.* (2015). Inhibition of PAD4 activity is sufficient to disrupt mouse and human NET formation. *Nat Chem Biol.* **11**:189–191.
230. Berger-Achituv S *et al.* (2013). A proposed role for neutrophil extracellular traps in cancer immunoediting. *Front Immunol.* **4**:48.
231. Krautgartner WD *et al.* (2010). Fibrin mimics neutrophil extracellular traps in SEM. *Ultrastructural Pathol.* **34**:226–231.
232. Nakashima K *et al.* (2013). PAD4 regulates proliferation of multipotent haematopoietic cells by controlling c-myc expression. *Nat Communications.* **4**:1836.
233. Dwivedi N *et al.* (2014). Deimination of linker histones links neutrophil extracellular trap release with autoantibodies in systemic autoimmunity. *FASEB Journal: Official Publication of the Federation of American Societies for Experimental Biology.* **28**:2840–2851.
234. Lin AM *et al.* (2011). Mast cells and neutrophils release IL-17 through extracellular trap formation in psoriasis. *J Immunol.* **187**:490–500.
235. Ueki S *et al.* (2013). Eosinophil extracellular DNA trap cell death mediates lytic release of free secretion-competent eosinophil granules in humans. *Blood.* **121**:2074–2083.
236. Ermert D *et al.* (2009). Mouse neutrophil extracellular traps in microbial infections. *J Innate Immunity.* **1**:181–193.
237. Chuammitri P *et al.* (2009). Chicken heterophil extracellular traps (HETs): novel defense mechanism of chicken heterophils. *Veterinary Immunol immunopathol.* **129**:126–131.

238. Palic D, Ostojic J, Andreasen CB, Roth JA. (2007). Fish cast NETs: neutrophil extracellular traps are released from fish neutrophils. *Develop Comparative Immunol.* **31**:805–816.
239. Altincicek B, Stotzel S, Wygrecka M, Preissner KT, Vilcinskas A. (2008). Host-derived extracellular nucleic acids enhance innate immune responses, induce coagulation, and prolong survival upon infection in insects. *J Immunol.* **181**:2705–2712.
240. Wen F, White GJ, VanEtten HD, Xiong Z, Hawes MC. (2009). Extracellular DNA is required for root tip resistance to fungal infection. *Plant Physiol.* **151**:820–829.

Chapter 7
Sepsis

Jamison J. Grailer*, Matthew J. Delano†
and Peter A. Ward*

1. Introduction

1.1. *Epidemiology of sepsis*

Sepsis is the constellation of symptoms occurring when an infection leads to a systemic inflammatory response,[1] including fever, leukocytosis or leukopenia, and decreased vascular resistance, frequently leading to hypotension (septic shock), organ failure (severe sepsis), and death.[2] Severe sepsis occurs in about 2% of patients admitted to the hospital. Of these patients, over one-half are treated in the intensive care unit (ICU), representing over 10% of all ICU admissions.[3] The number of cases of severe sepsis in the United States exceeds 1,000,000 per year and is steadily rising.[4] Even more alarming is the escalating cost of sepsis-associated medical care, which is estimated to be $17 billion annually.[5] Given the expanding elderly and

*University of Michigan Medical School, Department of Pathology, Ann Arbor, MI 48109, USA.
†University of Michigan, Department of Surgery, Division of Acute Care Surgery, Ann Arbor, MI 48109, USA.

comorbidly challenged population,[6] overall sepsis mortality is expected to grow at an alarming rate during the next two decades.[7]

1.2. *History of experimental and clinical sepsis studies*

Despite over 100 therapeutic clinical sepsis trials, no FDA-approved treatment options currently exist. Historically, most research has focused on ameliorating the hyper-inflammatory response by blocking TNF or IL-1.[8] However, steady improvements in clinical treatment protocols[9] have resulted in better patient survival during the initial features of severe sepsis, only to manifest varying states of prolonged immune dysfunction, immune suppression, and persistent inflammation and catabolism,[10] all of which are characterized by nosocomial infections, immune paralysis, and protracted events leading to death.[11] This realization has prompted many investigators to explore long-term options for immune cell modulation and augmentation expected to mitigate complications that hinder long-term sepsis survival.[12]

2. Brief overview of pathophysiology

2.1. *Hyperinflammation*

The inflammatory response initiating sepsis and leading to septic shock begins by the recognition of pathogens or tissue damage by pattern recognition receptors (PRRs). PRRs are expressed primarily on immune and phagocytic cells (with high levels on the latter), but also in many somatic tissues. Microbial infections are recognized by pathogen-associated molecular patterns (PAMPs) that are expressed by both pathogenic and harmless microbes. PAMPs are recognized by PRRs such as Toll-like receptors (TLRs, e.g., TLR-4 which recognizes Gram-negative bacterial lipopolysaccharide, LPS).[13] Proteins and other products (crystals) released by tissue damage are similarly recognized as damage-associated molecular patterns (DAMPs). During sepsis, systemic activation of the innate immune system by

PAMPs and/or DAMPs often results in a severe inflammatory response and subsequent overstimulation of inflammatory cells. As a result, sepsis is often characterized by an excessive release of cytokines (e.g., interleukin (IL)-17, tumor necrosis factor (TNF), IL-1β, etc.) known as the "cytokine storm" or systemic inflammatory response syndrome (SIRS). The release of excessive amounts of cytokines occurs over a relatively short period of time, along with intense complement activation and inflammatory cell stimulation, altering what should be a normal physiological response to infection into an excessive systemic inflammatory response causing host tissue damage and cellular and molecular dysregulation, the result being organ dysfunction and multi-organ failure.

2.2. *Immunosuppression*

Until fairly recently, most therapeutic strategies to treat sepsis have focused on inhibiting the hyperinflammatory phase. However, it is now clear that a phase of immunosuppression follows septic hyperinflammation and may be important to clinical outcomes (for a recent review, see Ref. 14). Immunosuppression during sepsis is characterized by defects in both innate and adaptive immune cells. Neutrophils, essential for early responses to pathogens, display defects in chemotaxis and recruitment to infected tissues during sepsis.[15,16] Furthermore, production and release of inflammatory effector molecules during sepsis, such as reactive oxygen species (ROS), may be significantly impaired.[16–18] Finally, myeloid cell production of pro-inflammatory cytokines is reduced, but anti-inflammatory cytokine (e.g., IL-10) release is elevated.[17] Adaptive immunity is similarly impaired. Defects in antigen-presenting cell (APC) function, including reduced HLA-DR expression and impaired cytokine production, occurs during sepsis.[19–22] Apoptosis of both lymphocytes and APCs (dendritic cells, especially) is also a hallmark of septic immunosuppression.[23,24] Taken together, the immunosuppressive phase of sepsis is detrimental to clearance of infectious organisms or their products and favors nosocomial and/or opportunistic secondary infections, thus increasing morbidity and mortality rates during sepsis.

2.3. *Long-term defects associated with sepsis*

Survivors of an acute septic episode often show sustained chronic health effects, leading to increased long-term morbidity and mortality rates.[25,26] Acute illness, such as sepsis, has been associated with long-term polyneuropathy and myopathy,[27] and an increased risk of dementia and cognitive impairments,[28,29] among the various potential hazards following "recovery" from sepsis.[30] The etiology of these effects is not known, outside of surviving the initial acute critical illness.

3. Cellular and molecular consequences of sepsis

Current observations about sepsis suggest that multiple organ failure occurs even in the context of preserved cell morphology and in the absence of significant cell injury. In addition, organ dysfunction is often times reversible, even in organs that regenerate poorly (heart, central nervous system, kidneys). Therefore, it is apparent that sepsis-induced organ dysfunction occurs primarily though cellular and molecular dysregulation, as opposed to gross tissue damage. Below, we outline several important pathways of cellular dysfunction that are perturbed during sepsis.

3.1. *Redox imbalance*

Clinical and experimental evidence has been generated that demonstrates septic patients exhibit severe oxidative stress.[31–33] Such oxidative stress is the result of uncontrolled production of reactive oxygen and nitrogen species (ROS and RNS, respectively) by activated immune or epithelial cells (oxidative burst), overexpression of oxide synthases (e.g., inducible nitric oxide synthase (iNOS)), or via mitochondrial production of ROS.[33–35] ROS and RNS play critical roles in the progression of sepsis via interference with signaling cascades (e.g., nitric oxide (NO) as a signaling mediator) or oxidation/nitrosylation of proteins or nucleic acid substrates resulting in deleterious molecular function.[34,36] Anti-oxidant therapies have shown benefit during animal models of sepsis, but this has not necessarily translated into successes during human clinical trials.[37]

3.2. *Defective Ca^{2+} homeostasis*

Hypocalcemia is common in sepsis and correlates with disease scores during critical illness.[38–41] It is hypothesized that there is altered intracellular calcium handling that underlies systemic hypocalcemia.[41] In other words, although systemic (plasma) Ca^{2+} levels are reduced during sepsis, there is increased Ca^{2+} inside cells. Indeed, intracellular calcium is elevated in a variety of tissues and cell types during sepsis.[42–44] The specific mechanisms underlying altered Ca^{2+} handling remain unclear. Buildup of $[Ca^{2+}]i$ in organs during sepsis can lead to significant organ dysfunction. Nevertheless, heightened intracellular calcium leads to elevated inflammatory responses, cellular dysfunction, and can even be cytotoxic.

3.3. *PARP1, PARP2 activation*

Poly(ADP-Ribose) Polymerase 1 (PARP1) and PARP2 are enzymes that catalyze poly(ADP-robosyl)ation of proteins. Catalytic activity of these enzymes is stimulated by DNA strand breaks. Thus, PARP activity is viewed as a sensor of DNA damage. PARP1 activation and initiation of the inflammatory response have been shown to occur simultaneously.[45] PARP1 activity upregulates proinflammatory gene expression,[46] which is thought to be due to PARP1-induced alterations in chromatin structure and in transcriptional regulation,[45,47] PARP1 may also directly contribute to cell death in affected tissues.[45] Therefore, it was hypothesized that PARP1 may play a role during sepsis. Indeed, PARP1 genetic deficiency was shown to be protective during cecal ligation and puncture (CLP) sepsis in mice and was associated with significantly lowered plasma cytokine levels and reduced tissue/organ dysfunction.[48] Inhibitors of PARP1 have been used in clinical trials as cancer therapeutics, but trials for sepsis have not been initiated. Therefore, it is not clear whether inhibitors of PARP1 will be beneficial during the treatment of human sepsis.

3.4. *Mitochondrial dysfunction*

Mitochondria are critical for maintaining an adequate supply of ATP for cellular processes. In addition, damaged mitochondria can trigger cell death pathways through the release of mitochondrial cytochrome c.[49] Mitochondria are affected in several ways during sepsis. The generation of excessive amounts of ROS and RNS can directly inhibit respiration and damage respiratory chain components in mitochondria.[50–52] In addition, impaired tissue perfusion (due to fluid loss, both intrinsic and extrinsic, as well as reduced vascular tone) leads to tissue hypoxia. Loss of tissue oxygenation significantly impairs oxidative phosphorylation and may trigger cell death pathways.[53] Mitochondrial dysfunction, or direct damage of mitochondria, can directly affect the generation of ATP. Not only will the drop in ATP negatively affect cellular processes, but severe lack of ATP can trigger cellular anergy, whereby the cell will not necessarily die, but instead acquire a hibernation-like state resulting in tissue dysfunction and organ failure.[54] The importance of mitochondrial dysfunction during sepsis is highlighted by the observations that cellular ATP levels are correlated with survival in both human sepsis and animal sepsis models.[52,55]

3.5. *Apoptosis of lymphoid cells and immunosuppression*

In the majority of septic patients, circulating lymphocytes and gastrointestinal epithelial cells undergo significant apoptosis, while apoptosis/necrosis in the heart, kidneys, and lungs is not apparent.[56] Lymphocyte apoptosis has now been accepted as an important step in the pathogenesis of sepsis and contributes to septic immunosuppression.[57] Indeed, lymphocyte apoptosis has been described in both septic patients as well as animal sepsis models.[58,59] Importantly, lymphocyte apoptosis was shown to occur through both the intrinsic

(Fas, FasL) and extrinsic (TNF, etc.) pathways.[59] Although the defining factors for this phenomenon are still not clear, recent evidence has suggested that the release of extracellular histones during sepsis may drive lymphocyte apoptosis.[60,61] Therapeutic blockade of lymphocyte apoptosis and/or restoring lymphocyte function have generated promising preclinical data that may lead to new treatments for sepsis in humans.[56,62,63]

3.6. *Extracellular histones*

Histones, normally restricted to the nucleus, are found in the extracellular space in significant amounts during sepsis. Histones have been shown to be important contributors to septic pathology.[64,65] Histones are released by damaged tissue, but also by activated neutrophils in the form of neutrophil extracellular traps (NETs).[61,66–68] Extracellular histones formed during sepsis have several severe deleterious effects. They can directly activate TLRs (2, 4) leading to increased inflammatory cytokine release.[69,70] In addition, histones are known to be potent activators of the NLRP3 inflammasome, resulting in significantly elevated release of IL-1β and IL-18.[68,71–73] Histones also have strong procoagulant activities.[73] As described earlier, histones can potently induce lymphocyte apoptosis.[60,61] Extracellular histones can also induce dysfunction of cardiomyocytes, leading to septic cardiomyopathy.[74] Histones are naturally degraded by activated protein C[64] However, administration of activated protein C has not shown any survival benefit during sepsis clinical trials.[75] It remains to be seen whether other histone-targeted therapies will be useful for improving clinical outcomes from sepsis.

4. Role of complement in sepsis

4.1. *Complement activation in sepsis*

It has long been known in human or rodent sepsis that robust consumptive depletion of complement occurs, resulting in a sharp drop in hemolytic plasma complement (CH50 units) and in the appearance in plasma of complement activation products.[76] There is also evidence human sepsis causes release (shedding) of the C5a receptor into plasma, likely due to release of microparticles from neutrophils.[77] Similar events occur in rats and mice with polymicrobial sepsis following CLP.[78] In addition to complement activation in septic rats and mice, there is robust activation of both the fibrinolytic and clotting systems.[79] There is also evidence for activation of several clotting factors, some of which have C3 and C5 convertase activities, generating C3a and its downstream degradation products as well as activation of thrombin which has C5 convertase activity and generates C5a and the terminal membrane attack complex (MAC).[80] There is well-established evidence that activation of the complement system is often linked to activation of both the clotting and the fibrinolytic systems.

4.2. *Role of C5a and its receptors in experimental sepsis*

In the late 1990s, we set out to define the role of C5a and, later, its receptors in the setting of polymicrobial sepsis in rats and mice. The going was quite slow, because there were virtually no reagents available for rat or mouse complement proteins and activation products, requiring us to generate our own reagents (neutralizing rabbit antibody to rat or mouse C5a). Development of those antibodies and their infusion into CLP rodents dramatically attenuated the intensity of CLP-induced sepsis, including greatly improved 7-day survival, reduced levels of plasma cytokines, and reduced evidence of multiorgan failure.[78,79,81] These neutralizing antibodies had the attribute that they did not block C5, which, if it occurred, would complicate interpretation of the results. Our results were somewhat similar to those of a group at Stanford University, who found their antibody to human C5a appeared to diminish some of the biochemical parameters (ARDS) of sepsis in monkeys, although the number of animals was too small to allow statistical significance.[82] On the basis of all of the findings described above, access to mice with knockout of either C5aR1 or C5aR2 allowed us to determine that blockade or deletion of either receptor greatly improved survival after CLP and that both receptors participate in the harmful effects of sepsis.[83–85]

4.3. *Role of complement and extracellular histones in sepsis*

There is extensive recent literature suggesting that in sepsis extracellular histones appear in plasma and are linked to cell and tissue damage.[64,86,87] Also, infusion of a histone mix into mice induces many of the features of experimental sepsis (multiorgan damage, hypothermia, etc.). We have recently shown that, after CLP in mice, the appearance of extracellular histones in plasma requires both C5aR1 and C5aR2, as well as the NLRP3 inflammasome, caspase 1, and availability of neutrophils,[74] Figure 1. These events suggest that extracellular histones derive from neutrophils (PMNs) after C5a interacts with C5a receptors on PMNs, causing formation of extracellular traps (NETs) from PMNs. These NETs contain spider web-like DNA strands, together with myeloperoxidase, histones, and various products of PMN granules. Histones appear as extracellular, soluble products which can gain entry into the circulation and have been associated with multiorgan dysfunction. PMNs also contain an enzyme (peptidyl arginine deiminases, PAD4) which converts histone peptidyl arginine to peptidyl citrulline. In autoimmune diseases, these citrullinated histones may cause autoantibodies which accentuate the inflammatory features. In the setting of sepsis, the extent to which peptidyl arginine products and peptidyl citrulline products each contribute to adverse outcomes is unknown.

As also shown in Fig. 1, distal pathway products include proteases and reactive oxygen species (ROS) which are generated by both PMNs and macrophages. These products, together with circulating cytokines and chemokines, likely contribute to the "physiological environment" that fosters the development of multiorgan dysfunction and lethality during the onset of sepsis.

Together, the events described in Fig. 1 underscore complement activation which occurs early in sepsis as a "driver" of events that have organ-damaging outcomes, often with lethality.

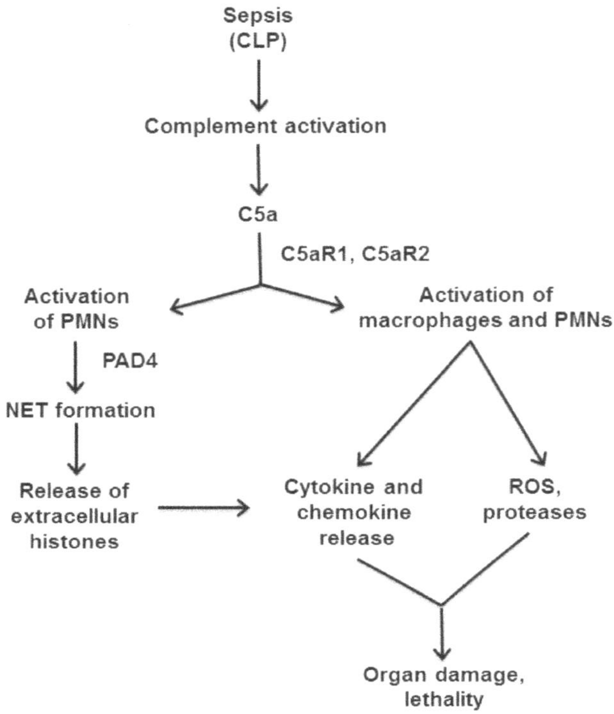

Fig. 1. Complement and extracellular Histones in sepsis. The figure shows the pathways in polymicrobial sepsis (mice) which leads to complement activation and generation of C5a, which interacts with its C5a receptors (C5aR1, C5aR2). This leads to PMN activation and NET formation, with release of extracellular histones. Simultaneously, there is activation of lung macrophages and PMNs which release cytokines and chemokines, proteins, and oxidants. The collective outcomes of these events are cell and organ damage and lethality.

5. Current concepts, problems, and controversies in animal sepsis models

The central aim of any animal disease model is to closely mimic clinically relevant pathogenesis observed in humans. Animal models of sepsis can generally fit into three categories: exogenous administration of a substance that triggers numerous pathways that cause cell, tissue, and organ damage (e.g., LPS); exogenous administration of a viable pathogen (e.g., bacteria); or alteration of the host natural innate immune defense barrier (e.g., CLP). Most animal models of sepsis have provided key information regarding the pathophysiology of sepsis. However, there is no one model that exemplifies the clinically relevant pathogenesis of human sepsis. Ergo, controversy remains about which model(s) to use when studying sepsis and how to best interpret and extrapolate the experimental results to the human condition. In this section, we will attempt to describe the differences and similarities between human sepsis and various animal models of sepsis.

5.1. *Heterogeneity of animal models of sepsis*

There is significant heterogeneity with regard to animal models of sepsis. Endotoxemia models typically entail a high-level, one-dose infusion of LPS. Such treatments induce a shock-like state in rodents (rodents are typically resistant to LPS treatment and require some 250 times higher dose than humans or rabbits to elicit similar cytokine responses[88]). Administration of an LPS bolus quickly produces sepsis-like symptoms including hypothermia, leukopenia, reduced cardiac output, and systemic vascular dilation.[89,90] Cytokine production peaks relatively early after endotoxin administration (1–5 h), then declines,[91] in contrast to human sepsis and other animal models in which high levels of circulating cytokines are sustained. The overall disease progression in the endotoxemia rodent model is much faster than in human sepsis.[92]

As opposed to the administration of a single toxic agent, injection of live Gram-negative bacteria (*E. coli*) can also elicit a sepsis-like state. The route of bacterial infection can vary according to the route (e.g., blood, peritoneal cavity), the bacterial strain and the number of microbes infected, and the frequency of administration (e.g., one-time dose vs. multiple doses or continuous infusion).[93] All of these parameters have important consequences for the host response. However, such models usually do not mimic important features of human sepsis.[94] Indeed, the injection of a large amount of a single species of bacteria (such as *E. coli*) does not mimic the natural course of human disease, which is often due to proliferation of polymicrobial species with distribution throughout the body over time.

Alteration of the body's natural barriers (e.g., surgical models of colonic perforation) has quickly become a relevant animal model of sepsis because such strategies are designed to mimic the natural course of events during human sepsis. CLP is considered by many to be the "gold standard" model of sepsis research because, among other features, it mimics many of the cardiovascular changes observed in septic humans.[93] In addition, in contrast to bolus injection of toxins or microbes, CLP mimics the progressive production of cytokines and other proinflammatory mediators seen in sepsis.[95,96] Animals that underwent CLP displayed the overt clinical presentation of sepsis: increased blood flow to organs, hyperglycemia during the early stages, followed by decreased vascular flow, and hypoglycemia and hypothermia in late stages.[93] Results from experiments employing the CLP model can be influenced by a number of procedural variables including the size and number of punctures and, especially, the mouse strain. Standardization of the CLP technical procedure was an important step in generating a reproducible animal CLP model for human sepsis.[97]

Besides the obvious species variation between human and rodent sepsis, there are significant factors about rodent sepsis models that need to be considered. For example, aged humans are much more susceptible to sepsis and septic shock and, therefore, the incidence of sepsis in these populations is higher. By contrast, most labs use juvenile or young adult rodents in their sepsis models. Studies have shown that aged mice are more susceptible to CLP (and effects of endotoxemia) than young mice.[98,99] In addition, humans with sepsis often have comorbidities (such as chronic kidney, cardiac or liver disease) which are not present in most aging rodents. Supportive care, in the form of fluids and/or antibiotics, is often lacking in animal models, or they are administered once, directly after surgery, and not on a continuous basis, contrasting to treatment of septic humans. Such differences can significantly alter the outcomes during rodent sepsis models and need to be considered during experimentation. Finally, in septic humans it seems that females have a better survival rate than males. Clearly, gender may substantially influence outcomes in sepsis studies.

5.2. *Endotoxemia studies*

Tight control over an experimental system is desirable in any experiment. Use of a specific agonist such as LPS at a specified dose provides the most reproducible animal model of sepsis. However, the use of a single dose does not necessarily mimic the clinically relevant condition. Endotoxemia studies are valuable because they are relatively straightforward to perform, and low-dose studies have been performed in humans.[100] Administration of LPS to activate TLR-4 is the most common agent used in these studies. Even with injections of LPS, there may be complications such as endotoxin "tolerance" which are usually dose-dependent. The mechanisms of tolerance are poorly understood. Bolus injections of other TLR agonists such as activated zymosan, poly I:C, or CpG DNA also induce a shock state in animals. As discussed above, there are many caveats for extrapolating the results of endotoxemia studies to human sepsis. As such, it is not surprising that therapeutic treatments that were promising in endotoxemia models were not found to be effective in human sepsis.[94,101]

5.3. *Use of rodents versus larger animals*

The choice of species is an important factor when devising a sepsis research study. Most sepsis research is performed in rodents. Rodents are popular because they are small, relatively inexpensive to house and breed, and they have well-defined genetics. However, rodents do provide some disadvantages, generally based on their size. For example, it is difficult to measure some hemodynamic parameters, such as cardiac output, without complex and expensive machinery, and large amounts of blood are difficult to obtain, especially if one wants to obtain cells such as PMNs which in mice are rather scant (<20% of all blood leukocytes). Differences in species physiology are also a consideration. For instance, when assessing cardiovascular physiology during sepsis, pigs as model animals have the advantage of being similar to humans with regard to cardiovascular anatomy and physiology. Nonhuman primates may represent the most relevant models for human sepsis due to their close phylogenetic relation. However, due to ethical concerns, high expense, and concerns regarding zoonotic disease transmission, primate models are generally reserved for preclinical studies.

6. Current concepts, problems and controversies in human sepsis studies

6.1. *Concerns about current clinical classifications of human sepsis*

Sepsis is the constellation of symptoms occurring when a pathologic infection leads to a systemic inflammatory response, including fever, leukocytosis or leukopenia, and decreased vascular resistance frequently leading to hypotension (septic shock), organ failure (severe sepsis) and death.[1] However, constraints in interpretation of data include vague clinical definitions, coding rules, confusion over the distinction between septicemia, severe sepsis, and septic shock, the capacity to provide intensive care, and increased awareness and surveillance. These factors have confounded attempts to better classify sepsis, severe sepsis and septic shock. Recently an international collaborative effort to better define individual aspects of sepsis was convened. The group defined "septic shock as a subset of sepsis in which underlying circulatory, cellular, together with metabolic abnormalities all are associated with a greater risk of mortality than sepsis alone. Adult patients with septic shock can be identified using the clinical criteria of "hypotension requiring vasopressor therapy to maintain mean BP 65 mm Hg or greater and having a serum lactate level greater than 2 mmol/L after adequate fluid resuscitation".[102]

6.2. *Failure in clinical trials, including recent clinical trials using antagonists of toll-like receptors*

One of the great disappointments during the past three decades has been the failure to convert advances in our understanding of the underlying biologic features of sepsis into effective new therapies.[103] Investigators have used both highly specific therapies and agents that exert pleiotropic effects. Generally, these agents can be divided into those designed to interrupt the initial cytokine cascade upswing (anti-lipopolysaccharide or anti-proinflammatory cytokine strategies) and agents designed to interfere with dysregulated coagulation (anti-thrombin or activated protein C).[104] The only agent that gained regulatory approval in the past few years was activated protein C. However, post-approval concerns about the safety and efficacy of activated protein C prompted the manufacturer to withdraw the drug from the market.[105] All of the other tested strategies thus far have not shown benefit or efficacy in the setting of sepsis. Moreover, with the recent decision to stop further development of a polyclonal anti-tumor necrosis factor antibody for use in sepsis,[106] there are no current large-scale trials of anti-cytokine strategies for the treatment of sepsis.

More recently, inhibition of TLR-4 with the antagonist, E5564 (Eritoran), was tested in septic humans. The ACCESS (A Controlled Comparison of Eritoran Tetrasodium and Placebo in Patients with Severe Sepsis) trial reported that among patients with severe sepsis, the use of Eritoran, compared with placebo, did not result in reduced 28-day mortality.[107] An earlier clinical trial that evaluated the inhibition of TLR-4 with another antagonist, TAK 242 (resatorvid), likewise found no statistically significant reduction in 28-day mortality.[108] These two failed clinical trials caused great consternation for clinical trialists and sugggested that endotoxin (LPS) may not play a major role in human sepsis based on North American clinical trials.

However, other agents may hold promise with broader immunomodulatory effects such as glucocorticoids, which have received the most attention. Intravenous immune globulin was also associated with what appeared to be potential benefit, but its routine use is not part of clinical practice.[106] A large number of observational studies have suggested that statins may improve outcomes during sepsis and severe infection. However these findings have not been substantiated in randomized, controlled trials, and statin use is not part of routine sepsis therapy.[109,110] Recent interest in drugs that have modulatory effects on immune cells following sepsis has gained traction; however, the benefits in treating sepsis with such a strategy remain to be identified.[12]

6.3. Concerns about clinical trial endpoints

In clinical studies, the enrollment criteria are typically very broad, the agent is administered on the basis of a standard formula for only a short period (a few days). There is little information on how an agent changes the host response and host–pathogen interactions, and the primary end point is death from any cause. Such a research strategy is probably overly simplistic in that it does not select patients who are most likely to benefit, cannot adjust therapy on the basis of the evolving host response and clinical course, and does not capture potentially important effects except for effects on 28-day mortality. A more advantageous strategy would be to implement an adaptive clinical trial design that evaluates a sepsis treatment by observing clinical outcomes and side effects on a routine schedule.[111] This information would then be used to modify the study protocols in accord with those newly acquired observations. The "adaptation process" would continue throughout the trial as described in the trial protocol. Modifications may include drug dosage, sample size, patient selection criteria, and drug cocktail administration. In some instances, trials have become an ongoing process that routinely adds and drops therapies and patient cohorts as more insight is gained.[112] Most importantly, the aim of an adaptive trial is to more quickly identify therapies that have a beneficial effect and the patient populations that are appropriate for such treatment.[113]

6.4. *The influence of age and co-morbidities in human sepsis*

Despite recent improvements in 30-day sepsis mortality, multiple reports demonstrate a dramatic increase in sepsis-associated mortality that escalates with time, especially in the elderly population after "recovery" from acute sepsis.[25] These data suggest that short-term gains in sepsis survival have been forfeited to escalating long-term sepsis mortality. These deaths may represent the consequence of more sophisticated ICU care that keeps elderly and co-morbidly challenged patients alive longer in spite of ongoing immune, physiologic, and biochemical aberrations.[114] Although the precise causes of long-term sepsis mortality are still uncertain, several reports suggest that advanced age, comorbidities, and persistent organ injury synergize to generate a deleterious state of chronic disease characterized by immune dysfunction, immune suppression, and persistent catabolism and inflammation.[12] A recent report suggests that hospital readmissions after "recovery" from sepsis may be related to development of new bacterial infections.[115] Furthermore, persistent inflammation coupled with chronic immobility, catabolic drugs, and extended paralytics, all contribute to a protracted state of immune dysregulation and chronic deterioration. Thus, investigators have been forced to refocus their efforts on the underlying innate and adaptive immune derangements that facilitate impaired sepsis recovery and survival, especially over the long term.[14]

6.5. *Genomic analysis of septic humans*

There is considerable interest and controversy in the contribution of host genetic characteristics to the incidence and outcome of sepsis, in part because of strong evidence of inherited risk factors.[116] Many studies have focused on polymorphisms in genes encoding proteins implicated in the pathogenesis of sepsis, including cytokines and other mediators involved in innate immunity, coagulation, and fibrinolysis. However, findings are often inconsistent, due at least in part to the heterogeneity of the patient populations studied.[117] Although a recent genome-wide association study explored drug responsiveness in sepsis, no such large-scale studies of susceptibility to or outcomes of sepsis have been published.[118]

6.6. *Human sepsis biomarkers*

Over 180 biomarkers have been evaluated for use in sepsis over the past 50 years. Most of the biomarkers had been tested clinically, primarily as prognostic markers in sepsis; relatively few have been used for sepsis diagnosis. Until recently, none of the markers has demonstrated sufficient specificity or sensitivity for application to clinical practice. Procalcitonin and C-reactive protein have been most widely used in the past, but possess a limited ability to distinguish sepsis from other inflammatory conditions or to predict outcome. However more recently, the use of serum lactate levels greater than 2 mmol/L (>18 mg/dL) in the absence of hypovolemia has become one of the clinical biomarkers used in the diagnosis of patients with septic shock.[119]

7. The current outlook on treatment of sepsis

The Surviving Sepsis Campaign, an international consortium of professional societies involved in critical care, treatment of infectious diseases, and emergency medicine, recently released a reiteration of clinical guidelines for the management of severe sepsis and septic shock. The fundamental elements of the guidelines were organized into two bundles of care. The initial management bundle was to be accomplished within the first 6 hours of the patient's presentation. The subsequent management bundle was to be accomplished during admission to the ICU.[110] Uniform implementation of these protocol and best practices bundles has been associated with improved sepsis outcomes.[120]

The principles of the initial management bundle have been to define best practice in cardiorespiratory resuscitation and to mitigate the sequela of uncontrolled infection. The initial resuscitation requires the use of intravenous fluids and vasopressors, with supportive oxygen therapy and mechanical ventilation provided, as necessary. The exact components required to optimize the initial resuscitation, such as the amount of fluids, type of hemodynamic monitoring, and role of vasoactive agents, remain the subject of ongoing debate. The initial management of infection requires forming a probable diagnosis, obtaining appropriate cultures, and initiating timely empirical antimicrobial therapy coupled with control of the source of infection, if appropriate.[110]

The choice of empiric antibiotic therapy depends on the suspected infection site, the clinical setting, medical history, and local microbial susceptibility patterns. Inappropriate or untimely delays in antibiotic treatment have been associated with increased mortality.[121] Intravenous antibiotic therapy should be initiated as early as possible and should cover likely pathogens. Current guidelines recommend combination antimicrobial therapy only for neutropenic patients with sepsis and sepsis caused by *Pseudomonas* species. Empirical antifungal therapy should be used only in patients at high risk for invasive candidiasis.[122]

The patient with sepsis should also be moved to an appropriate ICU setting for ongoing care focused on monitoring and support of organ function, avoidance of complications, and de-escalation of care as soon as possible. The only immunomodulatory therapy that is currently advocated is hydrocortisone (200 to 300 mg per day for up to 7 days or until vasopressor support is no longer required) in patients with refractory septic shock.[110]

Despite the advances in medical sciences, the morbidity and mortality due to sepsis remains high. There is a robust need for early and accurate identification of those patients who are genetically predisposed to develop severe sepsis or other complications that prompt poor outcomes. Over the past three decades, a vast amount of resources has been dedicated to developing a prediction model sensitive and specific enough to reasonably prognosticate which patients will develop progressive sepsis and which will not. Using a high-throughput genomic strategy, scientists were able to differentiate groups of patients with complications based on their genomic signatures.[123] Another report demonstrates the ability to differentiate between those patients at risk to develop in-hospital septicemia and ventilator-associated pneumonia based on individual patient genomic profiles.[124] If such prognostic programs are further developed and standardized, we might be able to proactively minimize the risk of sepsis from occurring in high-risk individuals.

References

1. Kaukonen KM *et al.* (2015). Systemic inflammatory response syndrome criteria in defining severe sepsis. *N Engl J Med.* **372**(17):1629–1638.

2. No Authors Listed, (1992). American College of Chest Physicians/Society of Critical Care Medicine Consensus Conference: definitions for sepsis and organ failure and guidelines for the use of innovative therapies in sepsis. *Crit Care Med.* **20**(6):864–874.
3. Rangel-Frausto MS *et al.* (1995).The natural history of the systemic inflammatory response syndrome (SIRS). A prospective study. *JAMA.* **273**(2):117–123.
4. Angus DC *et al.* (2001). Epidemiology of severe sepsis in the United States: analysis of incidence, outcome, and associated costs of care. *Crit Care Med.* **29**(7):1303–1310.
5. Coopersmith CM *et al.* (2012). A comparison of critical care research funding and the financial burden of critical illness in the United States. *Crit Care Med.* **40**(4):1072–1079.
6. Martin GS, Mannino DM, Moss M. (2006). The effect of age on the development and outcome of adult sepsis. *Crit Care Med.* **34**(1):15–21.
7. Kahn JM *et al.* (2015). The epidemiology of chronic critical illness in the United States. *Crit Care Med,.* **43**(2):282–287.
8. Tracey KJ *et al.* (1987). Anti-cachectin/TNF monoclonal antibodies prevent septic shock during lethal bacteraemia. *Nature.* **330**(6149):662–664.
9. Schorr CA, Dellinger RP. (2014). The Surviving Sepsis Campaign: past, present and future. *Trends Mol Med.* **20**(4):192–194.
10. Gentile LF *et al.* (2012). Persistent inflammation and immunosuppression: a common syndrome and new horizon for surgical intensive care. *J Trauma Acute Care Surg.* **72**(6):1491–1501.
11. Boomer JS *et al.* (2011). Immunosuppression in patients who die of sepsis and multiple organ failure. *JAMA.* **306**(23):2594–2605.
12. Delano MJ and Ward PA. (2016). Sepsis-induced immune dysfunction: can immune therapies reduce mortality? *J Clin Invest.* **126**(1):23–31.
13. Medzhitov R, and Janeway Jr, C. (2000). Innate immunity. *N Engl J Med.* **343**(5):338–344.
14. Hotchkiss RS, Monneret G, Payen D. (2013). Sepsis-induced immunosuppression: from cellular dysfunctions to immunotherapy. *Nat Rev Immunol.* **13**(12):862–874.
15. Cummings CJ *et al.* (1999). Expression and function of the chemokine receptors CXCR1 and CXCR2 in sepsis. *J Immunol.* **162**(4):2341–2346.
16. Kovach MA, and Standiford TJ. (2012). The function of neutrophils in sepsis. *Curr Opin Infect Dis.* **25**(3):321–327.
17. Grailer JJ *et al.* (2014). Persistent neutrophil dysfunction and suppression of acute lung injury in mice following cecal ligation and puncture sepsis. *J Innate Immun.* **6**(5):695–705.
18. Huber-Lang M *et al.* (2001). Role of C5a in multiorgan failure during sepsis. *J Immunol.* **166**(2):1193–1199.
19. Cavaillon JM, Adib-Conquy M. (2005). Monocytes/macrophages and sepsis. *Crit Care Med.* **33**(12 Suppl):S506–S509.

20. Benjamim CF *et al.* (2005). Reversal of long-term sepsis-induced immunosuppression by dendritic cells. *Blood.* **105**(9):3588–3595.
21. Pene F *et al.* (2008). Dendritic cells modulate lung response to Pseudomonas aeruginosa in a murine model of sepsis-induced immune dysfunction. *J Immunol.* **181**(12):8513–8520.
22. Grimaldi D, Llitjos JF, Pene F. (2014). Post-infectious immune suppression: a new paradigm of severe infections. *Med Mal Infect.* **44**(10):455–463.
23. Hotchkiss RS *et al.* (2002). Depletion of dendritic cells, but not macrophages, in patients with sepsis. *J Immunol.* **168**(5):2493–2500.
24. Hotchkiss RS *et al.* (1999). Apoptotic cell death in patients with sepsis, shock, and multiple organ dysfunction. *Crit Care Med.* **27**(7):1230–1251.
25. Winters BD *et al.* (2010). Long-term mortality and quality of life in sepsis: a systematic review. *Crit Care Med.* **38**(5):1276–1283.
26. Mayr FB, Yende S, Angus DC. (2014). Epidemiology of severe sepsis. *Virulence.* **5**(1):4–11.
27. Latronico N, Bolton CF. (2011). Critical illness polyneuropathy and myopathy: a major cause of muscle weakness and paralysis. *Lancet Neurol.* **10**(10):931–941.
28. Shah FA *et al.* (2013). Bidirectional relationship between cognitive function and pneumonia. *Am J Respir Crit Care Med.* **188**(5):586–592.
29. Iwashyna TJ *et al.* (2010). Long-term cognitive impairment and functional disability among survivors of severe sepsis. *JAMA.* **304**(16):1787–1794.
30. Guirgis FW *et al.* (2014). Persistent organ dysfunction after severe sepsis: a systematic review. *J Crit Care.* **29**(3):320–326.
31. Ogilvie AC *et al.* (1991). Plasma lipid peroxides and antioxidants in human septic shock. *Intensive Care Med.* **17**(1):40–44.
32. Cowley HC *et al.* (1996). Plasma antioxidant potential in severe sepsis: a comparison of survivors and nonsurvivors. *Crit Care Med.* **24**(7):1179–1183.
33. Santos SS *et al.* (2012). Generation of nitric oxide and reactive oxygen species by neutrophils and monocytes from septic patients and association with outcomes. *Shock.* **38**(1):18–23.
34. Andrades ME *et al.* (2011). Bench-to-bedside review: Sepsis — From the redox point of view. *Crit Care.* **15**(5):230.
35. Ojeda Ojeda M *et al.* (2011). Temporal trends of circulating nitric oxide and pro-inflammatory cytokine responses *ex vivo* in intra-abdominal sepsis: Results from a cohort study. *Inflamm Res.* **60**(3):289–297.
36. Dare AJ *et al.* (2009). A systematic review of experimental treatments for mitochondrial dysfunction in sepsis and multiple organ dysfunction syndrome. *Free Radic Biol Med.* **47**(11):1517–1525.
37. Mishra V. (2007). Oxidative stress and role of antioxidant supplementation in critical illness. *Clin Lab.* **53**(3–4):199–209.
38. Muller B *et al.* (2000). Disordered calcium homeostasis of sepsis: Association with calcitonin precursors. *Eur J Clin Invest.* **30**(9):823–831.

39. Zivin JR *et al.* (2001). Hypocalcemia: a pervasive metabolic abnormality in the critically ill. *Am J Kidney Dis.* **37**(4):689–698.
40. Desai TK, Carlson RW, Geheb MA. (1988). Prevalence and clinical implications of hypocalcemia in acutely ill patients in a medical intensive care setting. *Am J Med.* **84**(2):209–214.
41. Sayeed MM. (2000). Signaling mechanisms of altered cellular responses in trauma, burn, and sepsis: Role of Ca2+. *Arch Surg.* **135**(12):1432–1442.
42. Zaloga GP *et al.* (1993). Human sepsis increases lymphocyte intracellular calcium. *Crit Care Med.* **21**(2):196–202.
43. Thompson M *et al.* (2000). Increased cardiomyocyte intracellular calcium during endotoxin-induced cardiac dysfunction in guinea pigs. *Pediatr Res.* **47**(5):669–676.
44. Song SK *et al.* (1993). Increased intracellular Ca2+: A critical link in the pathophysiology of sepsis? *Proc Natl Acad Sci USA.* **90**(9):3933–3937.
45. Ba X, Garg NJ. (2011). Signaling mechanism of poly(ADP-ribose) polymerase-1 (PARP-1) in inflammatory diseases. *Am J Pathol.* **178**(3):946–955.
46. Liaudet L, Oddo M. (2003). Role of poly(adenosine diphosphate-ribose) polymerase 1 in septic peritonitis. *Curr Opin Crit Care.* **9**(2):152–158.
47. Wongsrichanalai C *et al.* (1992). Sensitivity of QBC malaria test. *Lancet.* **340**(8822):792–793.
48. Soriano FG *et al.* (2002). Resistance to acute septic peritonitis in poly(ADP-ribose) polymerase-1-deficient mice. *Shock.* **17**(4):286–292.
49. Hotchkiss RS *et al.* (2009). Cell death. *N Engl J Med.* **361**(16):1570–1583.
50. Larsen FJ *et al.* (2012). Regulation of mitochondrial function and energetics by reactive nitrogen oxides. *Free Radic Biol Med.* **53**(10):1919–1928.
51. Szabo C, Modis K. (2010). Pathophysiological roles of peroxynitrite in circulatory shock. *Shock*, **34** (Suppl 1):4–14.
52. Brealey D *et al.* (2002). Association between mitochondrial dysfunction and severity and outcome of septic shock. *Lancet.* **360**(9328):219–223.
53. Srinivasan S, Avadhani NG. (2012). Cytochrome c oxidase dysfunction in oxidative stress. *Free Radic Biol Med.* **53**(6):1252–1263.
54. Singer M. (2014). The role of mitochondrial dysfunction in sepsis-induced multi-organ failure. *Virulence.* **5**(1):66–72.
55. Brealey D *et al.* (2004). Mitochondrial dysfunction in a long-term rodent model of sepsis and organ failure. *Am J Physiol Regul Integr Comp Physiol.* **286**(3):R491–R497.
56. Hotchkiss RS, Coopersmith CM, Karl IE. (2005). Prevention of lymphocyte apoptosis — a potential treatment of sepsis? *Clin Infect Dis*, **41** (Suppl 7):S465–S469.
57. Lang JD, Matute-Bello G. (2009). Lymphocytes, apoptosis and sepsis: making the jump from mice to humans. *Crit Care.* **13**(1):109.

58. Hotchkiss RS *et al.* (1997). Apoptosis in lymphoid and parenchymal cells during sepsis: findings in normal and T- and B-cell-deficient mice. *Crit Care Med.* **25**(8):1298–1307.
59. Hotchkiss RS *et al.* (2005). Accelerated lymphocyte death in sepsis occurs by both the death receptor and mitochondrial pathways. *J Immunol.* **174**(8):5110–5118.
60. Liu ZG *et al.* (2013). Histones-mediated lymphocyte apoptosis during sepsis is dependent on p38 phosphorylation and mitochondrial permeability transition. PLoS One. **8**(10):e77131.
61. Grailer JJ *et al.* (2015). Cutting edge: critical role for C5aRs in the development of septic lymphopenia in mice. *J Immunol.* **194**(3):868–872.
62. Unsinger J *et al.* (2010). IL-7 promotes T cell viability, trafficking, and functionality and improves survival in sepsis. *J Immunol.* **184**(7):3768–3779.
63. Brahmamdam P *et al.* (2010). Delayed administration of anti-PD-1 antibody reverses immune dysfunction and improves survival during sepsis. *J Leukoc Biol.* **88**(2):233–240.
64. Xu J *et al.* (2009). Extracellular histones are major mediators of death in sepsis. *Nat Med.* **15**(11):1318–1321.
65. Hashiba M *et al.* (2015). Neutrophil extracellular traps in patients with sepsis. *J Surg Res.* **194**(1):248–254.
66. Brinkmann V *et al.* (2004). Neutrophil extracellular traps kill bacteria. *Science.* **303**(5663):1532–1535.
67. Fattahi F *et al.* (2015). Organ distribution of histones after intravenous infusion of FITC histones or after sepsis. *Immunol Res.* **61**(3):177–186.
68. Grailer JJ *et al.* (2014). Critical role for the NLRP3 inflammasome during acute lung injury. *J Immunol.* **192**(12):5974–5983.
69. Xu J *et al.* (2011). Extracellular histones are mediators of death through TLR2 and TLR4 in mouse fatal liver injury. *J Immunol.* **187**(5):2626–2631.
70. Yang X *et al.* (2016). Extracellular histones induce tissue factor expression in vascular endothelial cells via TLR and activation of NF-kappaB and AP-1. *Thromb Res*, **137**: 211–218.
71. Huang H *et al.* (2013). Histones activate the NLRP3 inflammasome in Kupffer cells during sterile inflammatory liver injury. *J Immunol.* **191**(5):2665–2679.
72. Allam R *et al.* (2013). Histones trigger sterile inflammation by activating the NLRP3 inflammasome. Eur *J Immunol,.* **43**(12):3336–3642.
73. Bosmann M *et al.* (2013). Extracellular histones are essential effectors of C5aR- and C5L2-mediated tissue damage and inflammation in acute lung injury. *FASEB J.* **27**(12):5010–5021.
74. Kalbitz M *et al.* (2015). Role of extracellular histones in the cardiomyopathy of sepsis. *FASEB J.* **29**(5):2185–2193.

75. Marti-Carvajal AJ *et al.* (2012). Human recombinant activated protein C for severe sepsis. *Cochrane Database Syst Rev.* **3**: CD004388.
76. Martin GS. (2012). Sepsis, severe sepsis and septic shock: changes in incidence, pathogens and outcomes. *Expert Rev Anti Infect Ther.* **10**(6):701–706.
77. Unnewehr H *et al.* (2013). Changes and regulation of the C5a receptor on neutrophils during septic shock in humans. *J Immunol.* **190**(8):4215–4225.
78. Czermak BJ *et al.* (1999). Protective effects of C5a blockade in sepsis. *Nat Med,.* **5**(7):788–792.
79. Huber-Lang MS *et al.* (2001). Protective effects of anti-C5a peptide antibodies in experimental sepsis. *FASEB J.* **15**(3):568–570.
80. Huber-Lang M *et al.* (2006). Generation of C5a in the absence of C3: A new complement activation pathway. *Nat Med.* **12**(6):682–687.
81. Ward PA. (2010). The harmful role of c5a on innate immunity in sepsis. *J Innate Immun.* **2**(5):439–445.
82. Stevens JH *et al.* (1986). Effects of anti-C5a antibodies on the adult respiratory distress syndrome in septic primates. *J Clin Invest.* **77**(6):1812–1816.
83. Ward PA, Bosmann M. (2012). A historical perspective on sepsis. *Am J Pathol.* **181**(1):2–7.
84. Ward PA. (2004). The dark side of C5a in sepsis. *Nat Rev Immunol.* **4**(2):133–142.
85. Rittirsch D *et al.* (2008). Functional roles for C5a receptors in sepsis. *Nat Med.* **14**(5):551–557.
86. Chaput C, Zychlinsky A. (2009). Sepsis: The dark side of histones. *Nat Med.* **15**(11):1245–1246.
87. Ekaney ML *et al.* (2014). Impact of plasma histones in human sepsis and their contribution to cellular injury and inflammation. *Crit Care.* **18**(5):543.
88. Copeland S *et al.* (2005). Acute inflammatory response to endotoxin in mice and humans. *Clin Diagn Lab Immunol.* **12**(1):60–67.
89. Brackett DJ *et al.* (1985). Evaluation of cardiac output, total peripheral vascular resistance, and plasma concentrations of vasopressin in the conscious, unrestrained rat during endotoxemia. *Circ Shock.* **17**(4):273–284.
90. D'Orio V *et al.* (1987). A comparison of Escherichia coli endotoxin single bolus injection with low-dose endotoxin infusion on pulmonary and systemic vascular changes. *Circ Shock.* **21**(3):207–216.
91. Remick DG *et al.* (2000). Comparison of the mortality and inflammatory response of two models of sepsis: lipopolysaccharide vs. cecal ligation and puncture. *Shock.* **13**(2):110–116.
92. Hollenberg SM. (2005). Mouse models of resuscitated shock. *Shock*, **24** (Suppl 1):58–63.
93. Nemzek JA, Hugunin KM, Opp MR. (2008). Modeling sepsis in the laboratory: Merging sound science with animal well-being. *Comp Med.* **58**(2):120–128.

94. Buras JA, Holzmann B, Sitkovsky M. (2005). Animal models of sepsis: Setting the stage. *Nat Rev Drug Discov.* **4**(10):854–865.
95. Ebong S *et al.* (1999). Immunopathologic alterations in murine models of sepsis of increasing severity. *Infect Immun.* **67**(12):6603–6610.
96. Ebong SJ *et al.* (1999). Immunopathologic responses to non-lethal sepsis. *Shock.* **12**(2):118–126.
97. Rittirsch D *et al.* (2009). Immunodesign of experimental sepsis by cecal ligation and puncture. *Nat Protoc.* **4**(1):31–36.
98. Sennett SH, Pomponi SA, Wright AE. (1992). Diterpene metabolites from two chemotypes of the marine sponge Myrmekioderma styx. *J Nat Prod.* **55**(10):1421–1429.
99. Saito H *et al.* (2003). Effects of aging on mortality, hypothermia, and cytokine induction in mice with endotoxemia or sepsis. *Mech Ageing Dev.* **124**(10–12):1047–1058.
100. Fink MP, Heard SO. (1990). Laboratory models of sepsis and septic shock. *J Surg Res.* **49**(2):186–196.
101. Deitch EA. (1998). Animal models of sepsis and shock: a review and lessons learned. *Shock.* **9**(1):1–11.
102. Shankar-Hari M *et al.* (2016). Developing a new definition and assessing new clinical criteria for septic shock: For the third international consensus definitions for sepsis and septic shock (Sepsis-3). *JAMA.* **315**(8):775–787.
103. Angus DC. (2011). The search for effective therapy for sepsis: back to the drawing board? *JAMA.* **306**(23):2614–2615.
104. Webster NR, Galley HF. (2009). Immunomodulation in the critically ill. *Br J Anaesth.* **103**(1):70–81.
105. Ranieri VM *et al.* (2012). Drotrecogin alfa (activated) in adults with septic shock. *N Engl J Med.* **366**(22):2055–2064.
106. Laupland KB, Kirkpatrick AW, Delaney A. (2007). Polyclonal intravenous immunoglobulin for the treatment of severe sepsis and septic shock in critically ill adults: A systematic review and meta-analysis. *Crit Care Med.* **35**(12):2686–2692.
107. Opal SM *et al.* (2013). Effect of eritoran, an antagonist of MD2-TLR4, on mortality in patients with severe sepsis: The ACCESS randomized trial. *JAMA.* **309**(11):1154–1162.
108. Rice TW *et al.* (2010). A randomized, double-blind, placebo-controlled trial of TAK-242 for the treatment of severe sepsis. *Crit Care Med.* **38**(8):1685–1694.
109. Yende S *et al.* (2011). Understanding the potential role of statins in pneumonia and sepsis. *Crit Care Med.* **39**(8):1871–1878.
110. Dellinger RP *et al.* (2013). Surviving sepsis campaign: international guidelines for management of severe sepsis and septic shock: 2012. *Crit Care Med.* **41**(2):580–637.

111. Coffey CS, Kairalla JA. (2008). Adaptive clinical trials: progress and challenges. *Drugs R D*. **9**(4):229–242.
112. Press WH. (2009). Bandit solutions provide unified ethical models for randomized clinical trials and comparative effectiveness research. *Proc Natl Acad Sci USA*. **106**(52):22387–22392.
113. Petroni GR *et al.* (2017). Implementation of adaptive methods in early-phase clinical trials. *Stat Med*. **36**(2): 215–224.
114. Yende S *et al.* (2008). Inflammatory markers at hospital discharge predict subsequent mortality after pneumonia and sepsis. *Am J Respir Crit Care Med*. **177**(11):1242–1247.
115. Sun A *et al.* (2016). Association between index hospitalization and hospital readmission in sepsis survivors. *Crit Care Med*. **44**(3):478–487.
116. Sorensen TI *et al.* (1988). Genetic and environmental influences on premature death in adult adoptees. *N Engl J Med*. **318**(12):727–732.
117. Namath A, Patterson AJ. (2011). Genetic polymorphisms in sepsis. *Crit Care Nurs Clin North Am*. **23**(1):181–202.
118. Man M *et al.* (2013). Beyond single-marker analyses: mining whole genome scans for insights into treatment responses in severe sepsis. *Pharmacogenomics J*. **13**(3):218–226.
119. Singer M *et al.* (2016). The third international consensus definitions for sepsis and septic shock (Sepsis-3). *JAMA*. **315**(8):801–810.
120. Levy MM *et al.* (2010). The surviving sepsis campaign: Results of an international guideline-based performance improvement program targeting severe sepsis. *Crit Care Med*. **38**(2):367–374.
121. Kumar A *et al.* (2006). Duration of hypotension before initiation of effective antimicrobial therapy is the critical determinant of survival in human septic shock. *Crit Care Med*. **34**(6):1589–1596.
122. Bochud PY *et al.* (2004). Antimicrobial therapy for patients with severe sepsis and septic shock: An evidence-based review. *Crit Care Med*, **32** (11 Suppl):S495–S512.
123. Cuenca AG *et al.* (2013). Development of a genomic metric that can be rapidly used to predict clinical outcome in severely injured trauma patients. *Crit Care Med*. **41**(5):1175–1185.
124. Cobb JP *et al.* (2009). Validation of the riboleukogram to detect ventilator-associated pneumonia after severe injury. *Ann Surg*. **250**(4):531–539.

Chapter 8

Granulomatous Inflammation

Marc Hilhorst*,**, Gene Hunder†, Jörg Goronzy*
and Cornelia Weyand*

1. Introduction

Granulomatous inflammation is a defined type of immune response characterized by focal tissue accumulation of macrophages mixed with other immune cells. Granuloma formation is a highly organized process, typically induced by certain infectious agents, but also occurs in some non-infectious chronic inflammatory diseases. The word granuloma originates from the Latin *granulum* meaning small grain or granule, probably referring to the microscopic appearance of the granuloma. The cellular organization of the inflammatory infiltrate is highly complex, involving many different cell types, and can occur in essentially every organ system.[1] The presence of granulomatous inflammation is generally assumed to be the result of a pathogen or particulate substance difficult for the body to eliminate. As such, most

*Division of Immunology and Rheumatology, Stanford University, Stanford, CA 94305, USA.
†Mayo Clinic College of Medicine, Rochester, MN, USA.
**Current address: Department of Internal Medicine, Academic Medical Center, Amsterdam, The Netherlands.

granulomatous disorders are chronic in nature. The formation of an area shielded off by the granuloma from healthy tissue may be an effective way of restoring or maintaining homeostasis despite the continuous presence of a pathogen or particle. As of yet, however, the ultimate functions and mechanisms of the granuloma remain enigmatic.[2]

In this chapter, we will first outline the general architecture and biology of the granuloma followed by a discussion of different types of granulomatous inflammation in the context of etiological factors or disease entities. The many diseases and conditions in which granulomatous inflammation occurs in humans are listed in Table 1.

Table 1. Diseases and conditions featuring granulomatous inflammation

Main group	Disease/condition
Bacterial	Tuberculosis
	Leprosy
	Brucellosis
	Syphilis
	Nocardiosis
	Bartonellosis
	Whipple's disease
Fungal	Histoplasmosis
	Coccidioidomycosis
	Cryptococcosis
	Zygomycosis
	Actinomycosis
	Aspergillosis
	Candidiasis
Viral	Hepatitis B virus
	Hepatitis C virus
	Varicella-Zoster virus
	Epstein–Barr virus
	Herpes simplex virus

(*Continued*)

Table 1. (*Continued*)

Main group	Disease/condition
	Cytomegalovirus
Other infectious	Helminthic
	Schistosomiasis
	Leishmaniasis
	Toxoplasmosis
	Pneumocystis jirovecii
Immune-related, idiopathic	Small-vessel vasculitis
	Large-vessel vasculitis
	Sarcoidosis
	Crohn's disease
Environmental	Berylliosis
	Silicosis
	Talc
	Zirconium
	Aluminium
Iatrogenic	Medication
	Sutures
Other	Chronic granulomatous disease
	Granuloma annulare
	Hodgkin lymphoma

1.1. *Architecture of the granuloma*

Granulomas consist of a core of highly activated, specialized macrophages, also termed histiocytes, which are believed to encapsulate and phagocytose a persistent stimulus, e.g., a pathogen or inert particles (Fig. 1). These macrophages can fuse to form multi-nucleated giant cells, a hallmark of some granulomatous diseases such as giant cell arteritis. Around the core of macrophages, T cells and other white blood cells — usually lymphocytes — accumulate, attracted by

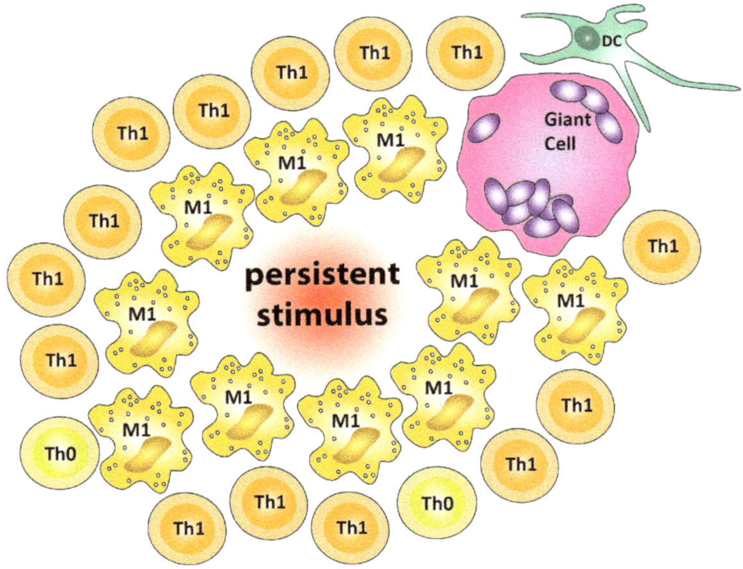

Fig. 1. Basic architecture of granulomatous inflammation: macrophages (M1) surround a persistent stimulus and are surrounded by T cells (Th1 and Th0). Macrophages sometimes fuse into multinucleated giant cells. Dendritic cells (DC) may participate in the reaction.

a variety of cytokines and chemokines produced by the macrophages, dendritic cells, and other surrounding cells. Depending on the type of granuloma, other cells including neutrophils, eosinophils, fibroblasts, and epithelial cells participate in the process. If the cells bordering the macrophage core form a single tightly packed row, the granulomatous inflammation is described as 'palisading'. This phenomenon is only seen in some disease states and is discussed in the corresponding sections.

1.2. *Basic principles of the granulomatous inflammation*

The immunologic response observed in a granulomatous inflammation is that of a delayed hypersensitivity reaction, in which different types of T cells play a pivotal role.[3,4] As a result of the accumulation of macrophages, T cells, and other cells in the granuloma, a complex micro-environment is created. Macrophages engaged in granulomatous inflammation are assumed not to leave the site and eventually to die there. Other cells are recruited over time, and some of them may recirculate.

A distinction between two types of granulomas can be made based on the macrophage turnover. In some granulomas, macrophages die continuously at a high rate and are replaced by newly arriving monocytes differentiating into macrophages. In the other type of granuloma, the macrophages live longer. The former type results in more tissue destruction, as seen in granulomatous inflammation in granulomatosis with polyangiitis and tuberculosis.

The macrophage forms the backbone in all granulomatous inflammatory reactions. At least in infectious models such as granulomas formed in response to *Mycobacterium bovis* and *Schistosoma mansoni* infection, macrophages are involved in antigen presentation since these granulomas do not form in MHC class II deficient mice.[5,6] As a result of macrophage activation, many cytokines and chemokines are produced that attract other immune cells into the inflammatory area and activate them. Cytokine and chemokine profiles differ between different causal agents.[7] As an example, one study found that IL-6 and IFNγ gene expression levels were higher in sarcoid granulomas and IL-13 and eotaxin-1 were higher in fungal granulomas,[8] clearly differentiating between Th1 and Th2 mediated granulomatous inflammation, discussed in further detail in the corresponding sections.

Little is known about the phenotype of macrophages. Many types of granulomatous inflammation have been termed Th1 mediated due to the presence of IFNγ and TNFα-producing $CD4^{+}CD45RO^{+}$ T cells. Their presence implies a signal from classically activated M1 macrophages. A different type of granulomatous inflammation regularly results in the activation of fibrotic pathways, often implicating alternatively activated M2 macrophages. The contribution of M1 and M2 cells to specific granulomas has not been studied in detail. Currently, only helminthic pathogens are known to result in granulomatous inflammation containing M2, in line with the presence of

Th2 cells. However, it cannot be excluded that Th1-mediated granulomatous inflammation also contains M2 that suppress excess inflammation. M1 and M2 macrophages can be distinguished based on their expression of NOS2 (M1) or arginase-1 (M2), both of which have L-arginine as their substrate. The expression of NOS2 is induced by Th1 cytokines (IFNγ, IL-12) whereas the expression of arginase-1 is induced by Th2 cytokines (IL-4, IL-13).[9]

The activation of macrophages found in areas of granulomatous inflammation results in higher levels of circulating vitamin D, specifically increased production of 1,25-$(OH)_2$ vitamin D. This may lead to hypercalcemia in patients with granulomatous disease such as sarcoidosis. Vitamin D is hypothesized to have immunomodulatory effects, and this may be the reason that activated macrophages increase the amount of enzyme to convert vitamin D into its active form.[10]

Osteopontin is produced by histiocytes within granulomatous inflammation.[11] It was demonstrated to function as a chemotactic factor for monocytes, macrophages, and T cells in granulomas in tuberculosis, sarcoidosis, Crohn's, ANCA associated vasculitis, primary biliary cirrhosis, and silicosis.[12–16] Osteopontin is therefore probably a general regulator of granulomatous inflammation by attracting monocytes and T cells to the inflammatory area. Chemotactic activity is likely mediated by its ability to bind various integrins and therefore involve a similar pathway as has been described for its role in extracellular matrix production in calcification processes. Osteopontin may be a therapeutic target to inhibit the buildup of granulomatous inflammation in non-infectious settings where anti-inflammatory treatment is needed.

Granulomas have been found to emerge and disappear in stages.[17] Initially, macrophages detect a pathogen or foreign body and center around it. During this initiation phase, there is significant tissue remodeling to protect the surrounding healthy tissue. Next, T cells respond to chemokines and cytokines produced by the activated macrophages. Following the accumulation of effector cells, the by now lymphoid organ will attempt to clear or at least diminish the pathogen load or foreign body. In some diseases, this process is associated with tissue necrosis. Once inflammation subsides as a result of less pathogenic stimuli or entry into the latent phase of the pathogen, cicatrization starts with resolution of the granuloma or scar formation.

2. Granulomatous inflammation of infectious origin

2.1. *Bacterial triggers*

2.1.1. *Tuberculosis*

The disease caused by *Mycobacterium tuberculosis* (Mtb) is the most frequent chronic human infectious disease and the most common cause of granulomatous inflammation.[18] Much has been learned from the human clinical syndrome as well as animal models of tuberculosis about granulomatous disease. Other mycobacteria, such as *Mycobacterium avium* induce similar pathology.

Patients with primary Mtb infections usually present with low-grade fever, lasting two to three weeks before the infection goes into latency. One-third of initial infections are in the lung, but any organ system can be affected. A large majority of immunocompetent patients enter the latent phase, in which the body is able to control further bacillus replication. The paradigm that granulomatous inflammation functions as a line of defense against further dissemination of the bacillus throughout the body is still plausible[2] and is supported by the finding of fibrosed sterile granulomas in asymptomatic patients. Importantly, not all patients are able to wall off the infection via granulomatous reactions, as is shown by the large number of deaths due to the disease.

Inflammatory cells form concentric layers around the center of the granuloma.[19] Necrosis develops in the center due to macrophages and other cells dying within the granuloma at a high rate. Around the layers of macrophages, epithelioid cells, giant cells, and lymphocytes are found. Peripheral to the cellular infiltrates, a fibrotic layer may develop. The inflammation seen in tuberculous granulomas

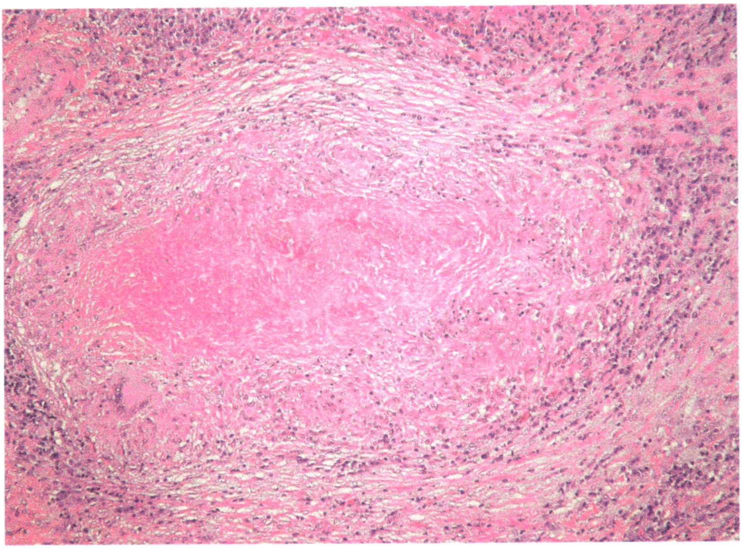

Fig. 2. Tuberculous granuloma; (courtesy of Yale Rosen).

induces the transformation of macrophages in so-called epithelioid histiocytes.[1,20] A typical characteristic of the tuberculous granuloma is that it may caseate, i.e., the granuloma disintegrates in the center. The term 'caseum' comes from Latin meaning cheese, probably because of the yellowish appearance. A disintegration of the granuloma's center results in bacilli spreading to nearby tissue and expanding the infection[21] (Fig. 2).

Many cytokines, chemokines, and other cellular products are produced in granulomatous inflammation. The most studied cytokine is TNFα.[22] Mtb elicits TNFα production at the site of infection, and patients with radiological findings of tuberculosis have increased circulating TNFα levels.[23–25] Macrophages and dendritic cells are the major source of TNF.[26,27] TNFα plays a bactericidal and therefore protective role in tuberculosis.[28,29] TNFα initiates formation and maintains granuloma integrity in a dose-dependent manner.[30] Mice deficient in TNFα fail to construct granulomas and show higher mortality rates.[31,32] Animals treated with anti-TNFα and infected with Mtb, fail to rid the infection due to disintegrated granulomas.[33–35] In patients, the use of TNFα antagonists is associated with a high risk of reactivation of Mtb, and screening for dormant mycobacterial infection is mandatory before treatment is initiated.[36–40] To defend itself, Mtb has been shown to release TNFα-R2, effectively binding and inactivating TNFα within the granuloma.[41] In addition to TNFα, many other members of the TNF superfamily, including CD40L, CD30L, OX40L, and LTα, play important roles in establishing granulomatous inflammation.[42]

Once TNFα is locally released, it regulates many complex processes and pathways. The production of TNFα inside the granuloma is crucial for the resistance against Mtb,[43] in part due to inducing local chemokine production by macrophages within the granulomatous inflammation, eventually leading to the recruitment of further immune cells.[44] Within areas of granulomatous inflammation, macrophages also produce nitric oxide synthase to combat the infection.[45] The programmed cell death of macrophages infected with *M. avium* results in the replenishment of macrophages to the site of granulomatous inflammation.[46] Besides attracting new monocytes and macrophages, cell death is important for cross-presentation of antigen to T cells.[47] In addition to macrophages, dendritic cells play a central role in fighting tuberculosis. Their recruitment to the area results in the production of IL-12 and IL-23 in response to TLR-2 stimulation,[48,49] cytokines driving T cell differentiation. In parallel, macrophages and dendritic cells produce anti-inflammatory cytokines to temper the inflammation to minimize damage to surrounding tissues, in particular IL-10.[50] Overproduction of IL-10 may impair the control and containment of the infection.[51]

T cells in the granuloma play a central role in fighting Mtb. Knocking out γδ T cells results in less granulomata in *M. avium* infections.[52] Both αβ and γδ T cells are involved in bacterial control as well as in curtailing the inflammation.[53,54] Besides TNFα, IFNγ and IL-17, typical T cell products, are required for mycobacterial granuloma formation.[55–57] $CD8^+$ T cells can also be found in granulomas, but their absence does not prevent the formation of granulomas.[58,59]

With the granuloma forming a closed entity inside the host, the pathogen can become dormant for many years. Paradoxically, the granuloma thus forms a protective area where the pathogen can survive until the infection is reactivated.[20] Granuloma formation may therefore even provide an evolutionary advantage for Mtb, and it has been hypothesized that Mtb induce granulomas, become dormant, and their granulomas serve as reservoirs for future dissemination.[60] As outlined above, immune failure can cause reactivation, but excess TNFα can also cause late Mtb dissemination by enhancing macrophage cell death.[61]

Interestingly, reinfection with Mtb shows that new mycobacteria home into already existing granulomas.[62] Current hypotheses do not incorporate all findings, and the discussion whether the tuberculous granuloma is protective or harmful is ongoing.

2.1.2. *Leprosy*

Leprosy is an infectious disease caused by *Mycobacterium leprae*. Its prevalence has decreased significantly over the last decades. The disease mainly affects the skin and the nervous system; a Th1 response to the bacteria is associated with granuloma formation, while a Th2 response causes lepromatous inflammation.[63] Not much is known about the nature of granulomas in leprosy. In a study of skin biopsies, granulomas were seen in half of leprosy patients. Cells in these granulomas were often HLA-DR positive and contained giant cells as well as $CD4^+$ T cells surrounding the core. Edema is frequently present in the granuloma, but central necrosis is not usual.[64]

A large genome-wide association study of leprosy patients found an association with polymorphisms in the HLA-DRB1 region, implicating the major histocompatibility complex in the disease. Other single-nucleotide polymorphisms (SNP) were mapped to genes of the NFκB pathway, possibly resulting in an ineffective buildup of an immune response in macrophages.[65] One of these was TNFSF15, a TNF-like molecule highly expressed in macrophages that induces a switch from Th1 to Th2 cells.[66] Another study found that patients with leprosy more often carry SNP in the PARK2 and PACRG genes which are expressed in Schwann cells and in monocyte-derived macrophages.[67] This finding points at a central role of macrophages in leprosy.

2.2. Other bacterial triggers

Brucella, Bartonella, and Whipple's disease (*Tropheryma whipplei*) cause granulomatous inflammation, but their incidences are infrequent and the specific inflammatory reactions have not been studied in depth.

2.3. Fungal triggers

2.3.1. Histoplasmosis

Histoplasma capsulatum is an opportunistic fungal pathogen endemic in regions of the United States, Africa, and Asia. The pathogen is mainly found in bird and bat droppings and in caves, hence the alternative name of "cave disease". Generally, infected patients are asymptomatic, but the disease can be devastating in immunocompromised patients such as those with AIDS or in patients on immunosuppressive treatment including TNF antagonists.[68,69]

H. capsulatum resides inside the macrophage, more specifically in the lysosomes.[70] The pathogen can enter the macrophage by being phagocytosed and also by binding to CD18 on the macrophage.[71] When mice are injected with *H.capsulatum* intraperitoneally, granulomatous inflammation is observed in the liver 7 days later.[72] Within these early granulomas, high levels of IL-10 and TGFβ are produced by macrophages. Granulomas reach a maximal size after 10 days, before contracting in size. The majority of the granuloma consists of macrophages (70%) that are activated and express MHC class II molecules on their cell surface. Dendritic cells — although few — can be found as well. Interestingly, among the T cells found within the granuloma, the TCR repertoire is very diverse.[73–76] These T cells produce high levels of IFNγ.[77] It has been shown in multiple studies that IFNγ supports a resistance to systemic histoplasmosis, implicating the importance of Th1 cells.[78] IFNγ knock-out mice succumb to the infection due to their inability to produce this vital cytokine.[79] Inside the granuloma, there is a high rate of apoptosis, especially when the size of the granuloma is large. This increase in apoptotic rate coincides with clearance of the pathogen.[80]

Patients with a $CD4^+$ T cell deficiency, such as HIV-infected patients, are unable to construct efficient granulomas and are therefore at higher risk of developing disseminated histoplasmosis. Also, patients receiving corticosteroids, anti-TNFα agents, or other immunosuppressive drugs are at a higher risk of complications of histoplasmosis.[81–85]

In summary, the formation of a granuloma is essential for containing histoplasma and preventing a symptomatic and systemic infection. Therefore, mainly immunocompromised patients, i.e., those who cannot construct efficient granulomas, are at high risk for dissemination.

2.3.2. *Other fungal pathogens*

Other fungal pathogens have been described to cause granulomatous inflammation. Examples are coccidioidomycosis, cryptococcosis,[86] candidiasis, zygomycosis, and aspergillosis. Cell players and cytokines have not been studied in detail but may be similar to histoplasmosis since comparable risk factors are associated with disseminated disease.

2.4. *Viral triggers*

2.4.1. *Hepatitis viruses*

The viruses causing hepatitis, particularly HBV and HCV known to cause chronic disease, infrequently induce granuloma formations, affecting especially the liver in 2–10% of chronically infected patients.[87,88] Interestingly, granulomas localize primarily close to the portal regions. The architecture of the granuloma appears to follow the general rules as in mycobacterial and fungal infection, however, at this time, no further information is available.

2.4.2. *Other viruses that can cause granulomatous inflammation*

The measles virus, Epstein-Barr virus (EBV), herpes simplex virus and cytomegalovirus have all been reported to cause granulomatous inflammation in rare instances. The evidence of the granulomatous processes is limited to case reports.

2.5. *Other infectious triggers*

2.5.1. *Schistosomiasis*

Schistosoma infections are common in endemic regions, especially in sub-Saharan Africa. The disease is caused by infection with parasitic blood fluke worms, initially carried by freshwater snails. Most endemic regions are therefore close to rivers such as the Nile and the Yangtze. The parasite can enter the body through the skin and homes in the mesenteric circulation, where eggs are produced. These eggs can enter the intestines where they are eventually excreted back into the river, completing the reproductive cycle. The disease usually remains asymptomatic, but in some patients advances to a life-threatening disease with hepatic fibrosis, splenomegaly, and portal hypertension.[89] Five species are known to infect humans: *S. mansoni*, *S. japonicum*, *S. haematobium*, *S. mekongi*, and *S. intercalatum*, with the first three species covering most of the incidence. Once infected, the immune response consists of a granulomatous inflammation around the eggs laid by the schistosomes[90] (Fig. 3).

These granulomas are predominantly localized in the liver. The architecture of the granuloma follows the general architecture with macrophages as a first line of defense together with dendritic cells, $CD4^+$ T cells around them, and eosinophils mixed within, indicating a Th2 component. The role of dendritic cells in the initiation of the granulomatous Th2 response has been shown to be crucial.[91] Interestingly, the initial reaction is Th1 mediated but switches to Th2 once eggs are produced by the parasite.[92] The eggs elicit a strong Th2 reaction as a result of their antigenic characteristics.[93] This switch may be mediated by T cells as IL-10-producing

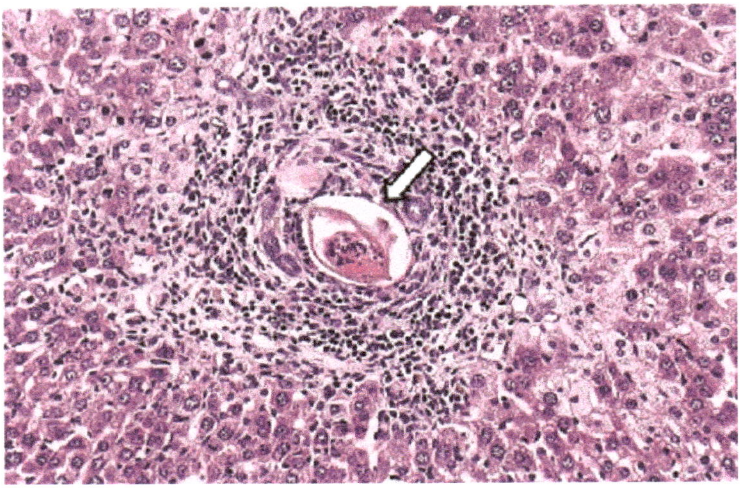

Fig. 3. Perioval granuloma (Hams *et al.*, 2013).

$CCR8^+CD4^+CD25^+FoxP3^-$ T cells have been identified to enhance the Th2 response, possibly preventing tissue damage as a result of Th1 reactions.[94] Both deficiency of the Th1-inducing cytokine IL-12 as well as neutralization of the Th2 cytokine IL-4 results in suppression of granuloma formation.[95] A failure to build up a Th2-dominant granulomatous inflammation is sometimes fatal for mice,[96] possibly due to a misbalance between IL-4 and TNFα.[97] One study showed that TNFα levels are higher in the acute infection when granulomatous inflammation develops, as compared to the chronic infection.[98] The balance between a Th1 and Th2 reaction depends on the type of helminth that infected the host. *Heligmosomoides polygyrus* mainly elicits a Th2 reaction, as opposed to *Schistosoma mansoni* and *Trichuris muris* which show mixed Th1/Th2 reactions.[90] Consequently, a granulomatous inflammation as a reaction to *H. polygyrus* shows more eosinophils and M2 or alternatively activated macrophages, induced by Th2 cells.[99] M2 macrophages in granulomatous infiltrates have been found to downregulate Th1 cells in the context of helminthic infection, calming down the overall inflammation.[100,101] Infection can become chronic with fibrotic features, probably mediated by IL-13.[102] M2 macrophages play a prominent role in producing collagen and enhancing fibrosis in response to IL-13 originating from Th2 cells.[103–105] The fibrosis is known to eventually cause portal hypertension in infected humans.

Correlative studies have identified several mediators that appear to be involved in influencing T cell and macrophage polarization in granulomas; for most of these mediators, their mode of action in the polarization process is undetermined. Schistosome granulomas have been shown to be regulated by neuropeptides.[106] Substance P is produced by eosinophils, which effectively downregulates the production of IFNγ by T cells without affecting IL-12 and TGFβ. In contrast, macrophages within the granulomatous inflammation produce somatostatin 14 (SST14), which signals T cells to produce more IFNγ. IFNγ and TNFα in turn stimulate macrophages to produce SST14. The predominantly M2 reaction in schistosomic granulomas is reflected by the abundant presence of arginase-1 in macrophages in response to high levels of IL-4 and IL-13. The M1 or NOS2 pathway counterbalances this to avoid excess fibrosis.[95,106]

Importantly, mice deficient in T cells fail to construct complete granulomas and succumb to the infection, indicating the protective role of granulomas in schistosoma infection.[107,108]

Besides preventing hepatotoxicity through granuloma formation, immunocompetence is also important for egg excretion. In mice, $CD4^+$ cells are needed for excretion of eggs into the feces, ridding the body of antigen but at the same time completing the parasitical life cycle.[108] Eosinophils are always present in granulomatous inflammation around schistosoma eggs but their role remains largely unknown.[109] Interestingly, in mice deficient for eosinophils, neither the infection nor the granuloma formation are affected.[110]

Overall, the granulomatous inflammation has a function of sealing off the pathogen in schistosoma infections, as well as ridding the body of eggs. In contrast to the mycobacterial and fungal infections, the schistosoma granulomas represent a complex interplay between Th1 and Th2 features regulated by mediators whose role in polarization processes are only beginning to be understood.

2.5.2. *Leishmaniasis*

Leishmaniasis is an infectious disease common in developing countries, caused by different strains of *Leishmania*. There are two types: cutaneous leishmaniasis (caused by *L. major, L. tropica, L. aethiopica, L. infatum-chagasi, L. mexicana,* or *L. braziliensis*) and visceral leishmaniasis (caused by *L. donovani* and *L. infantum-chagasi*). It is a round organism 1.5–4 μm in diameter with a rod-shaped kinetoplast. In this section, we will only consider visceral leishmaniasis because granulomatous inflammation is less common in cutaneous leishmaniasis. The parasite remains asymptomatic in most infected people[111] owing to the capacity of the human body to neutralize the pathogen. The most prominent symptom of visceral leishmaniasis is called kala-azar (Hindi for "black fever") with an average incubation period of two to six months. The disease is characterized by fever, weight loss, and splenomegaly. Enlargement of the liver is also observed in some cases. *Leishmania* invade and replicate within macrophages, placing one of the main cellular components of granulomatous inflammation at the center of *Leishmania* pathophysiology. Due to invasion of macrophages, the parasite is found in the spleen, the liver, and also the bone marrow, where it can cause bone marrow suppression, resulting in anemia. Kala-azar is almost always lethal, thus mandating treatment.[112]

It is known from mouse models that granulomatous inflammation develops within 2–6 weeks after infection.[113] Evidence points at granuloma formation supporting resistance against the pathogen.[114] Kupffer cells (KC), which are macrophage-like cells in the liver, play a central role in granuloma formation in leishmaniasis. These cells tend to migrate toward the source of the pathogen and often fuse, effectively forming giant cells. KC appear to form the basis of the granuloma, attracting other effector cells such as natural killer cells (NK) and T cells to the liver.[115] In addition, monocytes are attracted to the granulomatous inflammation to aid shielding off the pathogen.[116] Cell recruitment is likely facilitated by chemokines and cytokines, but these interactions need to be studied further. In a murine model of visceral leishmaniasis, CXCL10 has been shown to be protective, probably because more T cells can be attracted toward granulomatous inflammatory regions to close in on the pathogen.[117] *Leishmania* induces the production of IL-10 and TGFβ and depletes NO, probably to counter the inflammatory reaction. Production of IL-10 may indicate regulatory T cells which were found to suppress effector T cells in *Leishmania* infection, resulting in ineffective pathogen clearance.[118] In parallel, the pathogen diminishes the surrounding production of IL-12 and TNFα to inhibit granuloma formation.[117]

B cells are present in granulomatous inflammatory regions; their absence in mouse models has been associated with more efficient granuloma formation and more rapid pathogen clearance.[119] Although fibrotic processes are usually not observed in murine models of leishmaniasis, it is common in humans.[120] The process of fibrosis within granulomatous inflammation in leishmaniasis may be regulated by alternatively activated macrophages that are driven by Th2 products such as IL-13 and/or IL-4. Evidence points out that a deficiency of IL-13 or IL-4 results in delayed or absent granuloma maturation.[121] A balance between fibrosis and effective inflammation appears crucial.

3. Immune-related, idiopathic granulomatous inflammation

3.1. *Vasculitis*

3.1.1. *Small-vessel vasculitis*

Small-vessel vasculitides form a heterogeneous group defined by the Chapel Hill classification.[122] Within the group of small-vessel vasculitides, only the ANCA-associated vasculitides show granulomatous inflammation, specifically granulomatosis with polyangiitis (GPA; formerly known as Wegener's), microscopic polyangiitis (MPA), and eosinophilic GPA (EGPA; formerly known as Churg-Strauss syndrome).[123] ANCA associated vasculitis (AAV) is a rare disease (annual incidence 20/million) with a high mortality when left untreated.[124] The presence of anti-neutrophil cytoplasmic antibodies — discovered in the 1980s — forms a hallmark of the disease.[125,126] These antibodies are mainly directed against myeloperoxidase (MPO) and proteinase-3 (PR3). These enzymes are found in neutrophils and monocytes. MPO-AAV and PR3-AAV show differences in clinical characteristics and in pathophysiology.[127] Patients often present with ear, nose, and throat (ENT); pulmonary; and renal involvement, but due to involving small arteries and capillaries, any organ system in the body can be affected by destructive inflammation. Granulomatous inflammation is associated with particularly aggressive tissue destruction in the ENT region, the lungs, and the kidneys.[128] Treatment has improved the acute outcome considerably; however, the chronic disease manifestations remain difficult to manage[129,130] and are associated with many comorbidities.[131] Granulomatous inflammation is most common in GPA and less common in MPA and EGPA.[127] Granulomas in GPA are usually necrotizing, causing a lot of tissue damage. This is in contrast to EGPA, in which granulomas are not necrotizing.[132] In the kidney, the granulomatous inflammation is observed in a periglomerular pattern[124] (Fig. 4). Granulomatous inflammation in AAV is believed to start as microabscesses containing neutrophils that ultimately attract other immune cells.[133] The structure of the granuloma is similar to other (infectious) diseases with macrophages forming the core, often fusing to form giant cells. Around this core, T cells are found. Distinct from other granulomatous diseases is the presence of neutrophils, eosinophils, and B cells in the granuloma. Another important difference is that granulomas in AAV show features of palisading. Palisading implies that the immune cells surrounding the granulomatous inflammation position themselves tightly around, effectively fencing it off[134] but at the same time also inducing fibrotic processes which may be harmful for surrounding tissues.

Neutrophils play a central role in granulomatous inflammation in AAV and are the most prevalent cell in granulomatous lesions in AAV after macrophages.[135] When neutrophils become activated, they express the enzymes MPO and PR3 on the cell membrane, making them accessible for binding by circulating autoantibodies. Upon binding of the antibodies, neutrophils degranulate, releasing toxic

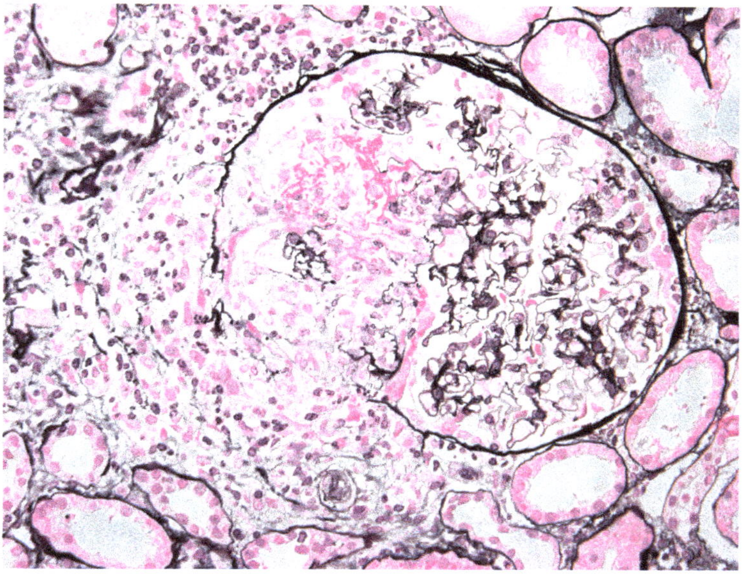

Fig. 4. Periglomerular granuloma with palisading features in a patient with GPA (courtesy of Dr. P. Van Paassen, Limburg Renal Registry, Maastricht, the Netherlands).

substances into their surroundings.[136] They also release neutrophil extracellular traps, physiologically designed to entrap pathogens, but in the setting of small-vessel vasculitis resulting in more damage.[137] Neutrophils can be "primed" by TNFα, placing the presence of TNFα at the center of pathophysiology.[138]

Besides granulocytes and macrophages, T cells are believed to play a pivotal role in AAV, with an increase in Th1 and Th17 cells during active disease[139] as well as lower numbers of regulatory T cells compared to healthy controls.[140] T cells are found within granulomatous inflammatory regions[141] and produce high levels of IFNγ, TNFα, and IL-17. The expansion and activation of T cells may be aided by the secretion of IL-12 by macrophages and dendritic cells in the lesions.

Granulomas in AAV function as lymphoid organs, differentiating naïve T cells and perhaps forming a basis for autoantibody production. B cells are found within the granulomatous inflammation and differentiate into plasma cells producing autoantibodies specifically against the neutrophilic enzymes.[142,143] The granuloma in AAV has therefore unique features distinct from that in infectious disease, although AAV has been frequently suspected to be caused by infectious organisms and cotrimoxazole — an antibiotic effective against *S. aureus* — significantly reduces the risk for disease relapse.[144] Certain drugs and medications may also elicit symptoms and histopathological characteristics mimicking AAV,[145] especially the use of levamisole-adulterated cocaine.

The presence of granulomatous inflammation, especially in PR3-ANCA positive patients, is associated with a higher risk for relapse, correlating persistent inflammation with refractory and/or relapsing disease, exemplified by patients with retro-orbital granulomatous masses, half of whom suffer from refractory disease.[146]

EGPA differs from GPA and MPA due to its eosinophilic component, including the presence of eosinophils in granulomatous lesions. While local destruction of bone in the ENT region is typical in GPA, it is rare in EGPA. However, patients with EGPA can develop eosinophilic myocarditis — sometimes granulomatous — with heart failure as a result.[147]

Treatment of ANCA-associated vasculitis consists of non-specific immunosuppression with cyclophosphamide and corticosteroids. B cell depletion has gathered popularity more recently. Surprisingly for a granulomatous disease, TNFα neutralization is not beneficial.[148,149]

3.1.2. *Large-vessel vasculitis*

Large and medium-size vessel vasculitides comprise the disease entities of giant cell arteritis (GCA), Takayasu arteritis (TA), and Kawasaki's syndrome, of which GCA and TA can share histopathological features of granulomatous inflammation.[150]

3.1.2.1. Giant cell arteritis

GCA is diagnosed exclusively in patients older than 50 years of age. Caucasians, particularly those of North European origin, are at highest risk.[151,152] Patients may present with malaise, anorexia, and night sweat, considered to be due to a systemic inflammatory response. Clinically more concerning are symptoms related to tissue ischemia caused by stenosis and/or occlusion of inflamed blood vessels. The disease mainly affects the thoracic aorta and its 2nd to 5th branches.[153] Granulomatous inflammation may cause destruction of the aortic wall and result in dissection, aneurysm formation, or rupture.

In GCA, granulomatous inflammatory infiltrates are located within the vessel wall[154,155] and consist of monocytes, macrophages, dendritic cells, and T cells. Granulomatous arrangements are mainly encountered in the medial layer, sometimes in the adventitia of affected vessels. About half of the cases have multinucleated giant cells which may typically be lined along the internal elastic lamina. Classical histopathologic findings will include fragmentation of the elastic membrane[4] (Fig. 5). B cells and neutrophils are infrequent.

Molecular studies have identified intra-lesional production of IL-12,[156,157] creating conditions to shape developing T cell responses.[158]

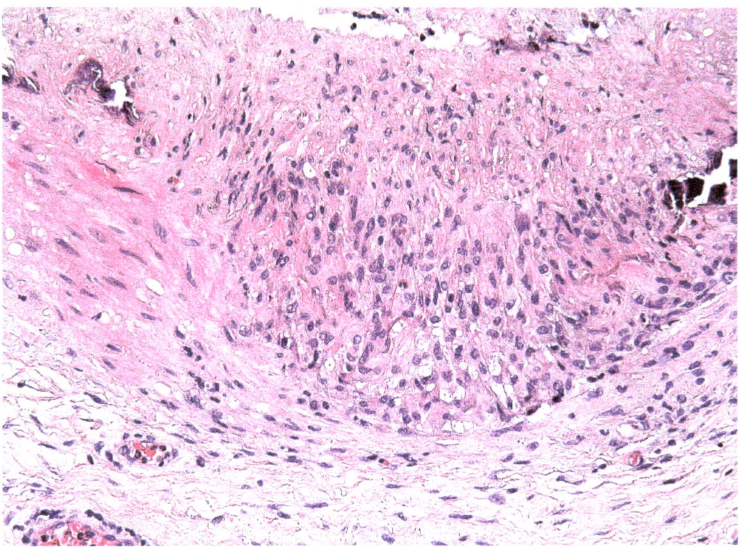

Fig. 5. Granulomatous inflammation in GCA (reproduced with permission from Hilhorst *et al.,* 2014).

GCA is a T cell-dependent disease, and both Th1 and Th17 cells have been found within the intramural lesions but also in the circulation of GCA patients. As a result, GCA is classified as a Th1-mediated disease, with Th2 responses essentially being non-contributory.

Circulating IFN-γ, IL-17, and IL-23 levels are increased in patients, and these cytokines are believed to originate within the inflammatory lesions.[37,159,160] These cytokines, possibly in conjunction with TGFβ,[161] are known to amplify the induction of T cells biased toward the Th1 and Th17 lineage.[162,163] High circulating levels of IL-32 have been reported in GCA patients. This T cell-derived cytokine has been implicated in T cell-macrophage interactions, regulating, among others, the induction of TNFα and IL-6.[164] IL-33 is also increased in patients with GCA and believed to derive from endothelial cells.[165] Functional studies have connected IL-33 to the differentiation of resting macrophages into M2 cells. The presence of IL-33 in the vascular lesions may thus reflect a negative feedback loop, intended to suppress the inflammatory response from M1 and dendritic cells in the granulomatous lesions.[166] Highly activated macrophages within the granulomatous infiltrates can fuse and form multi-nucleated giant cells, lending the disease its name. Such giant cells appear to participate in cytokine secretion and have been found to produce VEGF, FGF, and PDGF.[167,168] Elevated circulating levels of typical macrophage and dendritic cell products, including IL-12, IL-6, and IL-1β, are present in GCA patients.[37,169,170] There is direct evidence that IL-6 originates in the granulomatous inflammation.[171] Among the typical pro-inflammatory cytokines, TNFα appears to have the least pathogenic relevance. Well-designed treatment trials with anti-TNFα biologics have failed to show a steroid-sparing effect, and TNFα blockade has not found a place in managing GCA patients.[152,172]

Granuloma-residing Th17 cells have been shown to produce high levels of GM-CSF,[173] especially when IL-1β is present.[174] This cytokine may have lesion-stabilizing effects, as GM-CSF in turn can activate dendritic cells and promote the production of IL-6 and IL-21.[173] This mechanism could sustain a feed-forward loop, as IL-6 and IL-21 condition the microenvironment to enable Th17 lineage commitment.

Key players in GCA are the dendritic cells. Remarkably, dendritic cells are a constitutive population of vessel wall cells and are localized in the media–adventitia border. Dendritic cells are a consistent partner in the inflammatory infiltrates, increase massively in numbers, and are highly activated.[175,176] Studies in humanized mice have demonstrated that wall-residing DC respond to Toll-like receptor ligands and hold checkpoint functions in initiating and sustaining granulomatous vasculitis. Stimulation of vascular DC with different TLR ligands gives rise to distinct patterns of disease. Whereas TLR4 stimulation results in classical panarteritis, TLR5 ligands induce a perivasculitic infiltrate.[177] These data are compatible with a model in which wall-embedded DC receive stimulatory signals that eventually lead to the formation of a granulomatous reaction.

Placing DC at the heart of granuloma formation has nurtured the speculation that GCA is an infectious disease.[175,178] Multiple studies have attempted to identify triggering microorganisms, but no conclusive evidence has been provided that GCA granulomas represent anti-bacterial or anti-viral immune responses.[179]

3.1.2.2. Takayasu's arteritis

Takayasu's arteritis (TA) affects mainly young women, with the highest prevalence in Asia. The pathogenesis is less defined than that of GCA, but also has all the features of a T cell-driven delayed hypersensitivity reaction.[180] As in GCA, immune cells infiltrate the vessel wall and form a granulomatous network, forming giant cells. IL-12, IL-6, and IL-18 levels are found to be increased.[181,182] In contrast to GCA and distinct from most granulomatous diseases, cytotoxic T cells play an important role in TA, with $\gamma\delta$ T cells also present in granulomatous lesions in the vessel wall.[183,184] These cells exert a killer function, secreting perforin that directly damages arterial vascular cells. It has been postulated that these T cells target heat shock protein 65 (HSP-65).[185]

3.2. Sarcoidosis

Sarcoidosis is a systemic granulomatous disorder usually affecting young adults.[186] The granulomatous inflammation frequently involves the lymph nodes of the lung and elsewhere, lung parenchyma, eyes, skin, and liver, but may affect any organ. The infiltrate follows the general architectural rules of most granulomas with a core of macrophages and epithelioid cells surrounded mainly by $CD4^+$ cells. $CD8^+$ and B cells can also be found in sarcoid granulomas. How these cells interact within the granuloma remains unknown.[187] Macrophages in sarcoidosis produce high levels of TNFα, IL-1β, and IL-6 upon stimulation with TLR2 ligands.[188,189] Alveolar macrophages from patients have been shown to be highly activated, producing high levels of IL-1β and TNFα.[190,191] Macrophages and monocytes from patients also show an increased tendency to form multi-nucleated giant cells *in vitro* when compared with healthy controls.[192] These studies show that TNFα plays a pivotal role in granulomatous inflammation in sarcoidosis. TNFα is thought to initially attract monocytes and macrophages to the inflammatory site by inducing the production and release of CCL20, RANTES, MIP, and MCP-1, based on the presence of these chemokines in bronchoalveolar fluid from patients with active disease.[193,194] The chemokines CXCL9, CXCL10, CXCL11, and CXCL16 have been shown to be produced by alveolar macrophages from patients and presumably attract T cells carrying the CXCR3 and CXCR6 receptor, respectively, to the site of granulomatous inflammation.[195–197] Whether a distortion of the balance between pro-inflammatory M1 and anti-inflammatory M2 macrophages within sarcoid granulomatous inflammation plays an important role is hitherto unknown. The formation of the sarcoid granulomatous inflammation is driven by $CD4^+$ T cells that attract monocytes from the periphery.[198] Besides macrophages, dendritic cells have been implicated in granulomatous inflammation in sarcoidosis as well.[199] Granulomatous inflammation in sarcoidosis may drive the formation of Th1 and Th17 cells that characterizes the pathogenesis of this disease.[200,201]

Like any of the idiopathic granulomatous diseases, a causal antigen, either of environmental or infectious origin, has been suspected.[202] Several antigens have been explored, but convincing evidence is lacking.

Granulomatous inflammation in sarcoidosis has been associated with hypervitaminosis D, causing comorbidity in patients. The vitamin D is likely to originate from activated macrophages within the lesions.[203]

Sarcoidosis is a self-limiting disease in many patients, eventually leading to the disappearance of the granulomas. However, in some patients it becomes chronic with granulomatous inflammation transitioning into fibrotic processes. In patients with a chronic form of sarcoidosis, a treatment regimen that prevents granuloma formation or results in granuloma clearance would be promising. Regulatory T cells have been studied for their capacity to suppress granuloma formation but appear to fail to do so in sarcoidosis.[204–206]

3.3. *Crohn's disease*

Crohn's disease (CD) is an inflammatory panenteric disease with an incidence of 5/100,000 per year.[207,208] About 80% of patients have involvement of the small bowel and 50% have involvement of the ileum and colon. The main symptoms consist of fatigue, abdominal pain with diarrhea, fever, and weight loss. Extraintestinal involvement is common and ranges from joint to eye, skin involvement, and vasculitis.[209] Granulomatous involvement is usually limited to the intestines. The presence of granulomatous inflammation in the intestinal wall is one of the features that distinguishes the disease from ulcerative colitis[210] (Fig. 6).

Interestingly, corticosteroids do not have much effect on the number of granulomas.[211]

A meta-analysis showed that patients with granulomatous Crohn's disease are at higher risk of disease recurrence and therefore at a higher risk of surgical interventions.[212] A large longitudinal study, included in this meta-analysis, demonstrated that 25% of biopsies contained epithelioid granulomas at study entry which

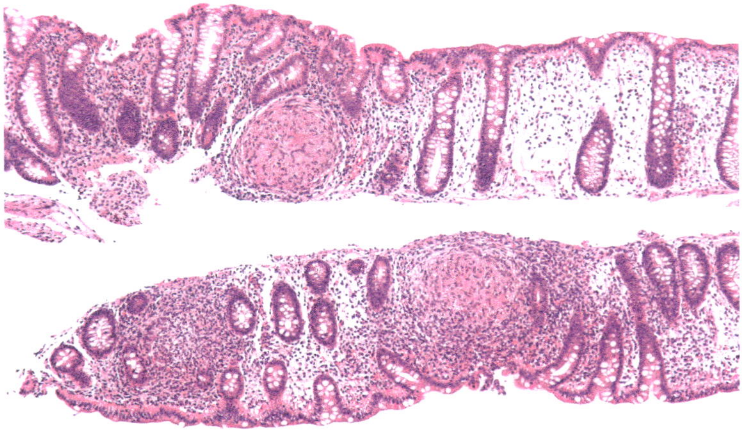

Fig. 6. Granulomatous inflammation in Crohn's disease (courtesy of "Nephron" [pseudonym] under the Creative Commons Attribution-Share Alike 3.0 Unported License).

increased to 37% of biopsies at last follow-up, confirming its chronic progressive nature.[213] Importantly, granulomas may be missed due to their location in the intestinal wall, which endoscopic biopsies may not reach.[214] Granulomas in CD are reported to be smaller than in tuberculosis and are sometimes termed microgranulomas, especially when compared to intestinal tuberculous granulomas.[215] Granulomatous inflammation in CD is never caseating. The granulomatous inflammation in CD is associated with lymphatic vessels.[216,217] The inflammation in CD obstructs regional lymph vessels and occasionally shows intralymphatic granulomas.[218] Granulomatous inflammation in CD has been hypothesized to have an infectious etiology. Granulomatous tissue has been found to contain mycobacteria[219,220] but contradictory data exist, and hitherto the evidence is insufficient to resolve the matter.[221] The presence of a luminal antigen in CD[222] has been postulated numerous times — both of infectious or of environmental origin — implicating an epithelial barrier dysfunction,[223,224] but also here the evidence is insufficient.[225] Co-stimulatory molecules CD80 and CD86 have been found in granulomatous inflammation in patients with active CD, indicating that the ability for antigen-induced T cell activation exists within the tissue.[226] The presence of different $CD4^+$ T cell receptors within the inflamed tissue as compared to non-inflamed tissue as well as the presence of CD68 macrophages in inflamed regions support this.[227,228] As a result of their interaction within the intestinal wall, T cells differentiate into Th1 and Th17, producing high levels of IFNγ[229,230] and IL-17.[231] The activated macrophages produce increased levels of TNFα and IL-12.[232]

Interestingly, neutralizing TNFα in Crohn's disease forms an effective treatment, as opposed to AAV or GCA where anti-TNFα treatments have failed. This probably points to a different composition of granulomas and a different pathophysiology.

3.4. *Primary biliary cirrhosis*

Primary biliary cirrhosis (PBC) is a rare disease, mainly affecting women, in which the intralobular bile ducts are destroyed due to an apparently autoimmune process. The T cell-mediated disease leads to cholestasis and eventually cirrhosis. Due to cholestasis, patients often present with jaundice or hyperpigmentation. Hepatosplenomegaly may be present.[233] Many patients show high levels of circulating polyclonal IgM and a positive test for antimitochondrial antibodies.[234]

Histologically, PBC presents as a non-suppurative cholangitis affecting the interlobular bile ducts, often with necrosis. The infiltrates are composed of plasma cells, macrophages, eosinophils, and sometimes, epithelioid cells. Granulomatous inflammation in PBC occurs mainly in the early course of disease.[235] CD11c-expressing dendritic cells, the major antigen-presenting cells, are present in PBC granulomas. Increased CD1d expression — a molecule that presents non-peptide antigens to T cells — on bile duct epithelial cells within the inflammatory areas during the early stages of PBC has led to the assumption that recognition of non-convential antigens is involved. CD1d was also found on epithelioid granuloma cells later in the course of PBC.[236] A possible antigenic candidate is *Propionibacterium acnes*, of which the ribosomal 16S rRNA has been found in tissue of PBC patients.[237] However, this study, as is the case for most claims on the presence of antigens in idiopathic granulomatous inflammation, awaits confirmation. The abundant presence of B cells and plasma cells within the granulomatous inflammation may form the basis for the high levels of circulating polyclonal IgM in PBC patients.[238]

Granulomatous inflammation in PBC resolves over time, giving way for fibrotic processes that can be detrimental for patients. Whether this transformation involves a transition from a Th1 to a Th2- mediated inflammation, as has been discussed for schistosomiasis, or whether a different mechanism is involved, remains to be seen.

3.5. *Common variable immune deficiency*

Common variable immune deficiency (CVID) is a condition characterized by impaired B cell function resulting in defective immunoglobulin production.[239] Its manifestations vary widely. Clinically, patients present with recurrent bacterial infections, autoimmune disorders, and an increased susceptibility to lymphoma. CVID patients are characterized by reduced immunoglobulin levels (IgA, IgG, and IgM) and a decreased reaction to vaccinations. The annual incidence is estimated at 1 in 25,000 per year. CVID is most common in Caucasian populations.[240] Granulomatous inflammation is observed in around 10% of CVID patients.[241,242] This number may be an underestimate since most patients are never biopsied. These granulomas are usually found in the lungs, lymph nodes, liver, spleen, intestines, brain, eyes, and the skin.[243,244] In some patients, the granulomas are found long before the diagnosis of CVID had been made. Some researchers have considered the granulomatous inflammation in CVID a presentation of sarcoidosis, but the presence of hypogammaglobulinemia contests this.[245] The sarcoidosis specific Kveim test may be inconclusive in CVID, and a chest X-ray showing perihilar granulomatous infiltrates cannot rule out one or the other. Recently, a comparative study concluded that, in general, CVID and sarcoidosis can be distinguished based on biochemical and radiological characteristics.[246]

Although the major problem in CVID is the hypogammaglobulinemia, T cell function is also impaired with decreased numbers of circulating regulatory T cells[247] and $CD4^+$ cells but increased $CD8^+$ cells.[248] Hitherto, the specific interactions between these cells in the context of granulomatous inflammation are unknown.

4. Granulomatous inflammation associated with environmental and iatrogenic triggers

4.1. *Berylliosis*

Berylliosis or chronic beryllium disease is caused by exposure to beryllium, an alkaline earth metal with varying industrial uses. In the past, it was used in fluorescent lamps, but this has since been prohibited based on the clear association with chronic granulomatous inflammation, particularly in the lungs.[249] An acute reaction to beryllium results in pneumonitis. Chronic exposure eventually leads to granulomatous inflammation.

T cells isolated from the lungs of berylliosis patients were found to be Be^{2+}-specific[250] and HLA-DP2 restricted. Be^{2+} can bind within the groove of the MHC molecule, specifically HLA-DP2, causing a conformational change recognized by the T cell receptor leading to T cell activation.[251] Accordingly, HLA-DP polymorphisms constitute a risk factor for developing berylliosis.[252] Activated T cells differentiate into Th1 cells producing IFNγ and TNFα. Regulatory T cells have been found to suppress excess granulomatous inflammation in a murine model of berylliosis.[253] Such regulatory T cells have been found to be decreased as well as dysfunctional in humans.[254]

Macrophages are clearly activated in berylliosis, perhaps phagocytosing beryllium to avoid systemic harm. This is supported by the finding of high levels of beryllium within pulmonary granulomas.[255] Berylliosis follows the classical paradigm of granulomatous inflammation with high levels of neopterin.[256] Persistent presence of beryllium leads to macrophage apoptosis[257] as well as to their fusion and the creation of multinucleated giant cells containing beryllium.[258]

Beryllium shares with other metals, such as nickel and copper, the ability to elicit T cell responses. However, the exposure to these metals does not result in granulomatous inflammation with macrophage activation and giant cell formation.

4.2. *Silicosis*

Silicosis comprises multiple pulmonary diseases that are the result of crystalline silica inhalation. The disease is mainly due to occupational exposures in the mining, glass manufacturing, and construction industries.[259] Although the incidence of silicosis has decreased due to preventive measures, many cases, especially in developing countries, continue to be diagnosed. The crystalline silica (quartz, cristobalite, tridymite) are the most harmful because they facilitate the production of reactive oxygen species that cause tissue damage and subsequent fibrosis.[260] Initially, macrophages phagocytose the silica particles and aggregate to form nodules (Fig. 7).

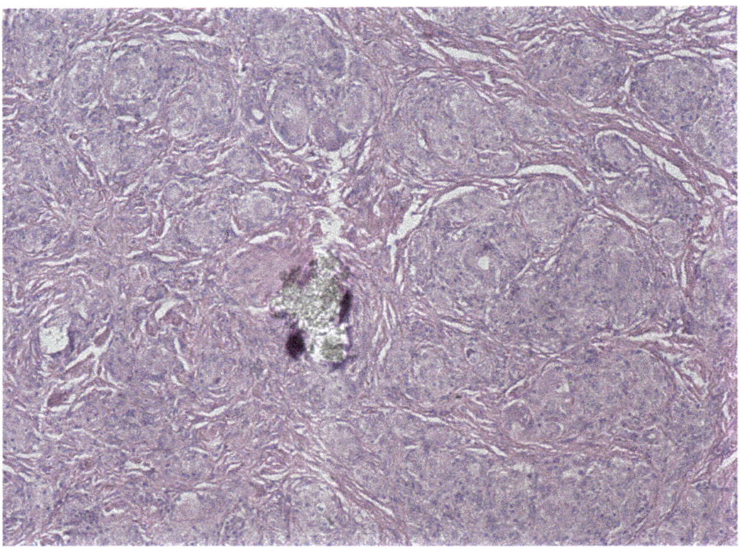

Fig. 7. Granulomatous inflammation in the skin induced by silica (courtesy of Dr. Peter L. Reisfeld, Long Island Dermatologic Society, NY).

These nodules grow in size and cause damage to the lung parenchyma. An ongoing cycle of phagocytosis and apoptosis induces a persistent inflammatory reaction with production of IL-1β and TNFα, attracting T cells and other immune cells.[261] Blocking IL-1β or TNFα prevents fibrosis associated with silicosis.[262,263] Activated macrophages also produce high levels of neopterin, which may function as a chemoattractant for monocytes and T cells.[12,264] After the acute phase of silicosis, fibrotic processes gradually increase under the influence of TGFβ. The fibrosis is presumably triggered by macrophages that deposit fibrous material in the extracellular matrix, mainly collagen 1 and elastin.[265]

Since the most severe complications of silicosis are fibrosis and the associated respiratory failure, research mainly focuses on slowing down the fibrotic processes, however, with little clinical translation. Until now, prevention remains the ultimate goal.

4.3. *Foreign bodies and topical medication*

Foreign bodies enter the human skin all the time, ranging from tattoo ink and cosmetic material to medication and accidental entry due to trauma. Some medications, when injected, can cause granulomatous inflammation. Examples are IFNβ and IFNα, used in the treatment of multiple sclerosis and the treatment of certain types of cancer, respectively.

The granulomatous inflammation which follows entry of a foreign body into the skin usually takes place in the dermis, with subcutaneous extension sometimes. Upon entry, the foreign body is first surrounded by neutrophils that provide a first signal to attract monocytes and macrophages. These macrophages go through a cycle of phagocytosis and apoptosis while attracting T cells that surround the macrophage core. Most foreign bodies elicit similar pathologies. Generally, reactions remain localized, and therefore not much is known about the inflammatory processes. The treatment usually consists of waiting to see if the foreign body is expelled or removing the foreign body surgically.[266]

4.4. Other triggers

4.4.1. Chronic granulomatous disease

Chronic granulomatous disease (CGD) is a genetic illness characterized by recurrent bacterial and fungal infections due to phagocytic dysfunction of macrophages. These defects lead to granulomatous inflammation in the context of a general hyperinflammatory reaction.[267] It has been estimated that 1 in 200,000 children are born with CGD.[268] The disease has a high mortality due to recurring infections. Granulomatous inflammation in CGD can affect all organ systems but is most common in hollow viscera such as the gastrointestinal and the genitourinary tract.[269] Due to the presence of granulomas in the gastrointestinal tract, sarcoidosis is always in the differential diagnosis. Patients can also present with lupus-like symptoms.

CGD is caused by defects in the nicotinamide adenine dinucleotide phosphate (NADPH) oxidase complex as a result of mutations in gp91phox, p47phox, p22phox, p67phox, and/or p40phox. gp91phox is X-linked, while the other genetic defects are autosomal recessive.[268] In order to form NADPH oxidase, the cytoplasmic proteins p47phox, p67phox, p40phox, and Rac2 combine with the cytochrome complex (gp91phox and p22phox). If any of these components has been mutated, the complex does not assemble correctly,[270] and the generation of superoxide and the subsequent generation of other reactive oxygen species such as HOCl in phagocytes is impaired. The deficiency in reactive oxygen species causes an ineffective bactericidal and antifungal response by the innate immune system. It is unclear why CGD patients develop granulomatous disease. Most granulomatous inflammatory areas were found to be sterile, ruling out infections. Reactive oxygen species are not only bactericidal but are also involved in a plethora of cellular and immunological processes. Earlier studies have shown that ROS can catabolize chemoattractants such as leukotrienes and activated complement factor 5 (C5a).[271–273] If these molecules are not catabolized, monocytes and macrophages are continuously attracted to the granulomatous lesion, resulting in a perpetuating inflammation.

A recent study in $p47^{phox-/-}$ mice infected with aspergillus fumigatus demonstrated that indoleamine 2,3-dioxygenase (IDO) cannot function properly due to the absence of superoxide. IDO uses superoxide as a cofactor to cleave tryptophan. Since IDO has broad immunoregulatory function, the infection caused a disproportional inflammatory response with an overstimulation of γδ T cell and Th17 cells.[274] Given the complexity of ROS function in immune cells, the current models have likely only scratched the surface to explain the granulomatous response in CGD.

The treatment of CGD patients remains challenging and consists of fighting infections and excess granulomatous inflammation. Since the latter requires broad and non-specific immunosuppression, it increases the risk for infections.

4.4.2. *Granuloma annulare*

Granuloma annulare (GA) is a granulomatous skin disorder that is usually self-limited. It is relatively common, and only in rare cases the disease extends into the subcutaneous layers of the skin. The cause of GA is unknown, and no clear associations with systemic granulomatous diseases have been found. Implicated causes range from insect bites, vaccinations, and viruses to diabetes and malignancies. GA is characterized by a lymphohistiocytic infiltrate with mucin deposition. In approximately 25% of patients, it presents as a palisading granulomatous inflammation.[275] Whereas the early GA lesion shows an infiltrate with intact collagen, advanced lesions show disintegration of collagen, necrobiosis, and extension toward the subcutis. The perforating type of GA is usually accompanied by palisading granulomas including multinucleate giant cells. At that point, other lymphocytes such as T cells are usually low in number.[276] T cells present in the granulomatous inflammation in GA are usually $CD4^{+}CD45^{RO+}$ and express high levels of TNF as well as IFNγ. Macrophages present in the palisading granuloma express high levels of TNF as well, along with high expression of MMP2 and MMP9.[277] In summary, the granulomatous inflammation in GA is a typical example of a Th1-mediated inflammation resulting in tissue damage. The etiology of GA is unknown.

5. Conclusions

Granulomatous inflammation follows a persistent and chronic stimulus, be it of infectious, environmental, or idiopathic origin. Although granuloma formation may be considered as beneficial limiting tissue injury and maintaining homeostasis, it can in many cases lead to detrimental inflammatory consequences that may even be lethal. Tuberculous granuloma formation has long been hypothesized to keep the infection at bay, but newer studies indicate that the pathogen may be using granulomas as a hideout. A similar case for protecting the host and sealing off potential harm can be made for other infectious organisms causing granuloma or for environmental toxins such as beryllium. In case of vasculitis and other idiopathic inflammatory diseases, the presence of granulomatous inflammation remains largely enigmatic. Whatever the cause of granulomatous inflammation, the overall architecture is largely the same: a core of macrophages (and often dendritic cells) surrounded by lymphocytes and sometimes other cells. As described in detail for the different entities, the immunological pathways can differ depending on which cells are involved and how easily the stimulus can be managed. Interfering with granulomatous inflammation, perhaps enhancing granuloma formation in infectious causes and inhibiting the process in autoimmune disorders, can form an effective form of treatment, but such interventions are still in their infancy. Moreover, such interventions are not without risk, as is exemplified by anti-TNF treatment that can lead to the reactivation of tuberculous in patients with latent infection or the induction of sarcoid lesions in other patients, presumably by shifting the cytokine balance.

References

1. Williams G, Williams W. (1983). Granulomatous inflammation — a review. *J Clin Pathol.* 36:723–733.
2. Adams D. (1976). The granulomatous inflammatory response. *Am J Pathol.* 84:164–192.
3. Modlin R, Pirmez C, Hofman F, Torigian V, Uyemura K, Rea T *et al.* (1989). Lymphocytes bearing antigen-specific gamma delta T-cell receptors accumulate in human infectious disease lesions. *Nature.* 339:544–548.

4. Hilhorst M, Shirai T, Berry GJ, Goronzy J, Weyand C. (2014). T-cell macrophage interactions in vasculitis and granuloma formation. *Front Immunol.* **5**:432.
5. Ladel C, Daugelat S, Kaufmann S. (1995). Immune response to Mycobacterium bovis bacille Calmette Guérin infection in major histocompatibility complex class I- and II-deficient knock-out mice: contribution of CD4 and CD8 T cells to acquired resistance. *Eur J Immunol.* **25**:377–384.
6. Hernandez H, Wang Y, Tzellas N, Stadecker M. (1997). Expression of class II, but not class I, major histocompatibility complex molecules is required for granuloma formation in infection with Schistosoma mansoni. *Eur J Immunol.* **27**:1170–1176.
7. Qiu B, Frait K, Reich F, Komuniecki E, Chensue S. (2001). Chemokine expression dynamics in mycobacterial (type-1) and schistosomal (type-2) antigen-elicited pulmonary granuloma formation. *Am J Pathol.* **158**:1503–1515.
8. Christophi G, Caza T, Curtiss C, Gumber D, Massa P, Landas S. (2014). Gene expression profiles in granuloma tissue reveal novel diagnostic markers in sarcoidosis. *Exp Mol Pathol.* **96**:393–399.
9. Wynn T, Chawla A, Pollard J. (2013). Macrophage biology in development, homeostasis and disease. *Nature.* **496**:445–455.
10. Plum L, DeLuca H. (2010). Vitamin D disease and therapeutic opportunities. *Nat Rev Drug Discov.* **9**:941–955.
11. Carlson I, Tognazzi K, Manseau E, Dvorak H, Brown L. (1997). Osteopontin is strongly expressed by histiocytes in granulomas of diverse etiology. *Lab Invest.* **77**:103–108.
12. Nau G, Guilfoile P, Chupp G, Berman J, Kim S, Kornfeld H *et al.* (1997). A chemoattractant cytokine associated with granulomas in tuberculosis and silicosis. *Proc Natl Acad Sci.* **94**:6414–6419.
13. O'Regan A, Chupp G, Lowry J, Goetschkes M, Mulligan N, Berman J. (1999). Osteopontin is associated with T cells in sarcoid granulomas and has T cell adhesive and cytokine-like properties *in vitro*. *J Immunol.* **162**:1024–1031.
14. Sato T, Nakai T, Tamura N, Okamoto S, Matsuoka K, Sakuraba A *et al.* (2005). Osteopontin/Eta-1 upregulated in Crohn's disease regulates the Th1 immune response. *Gut.* **54**:1254–1262.
15. Harada K, Ozaki S, Sudo Y, Tsuneyama K, Ohta H, Nakanuma Y. (2003). Osteopontin is involved in the formation of epithelioid granuloma and bile duct injury in primary biliary cirrhosis. *Pathol Int.* **53**:8–17.
16. Lorenzen J, Lovric S, Krämer R, Haller H, Haubitz M. (2009). Osteopontin in antineutrophil cytoplasmic autoantibody-associated vasculitis: relation to disease activity, organ manifestation and immunosuppressive therapy. *Ann Rheum Dis.* **69**:1169–1171.
17. Co D, Hogan L, Il-Kim S, Sandor M. (2004). T cell contributions to the different phases of granuloma formation. *Immunol Lett.* **92**:135–142.
18. Zumla A, Raviglione M, Hafner R, Fordham von Reyn C. (2013). Tuberculosis. *N Engl J Med.* **368**:745–755.

19. Ulrichs T, Kaufmann S. (2006). New insights into the function of granulomas in human tuberculosis. *J Pathol.* **208**:261–269.
20. Ramakrishnan L. (2012). Revisiting the role of the granuloma in tuberculosis. *Nat Rev Immunol.* **12**:352–366.
21. Guirado E, Schlesinger L. (2013). Modeling the Mycobacterium tuberculosis granuloma — the critical battlefield in host immunity and disease. *Front Immunol.* **4**:1–7.
22. Dorhoi A, Kaufmann S. (2014). Tumor necrosis factor alpha in mycobacterial infection. *Semin Immunol.* **26**:203–209.
23. Barnes P, Fong S, Brennan P, Twomey P, Mazumder A, Modlin R. (1990). Local production of tumor necrosis factor and IFN-gamma in tuberculous pleuritis. *J Immunol.* **145**:149–154.
24. Casarini M, Ameglio F, Alemanno L, Zangrilli P, Mattia P, Paone G *et al.* (1999). Cytokine levels correlate with a radiologic score in active pulmonary tuberculosis. *Am J Respir Crit Care Med.* **159**:143–148.
25. Law K, Weiden M, Harkin T, Tchou-Wong K, Chi C, Rom W. (1996). Increased release of interleukin-1 beta, interleukin-6, and tumor necrosis factor-alpha by bronchoalveolar cells lavaged from involved sites in pulmonary tuberculosis. *Am J Respir Crit Care Med.* **153**:799–804.
26. Valone S, Rich E, Wallis R, Ellner J. (1988). Expression of tumor necrosis factor *in vitro* by human mononuclear phagocytes stimulated with whole Mycobacterium bovis BCG and mycobacterial antigens. *Infect Immun.* **56**:3313–3315.
27. Henderson R, Watkins S, Flynn J. (1997). Activation of human dendritic cells following infection with Mycobacterium tuberculosis. *J Immunol.* **159**:635–643.
28. Flynn J, Goldstein M, Chan J, Triebold K, Pfeffer K, Lowenstein C *et al.* (1995). Tumor necrosis factor-alpha is required in the protective immune response against Mycobacterium tuberculosis in mice. *Immunity.* **2**:561–572.
29. Kindler V, Sappino A, Grau G, Piquet P, Vassalli P. (1989). The inducing role of tumor necrosis factor in the development of bactericidal granulomas during BCG infection. *Cell.* **56**:731–740.
30. Bekker L, Moreira A, Bergtold A, Freeman S, Ryffel B, Kaplan G. (2000). Immunopathologic effects of tumor necrosis factor alpha in murine mycobacterial infection are dose dependent. *Infect Immun.* **68**:6954–6961.
31. Bean A, Roach D, Briscoe H, France M, Korner H, Sedgwick J *et al.* (1999). Structural deficiencies in granuloma formation in TNF gene-targeted mice underlie the heightened susceptibility to aerosol Mycobacterium tuberculosis infection, which is not compensated for by lymphotoxin. *J Immunol.* **162**:3504–3511.
32. Kaneko H, Yamada H, Mizuno S, Udagawa T, Kazumi Y, Sekikawa K *et al.* (1999). Role of tumor necrosis factor-alpha in Mycobacterium-induced

granuloma formation in tumor necrosis factor-alpha- deficient mice. *Lab Invest.* 79:379–386.
33. Senaldi G, Yin S, Shaklee C, Piquet P, Mak T, Ulich T. (1996). Corynebacterium parvum- and Mycobacterium bovis bacillus Calmette-Guerin-induced granuloma formation is inhibited in TNF receptor I (TNF-RI) knockout mice and by treatment with soluble TNF-RI. *J Immunol.* 157:5022–5026.
34. Egen J, Rothfuchs A, Feng C, Winter N, Sher A, Germain R. (2008). Macrophage and T cell dynamics during the development and disintegration of mycobacterial granulomas. *Immunity.* 28:271–284.
35. Chakravarty S, Zhu G, Tsai M, Mohan V, Marino S, Kirschner D *et al.* (2008). Tumor necrosis factor blockade in chronic murine tuberculosis enhances granulomatous inflammation and disorganizes granulomas in the lungs. *Infect Immun.* 76:916–926.
36. Garcia-Vidal C, Rodriguez-Fernandez S, Martinez-Lacasa J, Salavert M, Vidal R, Rodriguez-Carballeira M *et al.* (2005). Paradoxical response to antituberculous therapy in infliximab-treated patients with disseminated tuberculosis. *Clin Infect Dis.* 40:756–759.
37. Visvanathan S, Rahman M, Hoffman GS, Xu S, García-Martínez A, Segarra M *et al.* (2011). Tissue and serum markers of inflammation during the follow-up of patients with giant-cell arteritis — a prospective longitudinal study. *Rheumatology.* 50:2061–2070.
38. Wallis R. (2008). Tumour necrosis factor antagonists: structure, function, and tuberculosis risks. *Lancet Infect Dis.* 8:601–611.
39. Wallis R, Ehlers S. (2005). Tumor necrosis factor and granuloma biology: explaining the differential infection risk of etanercept and infliximab. *Sem Arthritis Rheum.* 34 (suppl 1):34–38.
40. Gardam M, Keystone E, Menzies R, Manners S, Skamene E, Long R *et al.* (2003). Anti-tumour necrosis factor agents and tuberculosis risk: mechanisms of action and clinical management. *Lancet Infect Dis.* 3:148–155.
41. Balcewicz-Sablinska M, Keane J, Kornfeld H, Remold H. (1998). Pathogenic Mycobacterium tuberculosis evades apoptosis of host macrophages by release of TNF-R2, resulting in inactivation of TNF-alpha. *J Immunol.* 161:2636–2641.
42. Saunders B, Britton W. (2007). Life and death in the granuloma: immunopathology of tuberculosis. *Immunol Cell Biol.* 85:103–111.
43. Fallahi-Sichani M, El-Kebir M, Marino S, Kirschner D, Linderman J. (2011). Multiscale computational modeling reveals a critical role for TNF-α receptor 1 dynamics in tuberculosis granuloma formation. *J Immunol.* 186:3472–3483.
44. Roach D, Bean A, Demangel C, France M, Briscoe H, Britton W. (2002). TNF regulates chemokine induction essential for cell recruitment, granuloma formation, and clearance of mycobacterial infection. *J Immunol.* 168:4620–4627.

45. MacMicking J, North R, LaCourse R, Mudgett J, Shah S, Nathan C. (1997). Identification of nitric oxide synthase as a protective locus against tuberculosis. *Proc Natl Acad Sci.* **94**:5243–5248.
46. Fratazzi C, Arbeit R, Carini C, Remold H. (1997). Programmed cell death of Mycobacterium avium serovar 4-infected human macrophages prevents the mycobacteria from spreading and induces mycobacterial growth inhibition by freshly added, uninfected macrophages. *J Immunol.* **158**:4320–4327.
47. Schaible U, Winau F, Sieling P, Fischer K, Collins H, Hagens K *et al.* (2003). Apoptosis facilitates antigen presentation to T lymphocytes through MHC-I and CD1 in tuberculosis. *Nat Med.* **9**:1039–1046.
48. Demangel C, Bean A, Martin E, Feng C, Kamath A, Britton W. (1999). Protection against aerosol Mycobacterium tuberculosis infection using Mycobacterium bovis Bacillus Calmette Guérin- infected dendritic cells. *Eur J Immunol.* **29**:1972–1979.
49. Hickman S, Chan J, Salgame P. (2002). Mycobacterium tuberculosis induces differential cytokine production from dendritic cells and macrophages with divergent effects on naive T cell polarization. *J Immunol.* **168**:4636–4642.
50. Demangel C, Bertolino P, Britton W. (2002). Autocrine IL-10 impairs dendritic cell (DC)-derived immune responses to mycobacterial infection by suppressing DC trafficking to draining lymph nodes and local IL-12 production. *Eur J Immunol.* **32**:994–1002.
51. Feng C, Kullberg M, Jankovic D, Cheever A, Caspar P, Coffman R *et al.* (2002). Transgenic mice expressing human interleukin-10 in the antigen-presenting cell compartment show increased susceptibility to infection with Mycobacterium avium associated with decreased macrophage effector function and apoptosis. *Infect Immun.* **70**:6672–6679.
52. Tanaka S, Itohara S, Sato M, Taniguchi T, Yokomizo Y. (2000). Reduced formation of granulomata in gamma(delta) T cell knockout BALB/c mice inoculated with Mycobacterium avium subsp. paratuberculosis. *Vet Pathol.* **37**:415–421.
53. Ladel C, Blum C, Dreher A, Reifenberg K, Kaufmann S. (1995). Protective role of gamma/delta T cells and alpha/beta T cells in tuberculosis. *Eur J Immunol.* **25**:2877–2881.
54. D'Souza C, Cooper A, Frank A, Mazzaccaro R, Bloom B, Orme I. (1997). An anti-inflammatory role for gamma delta T lymphocytes in acquired immunity to Mycobacterium tuberculosis. *J Immunol.* **158**:1217–1221.
55. Cooper A, Dalton D, Stewart T, Griffin J, Russell D, Orme I. (1993). Disseminated tuberculosis in interferon gamma gene-disrupted mice. *J Exp Med.* **178**:2243–2247.
56. Smith D, Hänsch H, Bancroft G, Ehlers S. (1997). T-cell-independent granuloma formation in response to Mycobacterium avium: Role of tumour necrosis factor-alpha and interferon-gamma. *Immunology.* **92**:413–421.

57. Okamoto Yoshida Y, Umemura M, Yahagi A, O'Brien R, Ikuta K, Kishihara K *et al.* (2010). Essential role of IL-17A in the formation of a mycobacterial infection-induced granuloma in the lung. *J Immunol.* **184**:4414–4422.
58. D'Souza C, Cooper A, Frank A, Ehlers S, Turner J, Bendelac A *et al.* (2000). A novel nonclassic beta2-microglobulin-restricted mechanism influencing early lymphocyte accumulation and subsequent resistance to tuberculosis in the lung. *Am J Respir Cell Mol Biol.* **23**:188–193.
59. Mogues T, Goodrich M, Ryan L, LaCourse R, North R. (2001). The relative importance of T cell subsets in immunity and immunopathology of airborne Mycobacterium tuberculosis infection in mice. *J Exp Med.* **193**:271–280.
60. Davis J, Ramakrishnan L. (2009). The role of the granuloma in expansion and dissemination of early tuberculous infection. *Cell.* **136**:37–49.
61. Roca F, Ramakrishnan L. (2013). TNF dually mediates resistance and susceptibility to mycobacteria via mitochondrial reactive oxygen species. *Cell.* **153**:521–534.
62. Cosma C, Humbert O, Ramakrishnan L. (2004). Superinfecting mycobacteria home to established tuberculous granulomas. *Nat Immunol.* **5**:828–835.
63. Walker SL, DNJ. (2006). The clinical and immunological features of leprosy. *Br Med Bull.* **77–78**:103–121.
64. Lockwood D, Lucas S, Desikan K, Ebenezer G, Suneetha S, Nicholls P. (2008). The histological diagnosis of leprosy type 1 reactions: identification of key variables and an analysis of the process of histological diagnosis. *J Clin Pathol.* **61**:595–600.
65. Zhang F, Huang W, Chen S, Sun L, Liu H, Li Y *et al.* (2009). Genomewide association study of leprosy. *N Engl J Med.* **361**:2609–2618.
66. Meylan F, Davidson T, Kahle E, Kinder M, Acharya K, Jankovic D *et al.* (2008). The TNF-family receptor DR3 is essential for diverse T cell-mediated inflammatory diseases. *Immunity.* **29**:79–89.
67. Mira M, Alcais A, Nguyen V, Moraes M, Di Flumeri C, Vu H *et al.* (2004). Susceptibility to leprosy is associated with PARK2 and PACRG. *Nature.* **427**:636.
68. Darling S. (1906). A protozoan general infection producing pseudotubercles in the lungs and focal necrosis in the liver, spleen and lymph nodes. *JAMA.* **46**:1283–1285.
69. Kauffman C. (2007). Histoplasmosis: a clinical and laboratory update. *Clin Microbiol Rev.* **20**:115–132.
70. Woods J. (2003). Knocking on the right door and making a comfortable home: Histoplasma capsulatum intracellular pathogenesis. *Curr Opin Microbiol.* **6**:327–331.
71. Long K, Gomez F, Morris R, Newman S. (2003). Identification of heat shock protein 60 as the ligand on Histoplasma capsulatum that mediates binding to CD18 receptors on human macrophages. *J Immunol.* **170**:487–494.

72. Heninger E, Hogan L, Karman J, Macvilay S, Hill B, Woods J *et al.* (2006). Characterization of the Histoplasma capsulatum-induced granuloma. *J Immunol.* **177**:3303–3313.
73. Deepe GJ, Gibbons R, Ward S. (2002). Discordance between T-cell receptor expression and effector function in mice infected with Histoplasma capsulatum. *Infect Immun.* **70**:1648–1652.
74. Scheckelhoff M, Deepe GJ. (2002). The protective immune response to heat shock protein 60 of Histoplasma capsulatum is mediated by a subset of V beta 8.1/8.2+ T cells. *J Immunol.* **169**:5818–5826.
75. Gomez F, Cain J, Gibbons R, Allendoerfer R, Deepe GJ. (1998). Vbeta4(+) T cells promote clearance of infection in murine pulmonary histoplasmosis. *J Clin Invest.* **102**:984–995.
76. Deepe GJ, Gibbons R. (2002). Functional properties of the T cell receptor repertoire in responding to the protective domain of heat-shock protein 60 from Histoplasma capsulatum. *J Infect Dis.* **186**:815–822.
77. Lin J, Wu-Hsieh B. (2002). Functional T cells in primary immune response to histoplasmosis. *Int Immunol.* **16**:1663–1673.
78. Clemons K, Darbonne W, Curnutte J, Sobel R, Stevens D. (2000). Experimental histoplasmosis in mice treated with anti-murine interferon-γ antibody and in interferon-γ gene knockout mice. *Microbes Infect.* **2**:997–1001.
79. Allendoerfer R, Deepe GJ. (1997). Intrapulmonary response to Histoplasma capsulatum in gamma interferon knockout mice. *Infect Immun.* **65**:2564–2569.
80. Allen H, Deepe GJ. (2005). Apoptosis modulates protective immunity to the pathogenic fungus Histoplasma capsulatum. *J Clin Invest.* **115**:2875–2885.
81. Zerbe C, Holland S. (2005). Disseminated histoplasmosis in persons with interferon γ receptor 1 deficiency. *Clin Infect Dis.* **41**:e38–e41.
82. Wood K, Hage C, Knox K, Kleiman M, Sannuti A, Day R *et al.* (2003). Histoplasmosis after treatment with anti-tumor necrosis factor α therapy. *Am J Respir Crit Care Med.* **167**:1279–1282.
83. Rosenberg J, Scheinfeld N. (2003). Cutaneous histoplasmosis in patients with acquired immunodeficiency syndrome. *Cutis.* **72**:439–445.
84. Giles J, Bathon J. (2004). Serious infections associated with anticy-tokine therapies in the rheumatic diseases. *J Intensive Care Med.* **19**:320–334.
85. Conant M. (1996). Fungal infections in immunocompromised individuals. *Dermatol Clin.* **14**:155–162.
86. Fairhurst R, Pegues D. (2002). Images in clinical medicine. Pulmonary cryptococcal granulomas. *N Engl J Med.* **347**:497.
87. Emile J, Sebagh M, Feray C, David F, Reynes M. (1993). The presence of epithelioid granulomas in hepatitis C virus-related cirrhosis. *Hum Pathol.* **24**:1095–1097.
88. Goldin R, Levine T, Foster G, Thomas H. (1996). Granulomas and hepatitis C. *Histopathology.* **28**:265–267.

89. Gryseels B, Polman K, Clerinx J, Kestens L. (2006). Human schistosomiasis. *Lancet.* **368**:1106–1118.
90. Anthony R, Rutitzky L, Urban JJ, Stadecker M, Gause W. (2007). Protective immune mechanisms in helminth infection. *Nat Rev Immunol.* 7:975–987.
91. Phythian-Adams A, Cook P, Lundie R, Jones L, Smith K, Barr T *et al.* (2010). CD11c depletion severely disrupts Th2 induction and development *in vivo*. *J Exp Med.* **207**:2089–2096.
92. Fallon P, Smith P, Dunne D. (1998). Type 1 and type 2 cytokine-producing mouse CD4+ and CD8+ T cells in acute Schistosoma mansoni infection. *Eur J Immunol.* **28**:1408–1416.
93. Hams E, Aviello G, Fallon P. (2013). The Schistosoma granuloma: friend or foe? *Front Immunol.* **4**:89.
94. Freeman C, Chiu B, Stolberg V, Hu J, Zeibecoglou K, Lukacs N *et al.* (2005). CCR8 is expressed by antigen-elicited, IL-10-producing CD4+CD25+ T cells, which regulate Th2-mediated granuloma formation in mice. *J Immunol.* **174**:1962–1970.
95. Wynn T, Cheever A. (1995). Cytokine regulation of granuloma formation in schistosomiasis. *Curr Opin Immunol.* 7:505–511.
96. MacDonald A, Patton E, La Flamme A, Araujo M, Huxtable C, Bauman B *et al.* (2002). Impaired Th2 development and increased mortality during schistosoma mansoni infection in the absence of CD40/CD154 interaction. *J Immunol.* **168**:4643–4649.
97. Brunet L, Finkelman F, Cheever A, Kopf M, Pearce E. (1997). IL-4 protects against TNF-alpha-mediated cachexia and death during acute schistosomiasis. *J Immunol.* **159**:777–785.
98. Joseph A, Boros D. (1993). Tumor necrosis factor plays a role in Schistosoma mansoni egg-induced granulomatous inflammation. *J Immunol.* **151**:5461–5471.
99. Anthony R, Urban JJ, Alem F, Hamed H, Rozo C, Boucher J *et al.* (2006). Memory T(H)2 cells induce alternatively activated macrophages to mediate protection against nematode parasites. *Nat Med.* **12**:955–960.
100. Flores-Villanueva P, Harris T, Ricklan D, Stadecker M. (1994). Macrophages from schistosomal egg granulomas induce unresponsiveness in specific cloned Th-1 lymphocytes *in vitro* and down- regulate schistosomal granulomatous disease *in vivo*. *J Immunol.* **152**:1847–1855.
101. Herbert D, Hölscher C, Mohrs M, Arendse B, Schwegmann A, Radwanska M *et al.* (2004). Alternative macrophage activation is essential for survival during schistosomiasis and downmodulates T helper 1 responses and immunopathology. *Immunity.* **20**:623–635.
102. Wynn T. (2004). Fibrotic disease and the Th1/Th2 paradigm. *Nat Rev Immunol.* **4**:583–594.
103. Chiaramonte MD, DD, Cheever A, Wynn T. (1999). An IL-13 inhibitor blocks the development of hepatic fibrosis during a T-helper type 2-dominated inflammatory response. *J Clin Invest.* **104**:777–785.

104. Fallon P, Richardson E, McKenzie G, McKenzie A. (2000). Schistosome infection of transgenic mice defines distinct and contrasting pathogenic roles for IL-4 and IL-**13**: IL-13 is a profibrotic agent. *J Immunol.* **164**:2585–2591.
105. Hesse M, Modolell M, La Flamme A, Schito M, Fuentes J, Cheever A *et al.* (2001). Differential regulation of nitric oxide synthase-2 and arginase-1 by type 1/type 2 cytokines *in vivo*: granulomatous pathology is shaped by the pattern of L-arginine metabolism. *J Immunol.* **167**:6533–6544.
106. Sandor M, Weinstock J, Wynn T. (2003). Granulomas in schistosome and mycobacterial infections: a model of local immune responses. *Trends Immunol.* **24**:44–52.
107. Byram J, von Lichtenberg F. (1977). Altered schistosome granuloma formation in nude mice. *Am J Trop Med Hyg.* **26**:944–956.
108. Doenhoff M, Pearson S, Dunne D, Bickle Q, Lucas S, Bain J *et al.* (1981). Immunological control of hepatotoxicity and parasite egg excretion in Schistosoma mansoni infections: stage specificity of the reactivity of immune serum in T-cell deprived mice. *Trans R Soc Trop Med Hyg.* **75**:41–53.
109. Moore D, Grove D, Warren K. (1977). The Schistosoma mansoni egg granuloma: quantitation of cell populations. *J Pathol.* **121**:41–50.
110. Swartz J, Dyer K, Cheever A, Ramalingam T, Pesnicak L, Domachowske J *et al.* (2006). Schistosoma mansoni infection in eosinophil lineage-ablated mice. *Blood.* **108**:2420–2427.
111. Singh O, Hasker E, Sacks D, Boelaert M, Sundar S. (2014). Asymptomatic Leishmania infection: a new challenge for Leishmania control. *Clin Infect Dis.* **58**:1424–1429.
112. Seaman J, Mercer A, Sondorp E. (1996). The epidemic of visceral leishmaniasis in western Upper Nile, southern Sudan: course and impact from 1984 to 1994. *Int J Epidemiol.* **25**:862–871.
113. Gutierrez Y, Maksem J, Reiner N. (1984). Pathologic changes in murine leishmaniasis (Leishmania donovani) with special reference to the dynamics of granuloma formation in the liver. *Am J Pathol.* **114**:222–230.
114. Moore J, Moyo D, Beattie L, Andrews P, Timmis J, Kaye P. (2013). Functional complexity of the Leishmania granuloma and the potential of in silico modeling. *Front Immunol.* **4**:1–7.
115. Beattie L, Peltan A, Maroof A, Kirby A, Brown N, Coles M *et al.* (2010). Dynamic imaging of experimental Leishmania donovani-induced hepatic granulomas detects Kupffer cell-restricted antigen presentation to antigen-specific CD8 T cells. *PLos Pathog.* **6**:e1000805.
116. Cervia J, Rosen H, Murray H. (1993). Effector role of blood monocytes in experimental visceral leishmaniasis. *Infect Immun.* **61**:1330–1333.
117. Gupta G, Bhattacharjee S, Bhattacharyya S, Bhattacharya P, Adhikari A, Mukherjee A *et al.* (2009). CXC chemokine-mediated protection against

visceral leishmaniasis: involvement of the proinflammatory response. *J Infect Dis*. **200**:1300–1310.

118. Belkaid Y, Piccirillo C, Mendez S, Shevach E, Sacks D. (2002). CD4+CD25+ regulatory T cells control Leishmania major persistence and immunity. *Nature*. **420**:502–507.
119. Smelt S, Cotterell S, Engwerda C, Kaye P. (2000). B cell-deficient mice are highly resistant to Leishmania donovani infection, but develop neutrophil-mediated tissue pathology. *J Immunol*. **164**:3681–3688.
120. Duarte M, De Andrade HJ, Takamura C, Sesso A, Tuon F. (2009). TGF-beta and mesenchymal hepatic involvement after visceral leishmaniasis. *Parasitol Res*. **104**:1129–1136.
121. McFarlane E, Carter K, McKenzie A, Kaye P, Brombacher F, Alexander J. (2011). Endogenous IL-13 plays a crucial role in liver granuloma maturation during Leishmania donovani infection, independent of IL-4Rα-responsive macrophages and neutrophils. *J Infect Dis*. **204**:36–43.
122. Jennette JC, Falk RJ, Bacon P, Basu N, Cid M, Ferrario F *et al*. (2013). 2012 revised international Chapel Hill consensus conference nomenclature of vasculitides. *Arthritis Rheum*. **65**:1–11.
123. Franssen C, Stegeman C, Kallenberg C, Gans R, De Jong P, Hoorntje S *et al*. (2000). Antiproteinase 3-and antimyeloperoxidase-associated vasculitis. *Kidney Int*. **57**:2195–2206.
124. Wegener F. (1939). Über eine eigenartige rhinogene Granulomatose mit besonderer Beteiligung des Arteriensystems und der Nieren. *Beitrage zur Path Anat*. **102**:36–68.
125. Cohen Tervaert J, Goldschmeding R, Elema J, Van der Giessen M, Huitema M, Van der Hem G. (1990). Autoantibodies against myeloid lysosomal enzymes in crescentic glomerulonephritis. *Kidney Int*. **37**:799–806.
126. Davies D, Moran J, Niall J, Ryan G. (1982). Segmental necrotizing glomerulonephritis with antineutrophil antibody: possible arbovirus etiology? *Br Med J*. **285**:606.
127. Hilhorst M, Van Paassen P, Cohen Tervaert JW. (2015). Proteinase 3-ANCA Vasculitis versus Myeloperoxidase-ANCA Vasculitis. *J Am Soc Nephrol*, **26**: 2314–2327.
128. Holle J, Gross WL, Latza U, Noelle B, Ambrosch P, Heller M *et al*. (2011). Improved outcome of 445 Wegener's granulomatosis patients in a German vasculitis center over four decades. *Arthritis & Rheum*. **63**:257–266.
129. Hilhorst M, Wilde B, Van Paassen P, Winkens B, Van Breda Vriesman P, Cohen Tervaert JW. (2013). Improved outcome in anti-neutrophil cytoplasmic antibody (ANCA)-associated glomerulonephritis: a 30-year follow-up study. *Nephrol Dial Transplant*. **28**:373–379.

130. Wilde B, Van Paassen P, Witzke O, Cohen Tervaert JW. (2011). New pathophysiological insights and treatment of ANCA-associated vasculitis. *Kidney Int.* **79**:599–612.
131. Little MA, Nazar L, Farrington K. (2004). Outcome in glomerulonephritis due to systemic small vessel vasculitis: effect of functional status and non-vasculitic co-morbidity. *Nephrol Dial Transplant.* **19**(2):356–364.
132. Mahr A, Moosig F, Neumann T, Szczeklik W, Taille C, Vaglio A *et al.* (2014). Eosinophilic granulomatosis with polyangiitis (Churg–Strauss): Evolutions in classification, etiopathogenesis, assessment and management. *Curr Opin Rheumatol.* **26**:16–23.
133. Holl-Ulrich K. (2013). L18. Granuloma formation in granulomatosis with polyangiitis. *Presse Med.* **42**:555–558.
134. Godman G, Churg J. (1954). Wegener's granulomatosis: pathology and review of the literature. *AMA Arch Pathol.* **58**:533–553.
135. Weidner S, Carl M, Riess R, Rupprecht HD. (2004). Histologic analysis of renal leukocyte infiltration in antineutrophil cytoplasmic antibody–associated vasculitis. *Arthritis Rheum.* **50**:3651–3657.
136. Falk RJ, Terrell R, Charles L, Jennette JC. (1990). Anti-neutrophil cytoplasmic autoantibodies induce neutrophils to degranulate and produce oxygen radicals *in vitro*. *Proc Natl Acad Sci.* **87**:4115–4119.
137. Sangaletti S, Tripodo C, Chiodoni C, Guarnotta C, Cappetti B, Casalini P *et al.* (2012). Neutrophil extracellular traps mediate transfer of cytoplasmic neutrophil antigens to myeloid dendritic cells toward ANCA induction and associated autoimmunity. *Blood.* **120**:3007–3018.
138. Jennette J, Falk R. (1997). Small-vessel vasculitis. *N Engl J Med.* **337**:1512.
139. Abdulahad W, Lamprecht P, Kallenberg C. (2011). T-helper cells as new players in ANCA-associated vasculitides. *Arthritis Res Ther.* **13**:236–244.
140. Berden A, Kallenberg C, Savage C, Yard B, Abdulahad W, De Heer E *et al.* (2009). Cellular immunity in Wegener's granulomatosis: characterizing T lymphocytes. *Arthritis Rheum.* **60**:1578–1587.
141. Komocsi A, Lamprecht P, Csernok E, Mueller A, Holl-Ulrich K, Seitzer U *et al.* (2002). Peripheral blood and granuloma CD4(+)CD28(–) T cells are a major source of interferon-gamma and tumor necrosis factor-alpha in Wegener's granulomatosis. *Am J Pathol.* **160**:1717–1724.
142. Voswinkel J, Mueller A, Lamprecht P. (2005). Is PR3-ANCA formation initiated in Wegener's granulomatosis lesions? Granulomas as potential lymphoid tissue maintaining autoantibody production. *Ann N Y Acad Sci.* **1051**:12–19.
143. Voswinkel J, Assmann G, Held G, Pitann S, Gross WL, Holl-Ulrich K *et al.* (2008). Single cell analysis of B lymphocytes from Wegener's granulomatosis: B cell receptors display affinity maturation within the granulomatous lesions. *Clin Exp Immunol.* **154**:339–345.

144. Stegeman C, Cohen Tervaert JW, De Jong P, Kallenberg C. (1996). Trimethoprim-sulfamethoxazole (co-trimoxazole) for the prevention of relapses of Wegener's granulomatosis. Dutch Co-Trimoxazole Wegener Study Group. *N Engl J Med.* **335**:16–20.
145. Pendergraft Wr, Niles JL. (2014). Trojan horses: drug culprits associated with antineutrophil cytoplasmic autoantibody (ANCA) vasculitis. *Curr Opin Rheumatol.* **26**:42–49.
146. Holle J, Voigt C, Both M, Holl-Ulrich K, Nölle B, Laudien M *et al.* (2013). Orbital masses in granulomatosis with polyangiitis are associated with a refractory course and a high burden of local damage. *Rheumatology.* **52**:875–882.
147. Comarmond C, Pagnoux C, Khellaf M, Cordier J, Hamidou M, Viallard J *et al.* (2013). Eosinophilic granulomatosis with polyangiitis (Churg-Strauss): clinical characteristics and long-term followup of the 383 patients enrolled in the French Vasculitis Study Group cohort. *Arthritis Rheum.* **65**:270–281.
148. WGET, Research, Group. (2005). Etanercept plus standard therapy for Wegener's granulomatosis. *N Engl J Med.* **352**:351–361.
149. Jarrot P, Kaplanski G. (2014). Anti-TNF-alpha therapy and systemic vasculitis. *Mediators Inflamm.* **2014**:493–593.
150. Bjornsson J. (2002). Histopathology of primary vasculitic disorders. In: Hoffman GS, Weyand C, editors. Inflammatory diseases of blood vessels. New York: *Marcel Dekker.* 255–265.
151. Salvarani C, Cantini F, Hunder GG. (2008). Polymyalgia rheumatica and giant-cell arteritis. *Lancet.* **372**:234–245.
152. Weyand C, Goronzy J. (2014). Clinical practice. Giant-cell arteritis and polymyalgia rheumatica. *N Engl J Med.* **371**:50–57.
153. Weyand C, Liao Y, Goronzy J. (2012). The immunopathology of giant cell arteritis: diagnostic and therapeutic implications. *J Neuroophthalmol.* **32**:259–265.
154. Weyand C, Goronzy J. (2013). Immune mechanisms in medium and large-vessel vasculitis. *Nat Rev Rheumatol.* **9**:731–740.
155. Ghosh P, Borg F, Dasgupta B. (2010). Current understanding and management of giant cell arteritis and polymyalgia rheumatica. *Expert Rev Clin Immunol.* **6**:913–928.
156. Weyand C, Younge B, Goronzy J. (2011). IFN-γ and IL-17: the two faces of T-cell pathology in giant cell arteritis. *Curr Opin Rheumatol.* **23**:43–49.
157. Nizzoli G, Krietsch J, Weick A, Steinfelder S, Facciotti F, Gruarin P *et al.* (2013). Human CD1c+ dendritic cells secrete high levels of IL-12 and potently prime cytotoxic T-cell responses. *Blood.* **122**:932–942.
158. Deng J, Younge B, Olshen R, Goronzy J, Weyand C. (2010). Th17 and Th1 T-Cell responses in giant cell arteritis. *Circulation.* **121**:906–915.

159. Espígol-Frigolé G, Corbera-Bellalta M, Planas-Rigol E, Lozano E, Segarra M, García-Martínez A *et al.* (2013). Increased IL-17A expression in temporal artery lesions is a predictor of sustained response to glucocorticoid treatment in patients with giant-cell arteritis. *Ann Rheum Dis.* **72**:1481–1487.
160. Samson M, Audia S, Fraszczak J, Trad M, Ornetti P, Lakomy D *et al.* (2012). Th1 and Th17 lymphocytes expressing CD161 are implicated in giant cell arteritis and polymyalgia rheumatica pathogenesis. *Arthritis Rheum.* **64**:3788–3798.
161. Weyand C, Wagner A, Björnsson J, Goronzy J. (1996). Correlation of the topographical arrangement and the functional pattern of tissue-infiltrating macrophages in giant cell arteritis. *J Clin Invest.* **98**:1642–1649.
162. Mangan P, Harrington L, O'Quinn D, Helms W, Bullard D, Elson C *et al.* (2006). Transforming growth factor-b induces development of the TH17 lineage. *Nature.* **441**:231–234.
163. Noack M, Miossec P. (2014). Th17 and regulatory T cell balance in autoimmune and inflammatory diseases. *Autoimmun Rev.* **13**:668–677.
164. Ciccia F, Alessandro R, Rizzo A, Principe S, Raiata F, Cavazza A *et al.* (2011). Expression of interleukin-32 in the inflamed arteries of patients with giant cell arteritis. *Arthritis Rheum.* **63**:2097–2104.
165. Ciccia F, Alessandro R, Rizzo A, Raimondo S, Giardina A, Raiata F *et al.* (2013). IL-33 is overexpressed in the inflamed arteries of patients with giant cell arteritis. *Ann Rheum Dis.* **72**:258–264.
166. Kurowska-Stolarska M, Stolarski B, Kewin P, Murphy G, Corrigan C, Ying S *et al.* (2009). IL-33 amplifies the polarization of alternatively activated macrophages that contribute to airway inflammation. *J Immunol.* **183**:6469–6477.
167. Kaiser M, Weyand C, Björnsson J, Goronzy J. (1998). Platelet-derived growth factor, intimal hyperplasia, and ischemic complications in giant cell arteritis. *Arthritis Rheum.* **41**:623–633.
168. Kaiser M, Younge B, Björnsson J, Goronzy J, Weyand C. (1999). Formation of new vasa vasorum in vasculitis. Production of angiogenic cytokines by multinucleated giant cells. *Am J Pathol.* **155**:765–774.
169. Dasgupta B, Panayi G. (1990). Interleukin-6 in serum of patients with polymyalgia rheumatica and giant cell arteritis. *British journal of rheumatology.* **29**:456–458.
170. Wagner A, Goronzy J, Weyand C. (1994). Functional profile of tissue-infiltrating and circulating CD68+ cells in giant cell arteritis. Evidence for two components of the disease. *J Clin Invest.* **94**:1134–1140.
171. Emilie D, Liozon E, Crevon M, Lavignac C, Portier A, Liozon F *et al.* (1994). Production of interleukin 6 by granulomas of giant cell arteritis. *Hum Immunol.* **39**:17–24.
172. Hoffman GS, Cid M, Rendt-Zagar K, Merkel PA, Weyand C, Stone JH *et al.* (2007). Infliximab for maintenance of glucocorticosteroid-induced remission

of giant cell arteritis: a randomized trial. *Annals of Internal Medicine.* **146**:621–630.

173. Terrier B, Geri G, Chaara W, Allenbach Y, Rosenzwajg M, Costedoat-Chalumeau N *et al.* (2012). Interleukin-21 Modulates Th1 and Th17 Responses in Giant Cell Arteritis. *Arthritis Rheum.* **64**:2001–2011.
174. El-Behi M, Ciric B, Dai H, Yan Y, Cullimore M, Safavi F *et al.* (2011). The encephalitogenicity of TH17 cells is dependent on IL-1- and IL-23-induced production of the cytokine GM-CSF. *Nat Immunol.* **12**:568–576.
175. Krupa W, Dewan M, Jeon M, Kurtin P, Younge B, Goronzy J *et al.* (2002). Trapping of misdirected dendritic cells in the granulomatous lesions of giant cell arteritis. *Am J Pathol.* **161**:1815–1823.
176. Ma-Krupa W, Jeon M, Spoerl S, Tedder T, Goronzy J, Weyand C. (2004). Activation of arterial wall dendritic cells and breakdown of self-tolerance in giant cell arteritis. *J Exp Med.* **199**:173–183.
177. Deng J, Ma-Krupa W, Gewirtz A, Younge B, Goronzy J, Weyand C. (2009). Toll-like receptors 4 and 5 induce distinct types of vasculitis. *Circ Res.* **104**:488–495.
178. Bhatt A, Manzo V, Pedamallu C, Duke F, Cai D, Bienfang D *et al.* (2014). Brief Report: In Search of a candidate pathogen for giant cell arteritis: sequencing-based characterization of the giant cell arteritis microbiome. *Arthritis & Rheumatology.* **66**:1939–1944.
179. Rodríguez-Pla A, Stone JH. (2006). Vasculitis and systemic infections. *Curr Opin Rheumatol.* **18**:39–47.
180. Weyand C, Goronzy J. (2003). Medium- and large-vessel vasculitis. *N Engl J Med.* **349**:160–169.
181. Verma D, Tripathy N, Verma N, Tiwari S. (2005). Interleukin 12 in Takayasu's arteritis: plasma concentrations and relationship with disease activity. *J Rheumatol.* **32**:2361–2363.
182. Park M, Lee S, Park Y, Lee S. (2006). Serum cytokine profiles and their correlations with disease activity in Takayasu's arteritis. *Rheumatology.* **45**:545–548.
183. Seko Y, Sato O, Takagi A, Tada Y, Matsuo H, Yagita H *et al.* (1996). Restricted usage of T-cell receptor Valpha-Vbeta genes in infiltrating cells in aortic tissue of patients with Takayasu's arteritis. *Circulation.* **93**:1788–1790.
184. Chauhan S, Tripathy N, Sinha N, Nityanand S. (2006). T-cell receptor repertoire of circulating gamma delta T-cells in Takayasu's arteritis. *Clin Immunol.* **118**:243–249.
185. Seko Y, Minota S, Kawasaki A, Shinkai Y, Maeda K, Yagita H *et al.* (1994). Perforin-secreting killer cell infiltration and expression of a 65-kD heat-shock protein in aortic tissue of patients with Takayasu's arteritis. *J Clin Invest.* **93**:750–758.
186. Rybicki B, Iannuzzi M. (2007). Epidemiology of sarcoidosis: recent advances and future prospects. *Semin Respir Crit Care Med.* **28**:22–35.

187. Broos C, Van Nimwegen M, Hoogsteden H, Hendriks R, Kool M, Van den Blink B. (2013). Granuloma formation in pulmonary sarcoidosis. *Front Immunol.* **4**:437.
188. Chen E, Song Z, Willett M, Heine S, Yung R, Liu M *et al.* (2010). Serum amyloid A regulates granulomatous inflammation in sarcoidosis through Toll-like receptor-2. *Am J Respir Crit Care Med.* **181**:360–373.
189. Gabrilovich M, Walrath J, Van Lunteren J, Nethery D, Seifu M, Kern J *et al.* (2013). Disordered Toll-like receptor 2 responses in the pathogenesis of pulmonary sarcoidosis. *Clin Exp Immunol.* **173**:512–522.
190. Hunninghake G. (1984). Release of interleukin-1 by alveolar macrophages of patients with active pulmonary sarcoidosis. *Am Rev Respir Dis.* **129**:569–572.
191. Bachwich PL, JP 3rd, Larrick J, Spengler M, SL. K. (1986). Tumor necrosis factor production by human sarcoid alveolar macrophages. *Am J Pathol.* **125**:421–425.
192. Mizuno K, Okamoto H, Horio T. (2001). Heightened ability of monocytes from sarcoidosis patients to form multi-nucleated giant cells *in vitro* by supernatants of concanavalin A-stimulated mononuclear cells. *Clin Exp Immunol.* **126**:151–156.
193. Capelli A, Di Stefano A, Lusuardi M, Gnemmi I, CF D. (2002). Increased macrophage inflammatory protein-1alpha and macrophage inflammatory protein-1beta levels in bronchoalveolar lavage fluid of patients affected by different stages of pulmonary sarcoidosis. *Am J Respir Crit Care Med.* **165**:236–241.
194. Car B, Meloni F, Luisetti M, Semenzato G, Gialdroni-Grassi G, AW. (1994). Elevated IL-8 and MCP-1 in the bronchoalveolar lavage fluid of patients with idiopathic pulmonary fibrosis and pulmonary sarcoidosis. *Am J Respir Crit Care Med.* **149**:655–659.
195. Agostini C, Cassatella M, Zambello R, Trentin L, Gasperini S, Perin A *et al.* (1998). Involvement of the IP-10 chemokine in sarcoid granulomatous reactions. *J Immunol.* **161**:6413–6420.
196. Agostini C, Cabrelle A, Calabrese F, Bortoli M, Scquizzato E, Carraro S *et al.* (2005). Role for CXCR6 and its ligand CXCL16 in the pathogenesis of T-Cell alveolitis in sarcoidosis. *Am J Respir Crit Care Med.* **172**:1290–1298.
197. Nishioka Y, Manabe K, Kishi J, Wang W, Inayama M, Azuma M *et al.* (2007). CXCl9 and 11 in patients with pulmonary sarcoidosis: a role of alveolar macrophages. *Clin Exp Immunol.* **149**:317–326.
198. Hunninghake G, Gadek J, Young RJ, Kawanami O, Ferrans V, Crystal R. (1980). Maintenance of granuloma formation in pulmonary sarcoidosis by T lymphocytes within the lung. *N Engl J Med.* **302**:594–598.
199. Zaba L, Smith G, Sanchez M, Prystowksy S. (2010). Dendritic cells in the pathogenesis of sarcoidosis. *Am J Respir Cell Mol Biol.* **42**:32–39.

200. Facco M, Cabrelle A, Teramo A, Olivieri V, Gnoato M, Teolato S *et al.* (2011). Sarcoidosis is a Th1/Th17 multisystem disorder. *Thorax.* **66**:144–150.
201. Ten Berge B, Paats M, Bergen I, Van den Blink B, Hoogsteden H, Lambrecht B *et al.* (2012). Increased IL-17A expression in granulomas and in circulating memory T cells in sarcoidosis. *Rheumatology.* **51**:37–46.
202. Eishi Y, Suga M, Ishige I, Kobayashi D, Yamada T, Takemura T *et al.* (2002). Quantitative analysis of mycobacterial and propionibacterial DNA in lymph nodes of Japanese and European patients with sarcoidosis. *J Clin Microbiol.* **40**:198–204.
203. Adams J, Gacad M. (1985). Characterization of 1 alpha-hydroxylation of vitamin D3 sterols by cultured alveolar macrophages from patients with sarcoidosis. *J Exp Med.* **161**:755–765.
204. Taflin C, Miyara M, Nochy D, Valeyre D, Naccache J, Altare F *et al.* (2009). FoxP3+ Regulatory T Cells suppress early stages of granuloma formation but have little impact on sarcoidosis lesions. *Am J Pathol.* **174**:497–508.
205. Rappl G, Pabst S, Riemann D, Schmidt AW, C, Schütte W, Hombach A *et al.* (2011). Regulatory T cells with reduced repressor capacities are extensively amplified in pulmonary sarcoid lesions and sustain granuloma formation. *Clin Immunol.* **140**:71–83.
206. Idali F, Wahlström J, Müller-Suur C, Eklund A, Grunewald J. (2008). Analysis of regulatory T cell associated forkhead box P3 expression in the lungs of patients with sarcoidosis. *Clin Exp Immunol.* **152**:127–137.
207. Loftus EJ, Silverstein M, Sandborn W, Tremaine W, Harmsen W, Zinsmeister A. (1998). Crohn's disease in olmsted county, minnesota. 1940–1993: Incidence, prevalence, and survival. *Gastroenterology.* **114**:1161–1168.
208. Ekbom A, Helmick C, Zack M, Adami H. (1991). The epidemiology of inflammatory bowel disease: a large, population-based study in Sweden. *Gastroenterology.* **100**:350–358.
209. Schwartz D, Loftus EJ, Tremaine W, Panaccione R, Harmsen W, Zinsmeister A *et al.* (2002). The natural history of fistulizing Crohn's disease in Olmsted County, Minnesota. *Gastroenterology.* **122**:875–880.
210. Abraham C, Cho J. (2009). Inflammatory bowel disease. *N Engl J Med.* **361**:2066–2078.
211. Chambers T, Morson B. (1979). The granuloma in Crohn's disease. *Gut.* **20**:269–274.
212. Simillis C, Jacovides M, Reese G, Yamamoto T, Tekkis P. (2010). Meta-analysis of the role of granulomas in the recurrence of Crohn disease. *Dis Colon Rectum.* **53**:177–185.
213. Heresbach D, Alexandre J, Branger B, Bretagne J, Cruchant E, Dabadie A *et al.* (2005). Frequency and significance of granulomas in a cohort of incident cases of Crohn's disease. *Gut.* **54**:215–222.

214. Denoya P, Canedo J, Berho M, Allende D, Bennett A, Rosen L *et al.* (2011). Granulomas in Crohn's disease: does progression through the bowel layers affect presentation or predict recurrence? *Colorectal Dis.* **13**:1142–1147.
215. Yu H, Liu Y, Wang Y, Peng L, Li A, Zhang Y. (2012). Clinical, endoscopic and histological differentiations between Crohn's disease and intestinal tuberculosis. *Digestion.* **85**:202–209.
216. Mooney E, Walker J, Hourihane D. (1995). Relation of granulomas to lymphatic vessels in Crohn's disease. *J Clin Pathol.* **48**:335–338.
217. Sura RC, JF, Van Kruiningen H. (2011). Lymphatics, tertiary lymphoid organs and the granulomas of Crohn's disease: an immunohistochemical study. *Aliment Pharmacol Ther.* **33**:930–939.
218. Van Kruiningen H, Hayes A, Colombel J. (2014). Granulomas obstruct lymphatics in all layers of the intestine in Crohn's disease. *APMIS.* **122**:1125–1129.
219. Fidler H, Thurrell W, Johnson N, Rook G, McFadden J. (1994). Specific detection of Mycobacterium paratuberculosis DNA associated with granulomatous tissue in Crohn's disease. *Gut.* **35**:506–510.
220. Sanderson J, Moss M, Tizard M, Hermon-Taylor J. (1992). Mycobacterium paratuberculosis DNA in Crohn's disease tissue. *Gut.* **33**:890–896.
221. Matsumoto T, Nakamura S, Jin-no Y, Sawa Y, Hara J, Oshitani N *et al.* (2001). Role of granuloma in the immunopathogenesis of Crohn's disease. *Digestion.* **63** (Suppl 1):43–47.
222. Hundorfean G, Zimmer K, Strobel S, Gebert A, Ludwig D, Büning J. (2007). Luminal antigens access late endosomes of intestinal epithelial cells enriched in MHC I and MHC II molecules: in vivo study in Crohn's ileitis. *Am J Physiol Gastrointest Liver Physiol.* **293**:G798–G808.
223. Schulzke J, Ploeger S, Amasheh M, Fromm A, Zeissig S, Troeger H *et al.* (2009). Epithelial tight junctions in intestinal inflammation. *Ann N Y Acad Sci.* **1165**:294–300.
224. Meddings J. (2000). Barrier dysfunction and Crohn's disease. *Ann N Y Acad Sci.* **915**:333–338.
225. D'Haens G, Geboes K, Peeters M, Baert F, Penninckx F, Rutgeerts P. (1998). Early lesions of recurrent Crohn's disease caused by infusion of intestinal contents in excluded ileum. *Gastroenterology.* **114**:262–267.
226. Hara J, Ohtani H, Matsumoto N, Nakamura S, Kitano A, Arakawa T *et al.* (1997). Expression of costimulatory molecules B7-1 and B7-2 in macrophages and granulomas of Crohn's disease: demonstration of cell-to-cell contact with T lymphocytes. *Lab Invest.* **77**:175–184.
227. Gulwani-Akolkar B, Akolkar P, Minassian A, Pergolizzi R, McKinley M, Mullin G *et al.* (1996). Selective expansion of specific T cell receptors in the inflamed colon of Crohn's disease. *J Clin Invest.* **98**:1344–1354.
228. Liu S, Russo P, Baldassano R, Sullivan K. (2009). CD68 expression is markedly different in Crohn's disease and the colitis associated with chronic granulomatous disease. *Inflamm Bowel Dis.* **15**:1213–1217.

229. Fais S, Capobianchi M, Silvestri M, Mercuri F, Pallone F, Dianzani F. (1994). Interferon expression in Crohn's disease patients: increased interferon-gamma and -alpha mRNA in the intestinal lamina propria mononuclear cells. *J Interferon Res.* **14**:235–238.
230. Fuss I, Neurath M, Boirivant M, Klein J, De la Motte C, Strong S *et al.* (1996). Disparate CD4+ lamina propria (LP) lymphokine secretion profiles in inflammatory bowel disease. Crohn's disease LP cells manifest increased secretion of IFN-gamma, whereas ulcerative colitis LP cells manifest increased secretion of IL-5. *J Immunol.* **157**:1261–1270.
231. Annunziato F, Cosmi L, Santarlasci V, Maggi L, Liotta F, Mazzinghi B *et al.* (2007). Phenotypic and functional features of human Th17 cells. *J Exp Med.* **204**:1849–1861.
232. Monteleone G, Biancone L, Marasco R, Morrone G, Marasco O, Luzza F *et al.* (1997). Interleukin 12 is expressed and actively released by Crohn's disease intestinal lamina propria mononuclear cells. *Gastroenterology.* **112**:1169–1178.
233. Koulentaki M, Ioannidou D, Stefanidou M, Maraki S, Drigiannakis I, Dimoulios P *et al.* (2006). Dermatological manifestations in primary biliary cirrhosis patients: a case control study. Am J *Gastroenterol.* **101**:541–546.
234. Lindor K, Gershwin M, Poupon R, Kaplan M, Bergasa N, Heathcote E. (2009). Primary biliary cirrhosis. *Hepatology.* **50**:291–308.
235. Kaplan M, Gershwin M. (2005). Primary biliary cirrhosis. *N Engl J Med.* **353**:1261–1273.
236. Tsuneyama K, Yasoshima M, Harada K, Hiramatsu K, Gershwin M, YN. (1998). Increased CD1d expression on small bile duct epithelium and epithelioid granuloma in livers in primary biliary cirrhosis. *Hepatology.* **28**:620–623.
237. Harada K, Tsuneyama K, Sudo Y, Masuda S, Nakanuma Y. (2001). Molecular identification of bacterial 16S ribosomal RNA gene in liver tissue of primary biliary cirrhosis: is Propionibacterium acnes involved in granuloma formation? *Hepatology.* **33**:530–536.
238. You Z, Wang Q, Bian Z, Liu Y, Han X, Peng Y *et al.* (2012). The immunopathology of liver granulomas in primary biliary cirrhosis. *J Autoimmun.* **39**:216–221.
239. Xiao X, Miao Q, Chang C, Gershwin M, Ma X. (2014). Common variable immunodeficiency and autoimmunity — an inconvenient truth. *Autoimmun Rev.* **13**:858–864.
240. Cunningham-Rundles C, Bodian C. (1999). Common variable immunodeficiency: clinical and immunological features of 248 patients. *Clin Immunol.* **92**:34–48.
241. Resnick E, Moshier E, Godbold J, Cunningham-Rundles C. (2012). Morbidity and mortality in common variable immune deficiency over 4 decades. *Blood.* **119**:1650–1657.

242. Mechanic L, Dikman S, Cunningham-Rundles C. (1997). Granulomatous disease in common variable immunodeficiency. *Annals of internal medicine.* **127**:613–617.
243. Ardeniz O, Cunningham-Rundles C. (2009). Granulomatous disease in common variable immunodeficiency. *Clin Immunol.* **133**:198–207.
244. Boursiquot J, Gérard L, Malphettes M, Fieschi C, Galicier L, Boutboul D *et al.* (2013). Granulomatous disease in CVID: retrospective analysis of clinical characteristics and treatment efficacy in a cohort of 59 patients. *J Clin Immunol.* **33**:84–95.
245. James D. (1992). Mimics of sarcoidosis. *Granulomatous hypogammaglobulinaemia. Sarcoidosis.* **9**:1–2.
246. Bouvry D, Mouthon L, Brillet P, Kambouchner M, Ducroix J, Cottin V *et al.* (2013). Granulomatosis-associated common variable immunodeficiency disorder: a case-control study versus sarcoidosis. *Eur Respir J.* **41**:115–122.
247. Genre J, Errante P, Kokron C, Toledo-Barros M, Câmara N, LV R. (2009). Reduced frequency of CD4(+)CD25(HIGH)FOXP3(+) cells and diminished FOXP3 expression in patients with common variable immunodeficiency: a link to autoimmunity? *Clin Immunol.* **132**:215–221.
248. Giovannetti A, Pierdominici M, Mazzetta F, Marziali M, Renzi C, Mileo A *et al.* (2007). Unravelling the complexity of T cell abnormalities in common variable immunodeficiency. *J Immunol.* **178**:3932–3943.
249. Hardy H, Tabershaw I. (1946). Delayed chemical pneumonitis occurring in workers exposed to beryllium compounds. *J Ind Hyg Toxicol.* **28**:197–211.
250. Saltini C, Winestock K, Kirby M, Pinkston P, Crystal R. (1989). Maintenance of alveolitis in patients with chronic beryllium disease by beryllium-specific helper T cells. *N Engl J Med.* **320**:1103–1109.
251. Clayton G, Wang Y, Crawford F, Novikov A, Wimberly B, Kieft J *et al.* (2014). Structural basis of chronic beryllium disease: linking allergic hypersensitivity and autoimmunity. *Cell.* **158**:132–142.
252. Fontenot A, Torres M, Marshall W, Newman L, Kotzin B. (2000). Beryllium presentation to CD4+ T cells underlies disease-susceptibility HLA-DP alleles in chronic beryllium disease. *Proc Natl Acad Sci.* **97**:12717–12722.
253. Mack D, Falta M, McKee A, Martin A, Simonian P, Crawford F *et al.* (2014). Regulatory T cells modulate granulomatous inflammation in an HLA-DP2 transgenic murine model of beryllium-induced disease. *Proc Natl Acad Sci.* **111**:8553–8558.
254. Mack D, Lanham A, Falta M, Palmer B, Maier L, Fontenot A. (2010). Deficient and dysfunctional regulatory T cells in the lungs of chronic beryllium disease subjects. *Am J Respir Crit Care Med.* **181**:1241–1249.
255. Sawyer R, Abraham J, Daniloff E, Newman L. (2005). Secondary ion mass spectroscopy demonstrates retention of beryllium in chronic beryllium disease granulomas. *J Occup Environ Med.* **47**:1218–1226.

256. Maier L, Kittle L, Mroz M, Newman L. (2003). Beryllium-stimulated neopterin as a diagnostic adjunct in chronic beryllium disease. *Am J Ind Med.* **43**:592–601.
257. Kittle L, Sawyer R, Fadok V, Maier L, Newman L. (2002). Beryllium induces apoptosis in human lung macrophages. *Sarcoidosis Vasc Diffuse Lung Dis.* **19**:101–113.
258. Butnor K, Sporn T, Ingram P, Gunasegaram S, Pinto J, Roggli V. (2003). Beryllium detection in human lung tissue using electron probe X-ray microanalysis. *Mod Pathol.* **16**:1171–1177.
259. Merget R, Bauer T, Küpper H, Philippou S, Bauer H, Breitstadt R *et al.* (2002). Health hazards due to the inhalation of amorphous silica. *Arch Toxicol.* **75**:625–634.
260. Vallyathan V, Shi X, Dalar N, Irr W, Castranova V. (1988). Generation of free radicals from freshly fractured silica dust. Potential role in acute silica-induced lung injury. *Am Rev Respir Dis.* **138**:1213–1219.
261. Rimal B, Greenberg A, Rom W. (2005). Basic pathogenetic mechanisms in silicosis: current understanding. *Curr Opin Pulm Med.* **11**:169–173.
262. Piguet P, Vesin C, Grau G, Thompson R. (1993). Interleukin 1 receptor antagonist (IL-1ra) prevents or cures pulmonary fibrosis elicited in mice by bleomycin or silica. *Cytokine.* **5**:57–61.
263. Piguet P, Collart M, Grau G, Sappino A, Vassalli P. (1990). Requirement of tumour necrosis factor for development of silica-induced pulmonary fibrosis. *Nature.* **344**:245–247.
264. Altindag Z, Baydar T, Sachin G. (2003). Neopterin as a new biomarker for the evaluation of occupational exposure of silica. *Int Arch Occup Environ Health.* **76**:318–322.
265. Mariani T, Roby J, Mecham R, Parks W, Crouch E, Pierce R. (1996). Localization of type I procollagen gene expression in silica-induced granulomatous lung disease and implication of transforming growth factor-beta as a mediator of fibrosis. *Am J Pathol.* **148**:151–164.
266. Molina-Ruiz A, Requena L. (2015). Foreign body granulomas. *Dermatol Clin.* **33**:497–523.
267. Rieber N, Hector A, Kuijpers T, Roos D, Hartl D. (2012). Current concepts of hyperinflammation in chronic granulomatous disease. *Clin Dev Immunol.* **2012**:252–460.
268. Winkelstein J, Marino M, Johnston RJ, Boyle J, Curnutte J, Gallin J *et al.* (2000). Chronic granulomatous disease. report on a national registry of 368 patients. *Medicine.* **79**:155–169.
269. Rosenzweig S. (2008). Inflammatory manifestations in chronic granulomatous disease (CGD). *J Clin Immunol.* **28** (Suppl 1):S67–S72.
270. Segal B, Leto T, Gallin JI, Malech H. Holland S. (2000). Genetic, biochemical, and clinical features of chronic granulomatous disease. *Medicine.* **79**:170–200.

271. Clark R, Klebanoff S. (1979). Chemotactic factor inactivation by the myeloperoxidase-hydrogen peroxide-halide system. *J Clin Invest.* **64**:913–920.
272. Hamasaki T, Sakano T, Kobayashi M, Sakura N, Ueda K, Usui T. (1989). Leukotriene B4 metabolism in neutrophils of patients with chronic granulomatous disease: phorbol myristate acetate decreases endogenous leukotriene B4 via NADPH oxidase-dependent mechanism. *Eur J Clin Invest.* **19**:404–411.
273. Henderson W, Klebanoff S. (1983). Leukotriene production and inactivation by normal, chronic granulomatous disease and myeloperoxidase-deficient neutrophils. *J Biol Chem.* **258**:13522–13527.
274. Romani L, Fallarino F, De Luca A, Montagnoli C, D'Angelo C, Zelante T *et al.* (2008). Defective tryptophan catabolism underlies inflammation inmouse chronic granulomatous disease. *Nature.* **451**:211–215.
275. Umbert P, Winkelmann R. (1977). Histologic, ultrastructural and histochemical studies of granuloma annulare. *Arch Dermatol.* **113**:1681–1686.
276. Samlaska C, Sandberg G, Maggio K, Sakas E. (1992). Generalized perforating granuloma annulare. *J Am Acad Dermatol.* **27**:319–322.
277. Fayyazi A, Schweyer S, Eichmeyer B, Herms J, Hemmerlein B, Radzun H *et al.* (2000). Expression of IFNgamma, coexpression of TNFalpha and matrix metalloproteinases and apoptosis of T lymphocytes and macrophages in granuloma annulare. *Arch Dermatol Res.* **292**:384–390.

Index

www.ingramcontent.com/pod-product-compliance
Ingram Content Group UK Ltd.
Pitfield, Milton Keynes, MK11 3LW, UK
UKHW020350150926
8624IPUK00004B/95

9 789813 109438